CHIROPRACTIC TEXT BOOK

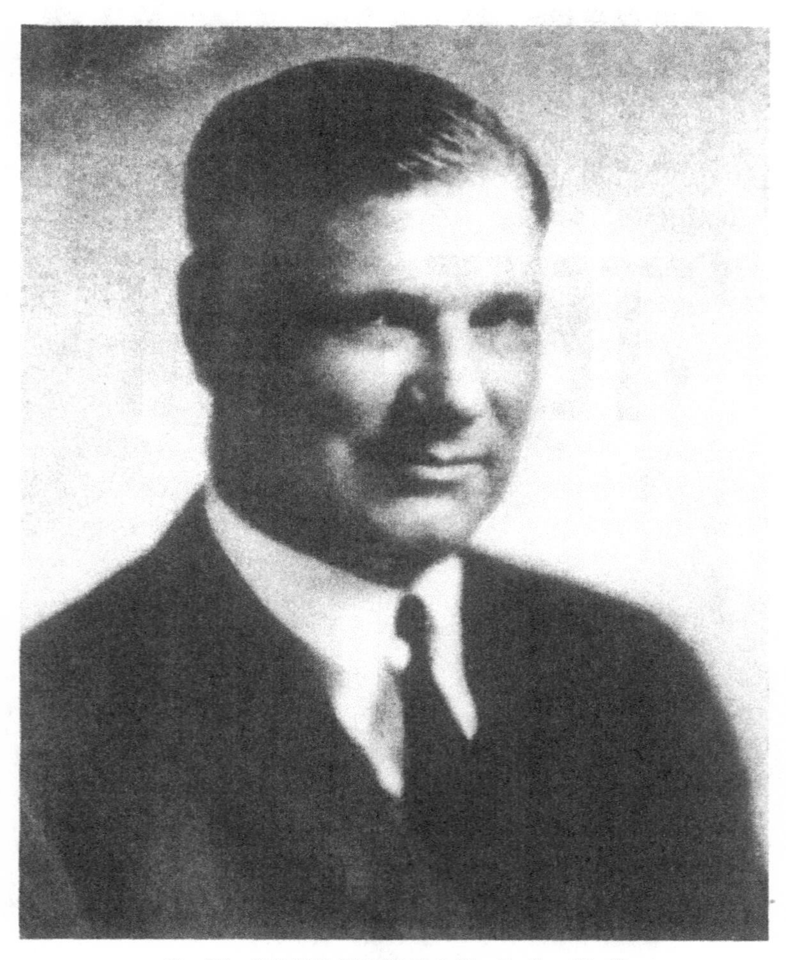

R. W. STEPHENSON, D.C., Ph.C.

CHIROPRACTIC TEXT BOOK

R. W. STEPHENSON

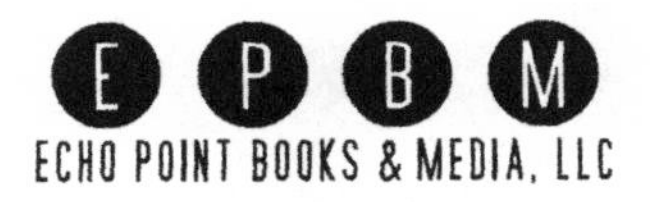

Published by Echo Point Books & Media
Brattleboro, Vermont
www.EchoPointBooks.com

ISBN: 978-1-62654-199-3

Cover design by Rachel Boothby Gualco,
Echo Point Books & Media

Editorial and proofreading assistance by Ian Straus,
Echo Point Books & Media

Dr. Palmer's Letter of Approval of Chiropractic Textbook

Dear "Stevie":

I could not blame you if you have grown impatient at my apparent silence in not giving you an expression of my opinion regarding your MSS. which you submitted for my approval or disapproval.

I have been doing some writing, taking my time to think it over carefully; and, between times when tired, I would go over another chapter of your book.

This is Sunday and I have just finished it. Of ALL *the books written and compiled on Chiropractic Philosophy, this is by far the best, not excepting my own. The one great, grand and glorious thing you* HAVE *done has been to compile the many principles which are in my writings, into a systematic, organized manner, building them up from simple to the higher forms, so that any layman inclined could investigate and find out what* CHIROPRACTIC IS, IS NOT; WHAT IT DOES AND DOES NOT; HOW AND WHY IT DOES WHAT IT DOES. *You have clearly, carefully and consistently compiled the many* PRINCIPLES *of Chiropractic into a readable, understandable book, simple enuf for the layman, deep enuf for the savant.*

My writings are many. They are in one form or another; either here or there. Each subject is exhaustive. If any person wanted full and complete information on a specific subject, then he should go to the special monograph on that subject; but, if he wants the working approximate principle then in your book he gets them all.

There has always been a void in Chiropractic literature. Assuming an understanding mind asks where he can get a book which would tell him what Chiropractic is—I have always felt that there was no one specific work that we could hand him for that purpose. WE NOW HAVE THAT BOOK. *It is your work. You have filled a niche that no other work has done. Here is a book that any chiropractor can hand to any investigating lay-mind and know that it will do him, Chiropractic and yourself justice. Your work can now be used as a handbook on that subject.*

I rejoice with you in its production. *As ever,*

B. J.

PREFACE

TO GAIN knowledge of Chiropractic I came to the Fountain Head. To me, then, the Fountain Head of Chiropractic was B. J. and not the school. To me, B. J. is still the Fountain Head of Chiropractic. I look to him for unsullied Chiropractic. I feel that the fundamental principles of Chiropractic, as given by this great teacher, are not to be tampered with by me or any one else, and in this book I merely serve as "Transmission from Source to Periphery."

I owe much to Dr. John H. Craven for more intimate instruction in Chiropractic and its Philosophy. I knew he never deviated from the teachings of Dr. Palmer. I am thankful for the great lessons in Philosophy and ideal Chiropractic and humanity, which I learned from this sincere teacher.

I have quoted freely from Dr. Palmer's books, and from Dr. Mabel Palmer and Dr. Craven; viz., Vol. V; Vol. IX; Vol. XV; Majors and Minors, (M&M).

This book has been prepared for class room use. Accordingly it is divided into sections for each semester. It has additional sections in etiology and thesis writing, for the convenience of the student. It is hoped that it will be a help to the field practitioner, who is still a student of Chiropractic, offering to him a review, as well as the later developments in the science of Chiropractic. It was the intention of the writer to make this book more than a Philosophy; it is intended to be a textbook of Chiropractic, conveying the more practical parts of Philosophy so that the student who pursues its subjects through, will have a comprehensive knowledge of Chiropractic. It is also hoped that it will prove interesting to the layman, should he choose to read it.

The book, with the exception of the section on thesis writing, is arranged in articles of varying lengths and numbered for reference and convenience. Each article is in two parts. The statements in bold faced type, contain the meat of the subject. They are the cardinal points—the high spots. If the student should learn these only, he would have a good knowledge of the subject of Chiropractic. The balance of the article is elaboration of the same.

The entire work is tied together by references, article to article, where it was deemed necessary; and proof given, by use of the fundamental principles, in the manner of deductive geometry.

Bold faced type is used for more important statements, italics for terms, and words or names are emphasized by capitalization, where necessary. Especially is this true of words entirely Chiropractic in character.

In the Introductory, Freshman, Sophomore, and Junior Section, are questions for review. These are intended to make the student think. Even if he is unable to answer some of them; if they set him to thinking; raise inquiry in the right direction, they have accomplished their purpose. There are no questions in the Senior Section, for by that time, the student should be able to ask his own question for the purpose of reviews.

Not until a student has reached the Senior Work is he able to question Chiropractic. The writer believes that no one is in a position to question Chiropractic with any justice, until he has studied it. Spencer says, "There is a principle which is a bar against information which is proof against all argument and which cannot fail to keep a man in everlasting ignorance. That principle is condemnation before investigation."

RALPH W. STEPHENSON, D.C., Ph.C.

List of Illustrations

INTRODUCTION

Art. 1. Remarks.

This book is written for use in the class room. It may, however, be studied just as easily by the field practitioner, and is not too technical in most of its parts to be readily grasped by the layman. It has grown, rather than having been written; it is the expansion of the notes which were tested in the class room for six years, and the writer believes that, with the constant arrangement and betterment to suit the requirements of the students of Chiropractic, this has created a real textbook, rendering easily understood a subject that students have always said was difficult.

Art. 2. Chiropractic Defined.

"Chiropractic is a philosophy, science and art of things natural; a system of adjusting the segments of the spinal column by hand only, for the correction of the cause of dis-ease."

"Chiropractic is defined, the science of palpating and adjusting the articulations of the human spinal column only."

"A system of adjustment consisting of palpation of the spinal column to ascertain vertebral subluxations followed by the adjustment of them by hand, in order to relieve pressure upon nerves at the intervertebral foramina, so that the nerve force may flow freely from the brain to the rest of the body."

The first definition is Dr. Palmer's and is the best. It tells exactly what Chiropractic is, without limiting its scope and without saying things which are not true, as the others are inclined to do. The second one is from the U.C.A. Model Bill, which is very limiting and therefore not exactly true. The third definition is from Dorland's Dictionary. After the student has mastered this book, if not before, he will see that this definition is too limited.

Art. 3. Science, Art and Philosophy.

The definition of Chiropractic quoted in the foregoing, states that it is a philosophy, science and art of things natural. Put simply, that means, "what it is, how it is done, and why." Science tells us what it is; art tells us how it is done, and philosophy, the "why" of the other two. According to that, then philosophy must tell us about both science and art; and that is the purpose of this book.

Art. 4. Science.

From Webster's International Dictionary: "Accumulated and accepted knowledge which has been systematized and formulated with reference to the discovery of general truths or the operation of general laws; knowledge classified and made available in work, life, or the search for truth; comprehensive, profound, or philosophical knowledge. **Any branch or department of systematized knowledge considered as a distinct field of investigation or object of study."** (Webster)

Though Chiropractic is young, comparatively, it is none the less, a well developed science with proven facts and plausible theories based upon those facts and precise art; all of them systematized knowledge, and a distinct field of investigation or object of study.

Art. 5. Art.

"Skill. dexterity, or the power of performing certain actions, acquired by experience, study or observation; knack."

"Skill in adaptation of things in the natural world to the uses of human life; human contrivance or ingenuity."

"The general principles of any branch of learning or of any developed craft; a system of rules or organized modes of operation serving to facilitate the performance of certain actions."

"Systematic application of knowledge or skill is effecting a desired result. Also, an occupation or business requiring such knowledge or skill." (These definitions are from Webster.)

The Art of Chiropractic consists of skill in analysis, palpation and adjusting vertebrae, most of it requiring dexterity with the hands. It requires many hours of drill and study; and since the chiropractor's hands are his only tools or instruments, they are of the same value to him as a musician's hands or voice are to the musician.

Art. 6. PHILOSOPHY.

"Literally the love of wisdom; in actual usage, the knowledge of phenomena as explained by, or resolved into, causes and reasons, powers and laws."

"Philosophy conceived as a branch of learning is, in the narrowest sense, nearly equivalent to metaphysics, but usually is understood as including all the mental and moral sciences, namely, logic, psychology, ethics, etc."

"In more general application, and usually with the or a, philosophy denotes a systematic body of general conceptions, ordinarily with the implication of their practical application." (Webster)

Art. 7. CHIROPRACTIC PHILOSOPHY.

Chiropractic Philosophy is the application of the foregoing definitions to Chiropractic as "the systematic body of conceptions . . . with the implication of their practical application."

It is the explanation of Chiropractic. It explains "the why" of everything Chiropractic. The explanation of cause and effect. It embraces the Chiropractic view of all the studies concerned in its science.

It should be noticed that general philosophy is a broad subject explaining all activities and natural phenomena. It is, with all its infinite branches, much too long to be learned in one lifetime. In the study of any philosophy, one must narrow his attention to the few philosophies that concern him most; and in the study of a given science, to specialize on that particular philosophy.

While Chiropractic philosophy is but one of the infinite number of philosophies and of one special science, it should be kept in mind that it is enough for a lifetime study. "A philosophy, science and art of things natural" is a broad field.

Chiropractic is a radical science. It is a right about face in method and in reasoning. It is contrary to the methods of healing in common use in the world. For that reason, it is misunderstood by those who have not had its benefits or are ignorant of its principles. Because of this wide difference, it is not always understood by all those who practice it and many of these persons doubt, because of their misunderstanding. However, all chiropractors who really adjust the cause of disease in the spine, do use philosophy to some extent, whether they believe it or not; whether they know it or not. Any one knowing the real meaning of philosophy as set forth by Webster's Dictionary, knows that any human activity has a philosophy.

Art. 8. Chiropractic Is a Deductive Science.

Chiropractic is a deductive science. The deductions are based upon a major premise that life is intelligent; that there is an Intelligent Creator, Who created matter, attends to its existence and gives to it all that it has. Many of the deductions are now proven facts because of thousands of clinical findings supporting them; and thousands of observations of the Laws of this Intelligence. The theories and hypotheses of Chiropractic are based upon these proven deductions which render them plausible, and nearly every year some of these theories become proven as solid facts of science.

Art. 9. Terminology.

Owing to the nature of the Science of Chiropractic, we believe it well to acquaint the student with the fact that Chiropractic has a terminology peculiarly its own. Many words commonly understood to have a certain meaning, have a different meaning when used in Chiropractic. Some of these are so frequently used that it is necessary to become acquainted with them early in the course, in order to understand the significance of the statements made descriptive of Chiropractic. The words and names will be given in the Text as needed.

Art. 10. Inductive Reasoning.

"Logic. Act or process of reasoning from a part to a whole, from particulars to generals, or from the individual to the universal; also, the result or inference so reached. By Aristotle's induction, epagoge, was treated as a subordinate form of reasoning, consisting, when perfect, of a complete enumeration of all the particulars comprised under the inferred generalization; hence called induction by a simple enumeration. The great advance over this view was the inductive method, or philosophical induction, of Bacon, which consists in the inferring that what has been observed or established in respect to a part, individual, or species, may, on the ground of analogy, be affirmed or received of the whole to which it belongs. Such inference ascends from the parts to the whole, and forms, from the general analogy of nature, or special presumptions in the case, conclusions which have greater or less degrees of force, and which may be strengthened or weakened by a subsequent experience and experiment, but which, in the long run, by reason of repeated observations will rectify themselves. This method is known also as ampliative inference. John Stuart Mill further elaborated the philosophy of induction, propounding as its basis the law of the uniformity of nature, and furnishing criteria for inference in these four methods, namely, of agreement, difference, residues, and concomitant variations. Later logicians have been concerned with the more exact determination of the nature of the universal element which enables an inference from particular to particular, and with the significance of Mill's doctrine of nature's uniformity." (Webster)

"Induction is a process by which we conclude that what is true of certain individuals of a class, is true of the whole class, or that what is true at certain times will be true in similar circumstances at all times." (Webster)

Thus it is seen from the foregoing definitions that inductive reasoning is really synthesis, that is to say, building a law instead of assuming it. It reasons that **the whole thing is like any of its parts, the conclusion being based upon a representative number of parts, going from the specific to the general.** It is accurate if all the data have been found; if all the parts have been observed. Sometimes the conclusion is arbitrary, disregarding some of the parts which are different from the rest, if they are far in the minority.

Inductive reasoning goes hand in hand with laboratory work because a laboratory is a place where parts of the whole are examined. For this reason it is unsuited to Chiropractic and applicable to the science of medicine.

Review Questions for Articles 2 to 10, inclusive.

1. Give Dr. Palmer's definition of Chiropractic.
2. Why is it the best definition?
3. What do you think is the reason that Chiropractic should not be limited to the human specie?
4. What is Art? Answer in your own words, or learn a pertinent part of Webster's definitions.

5. What is Science? Answer in your own words or learn a part of Webster's definitions that apply to a working science.
6. What field for Chiropractic does science, art and philosophy encompass?
7. What is philosophy? Answer in your own words or learn a definition.
8. What is Chiropractic Philosophy?
9. Which of Webster's definitions of philosophy is most applicable to Chiropractic? Why?
10. Tell why the Philosophy of Chiropractic is Chiropractic itself.
11. What is the Major Premise of Chiropractic?
12. Explain why Chiropractic is a well established science.
13. What is inductive reasoning?
14. What are the merits and the faults of inductive reasoning?
15. With what kind of work does inductive reasoning go hand in hand?

Art. 11. LABORATORY.

"Orig., the workroom of a chemist; hence a place devoted to experimental study in any branch of natural science, or to the application of scientific principles in testing and analysis or in the preparation of drugs, chemicals, explosives, etc.; as, a chemical, physical, or biological laboratory; by extension, a place where something is prepared or some operation is performed." (Webster)

The conclusions reached in a laboratory, based upon the laboratory findings, are necessarily synthetic. Laboratory work and inductions are very useful to the scientific world and the human race would be sadly impoverished without it, but chiropractors believe that while it is indispensable to industry, it is not suitable to healing the ills of living things."

Chiropractic definition, **"A laboratory is a room or series of rooms where every standard, and criterion or process of reasoning is denied to things being reasoned upon or upon which reason is used."** (Palmer)

"Men who conduct laboratorical experiments use reason in their process yet deny that process to things upon which they work." (Palmer)

From the foregoing it is evident that laboratory research with inductive reasoning cannot be used in Chiropractic except insofar as a chiropractor is obliged to study the material as material, such as, structure, chemical and physical laws.

We wish to make it clear that at no time does Chiropractic deny laboratory findings or discredit them as science, but Chiropractic reasons deductively instead of inductively upon them; seeing therein the action of intelligence, every finding being more proof of its Major Premise.

Art. 12. DEDUCTION.

Definition: "Act or process of deducing; mediate inference in which the conclusion follows necessarily from a full understanding of given data or proposition;—contrasted with induction."

"That which is deducted or drawn from premises by a process of reasoning; an inference; a conclusion."

"A withdrawing; a leading forth."

"Deduction as contrasted with induction, is reasoning from the general to the particular or from the implicit to the explicit, as contrasted with reasoning from particular facts to general truths or from a part to a whole. Deductions give explicit knowledge, as in geometrical demonstration; induction gives general principles, as in the formation of a natural law. Both processes appear in ordinary reasoning." (Webster)

Deductive reasoning is exactly suited to Chiropractic. By assuming a major premise, that there is a Universal Intelligence which governs all matter, every inference drawn from that major premise and subjected to specific scrutiny, stands the test. To prove the whole by specific examination of its parts is being exact; that is why geometry is exact. This exactness is suitable for Chiropractic, which rather than operate in a fog of generalities prefers the specific.

Deductive reasoning can be faulty if the propositions or premises are made unwisely; the examination of the details will quickly expose it. However, unlike induction, it is not necessary to see all the parts to be accurate, for the real premise was not made by man, but by a Higher Power. We wish to advise the student to watch for the passing from the general to the specific in every phase of Chiropractic, in both theory and practice, throughout the whole course.

Art. 13. Clinic.

Definition: "Instruction of a class of medical students by the examination and treatment of patients in the presence of pupils."

"The gathering of a number of students at a clinical lecture." (Webster)

"Definition of *clinical*: "*Surgery*, that part of medicine or surgery occupied with investigation of disease in a living subject." (Webster)

Chiropractic definition of *clinical*: "Clinical, by way of definition, **possesses all the contrasts of thought and introduces the opposite. Clinic is where immaterialism enters everything materialistic; where the very process of reasoning is admitted to be the method of procedure in elucidation."** (Palmer)

In Chiropractic, clinic means more than class instruction by investigation of dis-ease before a number of students. It means that merely a doctor alone with his patient, the reasoning of both being used, is a clinic. This is made clear by a quotation from B. J. Palmer:

"A patient comes, you don't know whether he is sick or not. He says he is, mental activity on his part, and faith upon yours. Just the opposite of what is done in the laboratory; there you take nothing for granted which can't be proven and seen. Ask the patient in the laboratory—there is none. The process of reasoning with the patient is the method used to illustrate facts. In the laboratory you have no patient to deduce with. In the clinic you use the ideas and facts of the patient as being of value and encompass your personal deductions in connections therewith. You and the patient do these things together. In the laboratory you are alone, except as you have something indirect." (Palmer)

Not only does Chiropractic recognize the co-operation of a patient in working upon his case, but the meaning of *clinic* or *clinical* goes still further. The Chiropractor's reasoning upon laboratory material, in which the physicist sees nothing but matter, is recognizing the intelligence that governs the matter in question and is therefore clinical. Also, the chiropractor does not treat matter with matter, in order to cure dis-ease; but calls upon the only power that can cure it—the inborn intelligence within the matter.

Therefore the true meaning of *clinic* in Chiropractic is the recognition of the intelligent guiding force in all "living things." The deductive study of life and abnormal life brings to the attention of the student, particular terms and principles which will be explained next.

Art. 14. Axioms.

Definition: "That which is thought worthy, that which is assumed, a basis of demonstration, a principle."

"A self evident truth, **a proposition whose truth is so evident that no reasoning or demonstration can make it plainer; a proposition which it is necessary to take for granted**; as, 'The whole is greater than a part,' 'A thing cannot at the same time, be and not be.' "

"An established principle in some art or science, which, though not a necessary truth, is universally received." (Webster)

There are many self-evident truths in Chiropractic; so many and such common evidences of the expression of Universal Intelligence everywhere about us, that they are overlooked because of their very simplicity and frequency. Everybody sees them daily; to attempt to prove them would be absurd if not impossible. These axioms are the foundation stones of Chiropractic. The self-evident truths of Chiropractic are so common and so simple that they seem paradoxical. For that reason, students sometimes think that Chiropractic Philosophy is difficult, when really it is quite simple.

Art. 15. Paradoxes.

Definition: **"A tenet or proposition contrary to received opinion; also an assertion or sentiment seemingly contradictory, or opposed to common sense, but that yet may be true in fact."** (Webster)

There are many paradoxes in Chiropractic; its enemies and people who do not know its principles, too readily condemn it as assertions or tenets opposed to common sense. A closer acquaintance with it, however, reveals the absolute truth of its principles. There is a reason for this first impression of the student or layman. It is because the method of modern education is nearly all inductive. We have all been educated that way—at home and in our schools. Most of our educational books are written inductively. Consequently, when we meet a science of, almost entirely, deductive reasoning and contrary to the existing mode of thinking, which we have seen by the preceding paragraphs; and which is exactly the reverse of induction, it is quite natural to fail to see the logic of Chiropractic at first.

Art. 16. Theories and Facts.

The tenets of Chiropractic, like those of other sciences, are made up of some well established facts with theories and hypotheses based upon them. These facts have been established by clinical findings. The theories and hypotheses have been deduced from general truths and their plausibility is supported by these clinically established facts.

Definition of *fact*: "The quality or character of being actual or of being made up facts; actuality; often, specific, physical actuality or practical experience as distinguished from imagination, speculation, theory, etc.; as, the realm of fact is distinct from fancy; a question of fact, that is, of actual evidence rather than hypothesis." (Webster)

Definition of *theory*: "The general or abstract principles of any body of facts real or assumed; pure, as distinguished from applied, science or art; as, the theory of music or medicine." (Webster)

"A general principle, formula, or **ideal construction, offered to explain phenomena and rendered more or less plausible by evidence in the facts or by the exactness and relevancy of the reasoning."**

"A plan or scheme theoretically constructed." (Webster)

Art. 17. Examples.

In order to explain the facts of a science more clearly it is often expedient to use examples; and to explain abstract principles and theories, it is often necessary to use analogies. While an example may be taken at its full value, the writer deems it advisable to caution the student, throughout the whole course, to avoid mistaking analogies for facts and examples; to remember that analogy is comparison and should not be used for actuality.

Definition of *example*: **"One or a portion taken to show the character or quality of all; a sample; a specimen; an instance."** (Webster)

An example is not a likeness but one of the things mentioned; an instance to show the working or application of a principle.

Art. 18. Analogy.

Definition: "Resemblance of relations; agreement or likeness between things in some circumstances or effects, when things are otherwise different. Thus, learning enlightens the mind because it is to the mind what light is to the eye, enabling it to discover things before hidden. Analogy is very commonly used to denote similarity or essential resemblance; but its specific meaning is a similarity of relations, and in this consists the difference between the argument from example and that from analogy. In the former, we argue from the mere similarity of two things; in the latter, from the similarity of their relations." (Webster)

The two things reasoned about may be utterly unlike, but the relations of the parts of one thing to each other, or the relations of the actions of its parts to each other, are the same as the relations of the parts or the actions of the other thing. For example, the conductivity of a nerve for mental impulses is often compared to the conductivity of a wire for electricity. Now, it is not desired to convey the idea that impulses are electricity, but the relationship of mental impulses to a nerve is similar to the relationship of electricity to a wire. It is the relationships that are being compared, rather than a comparison of the things themselves.

Art. 19. The Three Phases of Chiropractic Study.

1. **Study of the Immaterial.**
2. **Study of the Material.**
3. **Study of Art.**

The study of the Immaterial is the study of philosophy; that is to say, the study of intelligence, laws, causes, effects, rules, theories, functions and other abstractions. It is to gain a knowledge of the group of principles underlying the science.

The study of the Material is the study of anatomy, histology, chemistry, etc. In order that the chiropractor know something about the material and structure of the body, it is advisable for him to study the materials in order to understand the actions of structures in function; to better understand the effects of causes, and to trace to causes from the effects.

Also, in a broader sense, it increases his understanding of Chiropractic if he has a fair knowledge of the working of Universal laws in regard to matter, for Chiropractic is a study of Universal life as well as life in the human body. The subjects mentioned are taught at The P. S. C., always with the Chiropractic "slant" and at sufficient length and detail for Chiropractic needs. In the study of these subjects, the student should always be on the lookout for "the reason why"; the manifestations of intelligence and the *significance* of structure, rather than a purposeless observation of phenomena in structure and action. Effects are after all, only effects, and it avails the chiropractor nothing to make an endless classification of them.

The study of Art is learning how to do the things that every chiropractor must do, scientifically and skillfully; such as, analysis, palpation and adjusting. All of these require skill as well as mental work. The amount of skill required takes practice, since the chiropractor's only tools are his hands, for adjusting. As a musician begins with simple exercises and practices several hours a day, in order to become skilled with the hands, so a Chiropractic student is drilled daily in palpation and technic, and if he desires to become "professional" it will be necessary for him to be as diligent in practice as the professional musician. The study of Art is the study of how to restore the governed forces of intelligence to matter, when those forces are lacking in the dis-eased tissues of the body of a "living thing."

Art. 20. A Comparison.

It will be noticed all through the book that the immaterial, the material and the link between them are often mentioned. These terms apply to intelligence, matter and force; or mind, matter and the link between them. It will be noticed that all three of these phases are taken into consideration. Now, while all three are studied, Chiropractic as a science and art is based upon the link between mind and matter. To show the significance of this, the following comparison is quoted from Dr. Palmer.

Christian Science—based upon the immaterial—mind.

Medical Science—based upon the material—matter.

Chiropractic Science—based upon the link between the immaterial and the material.

B. J.'s pun:

Christian Science—always mind—never matter.

Medical Science—always matter—never mind.

Art. 21. "The Missing Link."

Since Chiropractic as a science and art is based upon the link between mind and matter, it naturally follows that the student is curious to know what that link is. Since Chiropractic science is based upon it, and since this book is explanatory of that science, the writer begs the patience of the student and he will find out in due time. Briefly, however, we can say that since all phenomena is the result of force in matter, and since the Major Premise of Chiropractic maintains that this force proceeds from intelligence, then the link is force. It is called the "missing link" because it was unrecognized, as the bond between the immaterial and material, until it was discovered by Chiropractic. Some sciences are a study of matter, as chemistry; some are studies of forces and energies, as physics; and some are studies of the mental or abstract realm entirely. But it never occurred to any of the sciences to get together on these, until Chiropractic put them together, and it is this embodiment of three things in one, that is implied in the Major Premise and the big fundamental of Chiropractic.

Aain we want to emphasize what Chiropractic Philosophy is and what it is not. It is the explanation of everything Chiropractic. That means the Chiropractic view of the material, as, anatomy, chemistry, etc. The Chiropractic view of abnormalities in anatomy and physiology. The Chiropractic view of the immaterial, as mind, force, function, etc., and of abnormalities of function. The Student should not make the mistake of believing that Chiropractic Philosophy is a sort of psychology, telepathy, occultism, or the classic philosophy of Plato and Socrates. It is not theology. While it may mention these things in passing it deals with them scarcely at all. Chiropractic Philosophy pertains more to the working principles of Chiropractic. The difference between a good chiropractor and a poor one is, that the good one has an ample supply of abstract principles in his head, and the poor one only a few. The difference between an electrical engineer and the lineman whom he commands, is that the engineer has more abstract principles and fewer wrenches and pliers. Poor chiropractors are apt to substitute machinery for knowledge.

Naturally, the statements of how Chiropractic deals with the things involved in it, or its tenets in regard to them, are principles.

Review Questions for Articles 11 to 21, inclusive.

1. What is a laboratory according to the Chiropractic view?
2. If a chiropractor works in a laboratory or uses laboratory findings, what interpretation does he put upon both?
3. What is deductive reasoning?
4. Why is deductive reasoning best suited to Chiropractic?
5. What is the Chiropractic idea of a clinic?
6. What does a chiropractor depend upon to do the work that he knows no man can do?
7. What is an axiom?
8. Why is Chiropractic so simple fundamentally?
9. Into what error does a chiropractor fall, who tries to add complications instead of keeping Chiropractic simple?
10. What is a paradox?
11. Why are people, who hear of Chiropractic the first time, so apt to discredit it?
12. What is a fact?

13. What is a theory?
14. Describe the origin of Chiropractic theories.
15. Where were Chiropractic facts obtained?
16. What is an example?
17. What is an analogy?
18. What is the difference between analogy and simile?
19. What very bad error is the misuse of analogy apt to produce?
20. What are the three phases of Chiropractic study?
21. What three factors of the Major Premise do these resolve themselves into?
22. What is "The Missing Link?"
23. What hitherto neglected application of the three phases of life does Chiropractic embody?
24. What is the value of principles in any science?
25. What is the difference between a poor chiropractor and a good one?

Art. 22. Principles.

Definition: "A source, or origin; that from which anything proceeds; fundamental substance or energy; primordial substance; ultimate element or cause."

"A fundamental truth; a comprehensive law or doctrine from which others are derived, or on which others are founded; a general truth; an elementary proposition; a maxim; an axiom; a postulate."

"A settled rule of action; a governing law of conduct; an opinion or belief which exercises a directing influence on the life and behavior; a rule (usually, a right rule) of conduct consistently directing one's actions." (Webster)

The principles of a science are its governing laws. These may be **the fundamental truths upon which it is founded, or the governing rules of conduct or operation.** Any human doctrine or belief has its fundamentals upon which it is based; and any human activity has its settled rules of action which guides these activities in the most expeditious and efficient manner.

Some examples: art (picture making) has its principles which are much the same as those of composition, as, unity, harmony, sequence, continuity, variation and the like. Design has unity, harmony, variation, balance, etc. Gardening has rules governing planting, cultivation, caretaking, etc.

Some of these principles stand out as more fundamental than others, which may be more or less working rules, or rules of more specific application than others. The number of rules or principles that a science may have is indeterminate and no positive number of principles can be set that is not arbitrary. The only sciences that might have, possibly, their principles numbered in any phase of it are sciences of abstract perfection.

Art. 23. The Principles of Chiropractic

Chiropractic like other sciences, has many principles. As in other sciences some of these principles are different from the rest; some being more fundamental than others. This fact can be seen by examining the foregoing definitions of principles. Some of the principles are basic, upon which others are founded or derived as going from the general to the specific; some are down to a part of the whole thing. These specific principles are of course derived principles. They are not limited to any given number. **A fundamental principle of Chiropractic is a statement of the quality or actions of intelligence in matter which will include any and all circumstances that may arise in study.**

Immediately following are a number of principles which have been chosen for discussion in this book. These are stated and numbered for convenience so that their application to things under discussion can be seen. They are arranged in an order which goes from the general to the specific. They are referred to by number in the text, of which each Article is supported by one or more principles, thereby giving the entire work unity and agreement.

Art. 24. A List of Thirty-Three Principles, numbered and named.

No. 1. The Major Premise.

A Universal Intelligence is in all matter and continually gives to it all its properties and actions, thus maintaining it in existence.

No. 2. The Chiropractic Meaning of Life.

The expression of this intelligence through matter is the Chiropractic meaning of life.

No. 3. The Union of Intelligence and Matter.

Life is necessarily the union of intelligence and matter.

No. 4. The Triune of Life.

Life is a triunity having three necessary united factors, namely, Intelligence, Force and Matter.

No. 5. The Perfection of the Triune.

In order to have 100% Life, there must be 100% Intelligence, 100% Force, 100% Matter.

No. 6. The Principle of Time.

There is no process that does not require time.

No. 7. The Amount of Intelligence in Matter.

The amount of intelligence for any given amount of matter is 100%, and is always proportional to its requirements.

No. 8. The Function of Intelligence.

The function of intelligence is to create force.

No. 9. The Amount of Force Created by Intelligence.

The amount of force created by intelligence is always 100%.

No. 10. The Function of Force.

The function of force is to unite intelligence and matter.

No. 11. The Character of Universal Forces.

The forces of Universal Intelligence are manifested by physical laws; are unswerving and unadapted, and have no solicitude for the structures in which they work.

No. 12. Interference with Transmission of Universal Forces.

There can be interference with transmission of universal forces.

No. 13. The Function of Matter.

The function of matter is to express force.

No. 14. Universal Life.

Force is manifested by motion in matter; all matter has motion, therefore there is universal life in all matter.

No. 15. No Motion without the Effort of Force.

Matter can have no motion without the application of force by intelligence.

No. 16. Intelligence in both Organic and Inorganic Matter.

Universal Intelligence gives force to both organic and inorganic matter.

No. 17. Cause and Effect.

Every effect has a cause and every cause has effects.

No. 18. Evidence of Life.

The signs of life are evidence of the intelligence of life.

No. 19. Organic Matter.

The material of the body of a "living thing" is organized matter.

No. 20. Innate Intelligence.

A "living thing" has an inborn intelligence within its body, called Innate Intelligence.

No. 21. The Mission of Innate Intelligence.

The mission of Innate Intelligence is to maintain the material of the body of a "living thing" in active organization.

No. 22. The Amount of Innate Intelligence.

There is 100% of Innate Intelligence in every "living thing," the requisite amount, proportional to its organization.

No. 23. The Function of Innate Intelligence.

The function of Innate Intelligence is to adapt universal forces and matter for use in the body, so that all parts of the body will have co-ordinated action for mutual benefit.

No. 24. The Limits of Adaptation.

Innate Intelligence adapts forces and matter for the body as long as it can do so without breaking a universal law, or Innate Intelligence is limited by the limitations of matter.

No. 25. The Character of Innate Forces.

The forces of Innate Intelligence never injure or destroy the structures in which they work.

No. 26. Comparison of Universal and Innate Forces.

In order to carry on the universal cycle of life, Universal forces are destructive, and Innate forces constructive, as regards structural matter.

No. 27. The Normality of Innate Intelligence.

Innate Intelligence is always normal and its function is always normal.

No. 28. The Conductors of Innate Forces.

The forces of Innate Intelligence operate through or over the nervous system in animal bodies.

No. 29. Interference with Transmission of Innate Forces.

There can be interference with the transmission of Innate forces.

No. 30. The Causes of Dis-ease.

Interference with the transmission of Innate forces causes incoordination of dis-ease.

No. 31. Subluxations.

Interference with transmission in the body is always directly or indirectly due to subluxations in the spinal column.

No. 32. The Principle of Coordination.

Coordination is the principle of harmonious action of all the parts of an organism, in fulfilling their offices and purposes.

No. 33. The Law of Demand and Supply.

The Law of Demand and Supply is existent in the body in its ideal state; wherein the "clearing house," is the brain, Innate the virtuous "banker," brain cells "clerks," and nerve cells "messengers."

These principles will be used for the concluding work of the Freshman Section of the book. They are discussed in detail in the Senior Section. The discussions are in advance of the Freshman work, but it is advisable to learn their names for reference.

Review Questions for Articles 22 to 24, inclusive.

1. What is a principle of a science?
2. What is a fundamental principle?
3. What are derived principles and what is their purpose?
4. How many principles has Chiropractic?
5. What is a fundamental principle of Chiropractic?
6. Could matter exist without the attention of Universal Intelligence?
7. Is the broad, general meaning of the term *life* confined to animals and plants in Chiropractic?
8. If one looks for it, what may he always perceive matter manifesting besides mere motion?
9. What very important combination of three elements is the basis of Chiropractic tenets?
10. What must this combination have, in order to be perfect?
11. Does anything ever happen so quickly that its duration is zero time?
12. How much intelligence or how much attention does any given amount of matter receive from intelligence?
13. What is the function of intelligence?
14. What is the character of Universal forces?
15. Can Universal forces be interfered with?
16. What is the function of matter?
17. Upon what evidence is based the tenet, that there is universal life?
18. Did any one ever see a force unless it was exhibited by matter?
19. Can you think of the existence of an effect without a cause?
20. What is Innate Intelligence?
21. What are signs of life?
22. Where do you find organic matter?
23. What is the mission of Innate Intelligence?
24. Is the wood of your pencil inorganic matter?
    Is it still actively organic or is it now inorganic matter?
25. What is the function of Innate Intelligence?
26. Has "she" any other function?
27. Does a flea have as much Innate Intelligence as an elephant?
28. What determines the limits to what Innate Intelligence can do in the way of adaptation?
29. What is the character of Innate forces?
30. Is Innate Intelligence ever sick or otherwise abnormal or imperfect?
31. What are the means of communication between mind and matter in the body?
32. If the Universal forces can suffer interference with transmission, could Innate forces be an exception to that law?
33. What does interference with transmission of Innate forces cause?
34. If we trace back to causes, where do we always find the cause of incoordination?

The Freshman Text

THE Freshman work consists of the foundation work of Chiropractic study; the consideration of the principles and fundamentals. This is principally the analysis of the Normal Complete Cycle. The student should take up his work progressively, instead of skipping all over the book.

Article 25. Chiropractic.

The Science of Chiropractic holds that a Universal Intelligence created and is maintaining everything in the universe. This is manifested by movement and is called Life. A specific, definite portion of this intelligence, localized in a definite portion of matter and keeping it actively organized, is called by Chiropractic, Innate Intelligence. The function of an inborn, localized intelligence is to adapt some of the forces and matter of the universe in a constructive manner. Organization points to centralization, or having a point of control. In animals, this point of control is in the brain. From this organ, Innate Intelligence sends its controlling forces via the spinal cord through the spinal column, thence through the nerve trunks emitting from the spinal cord and passing through the intervertebral foramina to nerve branches ramifying to all parts of the body. Perfect adaptation of universal elements for this body, depends upon perfect control by Innate Intelligence. Perfect adaptation results in health, and imperfect control results in dis-ease. Defective control by Innate Intelligence is never from any imperfection of Innate Intelligence, which is always perfect, and assembles perfect forces in the brain, but from interference with the transmission of those Innate forces through or over the nerves. Owing to the spinal column being the only segmented structure of bone through which the nerve trunks pass, and the possibility of the displacement of its segments, changing the size and shape of the intervertebral foramina, it is possible for subluxations to occur there and offer interference with the transmission of Innate forces indirectly, if not directly. All dis-ease is thus traceable to impingements of nerve tissue in the spinal column. Chiropractic is a science which consists in having scientific knowledge of this cause of dis-ease and the artistic ability to adjust and correct these displacements of the segments of the spinal column, thereby removing interference with the transmission of Innate forces. Adjustment does not add any material or forces to the body but allows Innate to restore to normal what it would have had, had there been no interference. In this manner, health is restored. Chiropractic includes the study of all life, but that of the human body in particular. At the present time adjustments are almost entirely confined to the human spine and restoring health to the human body. Therefore, our studies, with the exception of the fundamentals, will be in regard to the human Innate Intelligence, chiefly; the human body and the functioning of its parts; and incoordinations of the same in order to arrive at proficiency in ascertaining and removing the cause of dis-ease.

Art. 26. The Chiropractic Definition of Subluxation. (See Prin. 31.)

A subluxation is the condition of a vertebra that has lost its proper juxtaposition with the one above or the one below, or both; to an extent less than a luxation; which impinges nerves and interferes with the transmission of mental impulses.

All the factors of the foregoing definition must be given to make it complete and to make it Chiropractic. The student is advised to learn it verbatim.

Dislocations and fractures, also, can impinge nerves and interfere with the transmission of mental impulses, but fractures and dislocations are not in the realm of Chiropractic.

Art. 27. "THE CENTER."

"Center," has reference to the brain as the center of the organization, from which Innate Intelligence controls.

The brain in the central nervous system is called the *center*. The word, center, is used as opposed to *periphery*. Not only is it the center of the nervous system, anatomically, but it is the center of intelligence in the body.

Art. 28. "THE PERIPHERY." (See Prin. 13)

The tissues at the ends of efferent nerves; the tissue cells.

The word, *periphery*, is used as opposed to *center*. It means, the outside; the outer portion, away from the center.

Art. 29. EFFERENT NERVES. (See Prin. 28)

The nerves leading from the center to the periphery; from brain to tissue cell.

The word, *efferent*, refers to direction. The prefix *ef* is a change from *ex* for euphony, meaning *out*. The stem, from *ferre*, means, to bear. The ending, *ent*, is a participial affix. Literally, to bear out or bearing out. Of course this means to bear out from within.

Efferent nerves, then, are those which begin in the brain and lead out from the brain, through the spinal cord and branches to all parts of the body. There is no active part of the body without such nerve supply. If all the tissues of the body were removed, leaving nervous tissue only, the body would be fully outlined, having a fibrous appearance. If one doubts this, a pin prick will be convincing.

Art. 30. Afferent Nerves. (See Prin. 28)

The nerves leading from periphery to center; from tissue cells to the brain.

The word, *afferent,* also refers to direction. The *af* is a change from *ad* for euphony, meaning *to.* This, with the stem from *ferre,* and *ent* gives a word literally meaning *to bear to.* We use it, meaning to draw in from without.

Afferent nerves are those which begin at the tissues and lead to the brain. Anatomically, afferent nerves are not so well understood as the efferent, but it is not so difficult to trace the special sense nerves, which of course are afferent.

Art. 31. The Nerve Cycle. (See Prin. 28)

Efferent and afferent nerves form a material cycle from and to the brain.

The brain communicates with every tissue cell, by means of efferent nerves which are *distributed* from it as a center. All the tissues of the body have nerves—even bones and ligaments. Such tissues as hair, nails and outer cuticle have no nerves but while they are growing in their earlier life they have a supply of mental impulses.

Every tissue cell communicates with the brain by means of afferent nerves which are *collected* to it as a center. All tissues of the body in active organization are in communication with Innate Intelligence in order that "she" be fully aware of their condition.

Thus, there is a path from brain cell to tissue cell and back from tissue cell to brain cell for the mental current.

There are many material and functional cycles in the body which are not hard to understand; as, the digestive cycle, respiration cycle, cardiac cycle, and serous cycle. Perhaps the most obvious cycle is the blood circulation in its course from the heart as a center to all parts of the body, through arteries and back again to the heart as a center through the veins. There is a close similarity in the arrangement of blood vessels in the body to the arrangement of nerves. The purpose of the blood vessels is easily seen, for what they carry is a material thing and it can be seen coursing through them. Since the arrangement of the nerves is similar to the arrangement of blood vessels, it is obvious that they carry something, but what this is cannot be seen, for it is intangible. However, it is obvious that it is something necessary to the tissue cells, for its effects or lack of its effects can be perceived. This something is a mental force from Innate Intelligence.

REVIEW QUESTIONS FOR ARTICLES 25 to 31, inclusive.

1. Practice making a short description of Chiropractic, similar to that in Art. 25.
2. Give the Chiropractic definition of subluxation, verbatim.
3. Show why the lack of any of its statements would leave it incomplete and not Chiropractic.
4. Dislocations and fractures are in the realm of what profession?
5. What is meant by "center"?
6. What is meant by "periphery"?
7. What is meant by "efferent nerve"?
8. What is meant by "afferent nerve"?
9. Which nerves are better understood in anatomy and physiology, efferent or afferent nerves?
10. What is the arrangement of nerve tissue in the body?
11. Of what is this arrangement significant?

Art. 32. MENTAL FORCES.

A mental force is that something, transmitted by nerves, which unites intelligence with matter... (See Prin. No. 3)

Mental force is called mental impulse because it impels tissue cells to intelligent action.

Mental force is evidently a form of energy, or conveyed by a form of energy, for it can control forces that move matter physically or balance forces that do it.

Mental forces are necessary to the tissues of the body.

Mental force is not a physical or a chemical force; nor is it a stimulant.

If a nerve is impinged the function of a tissue is made abnormal and the tissue cells weakened in condition. If the nerve is severed the tissue cell loses function and dies. This is proof that the mental impulse is necessary to life. The condition of the tissue cell and its organization must be kept up to the point that it is able to function, and that function controlled.

Art. 33. Location of the Power in Organisms.

In animals, the headquarters or center of control of Innate Intelligence is the brain.

It is the place from which life force is distributed to the tissues of an organism. The intelligence is the power and is the source of mental force. The place from which it comes is the center. Condition and actions of tissue cells are reported to this center. Thus, mental force completes a cycle.

These statements are equivalent to saying that the brain is the seat of the mind. Although we do not know where Innate resides, we have plenty of proof that the seat of control is the brain. The ancients believed that the seat of mind was in the heart and some emotions, as anger, in the spleen; and some thought the home of the soul was in the sacrum.

We have no way of knowing whether Innate resides in the brain, in the body or outside of the body but as the locomotive engineer's place of control is the cab, so Innate's place of control is the brain.

Art. 34. Cycles.

Definition: "A ring; a circle; **a complete course of operations of some kind, returning into itself and restoring the original state."** (Webster)

Art. 35. Chiropractic Cycles.

The course of mental force from brain to tissue and back again and the consecutive places and operations in that course.

The explanation of the successive steps from cause to effect and back again to cause.

The story of what happens between cause and effect, and effect and cause.

The earnest student will notice that most phenomena of life and nature pass through a cyclic course, the cycle repeating itself countless times. The number of times these cycles repeat is infinite. The stars and planets travel in cycles; the processes of life and death are in cycles. The number of cycles in the body extends into infinity. Therefore, if we get a grasp of it at all, we select the story that we want told, thus going from the general to the specific, and confine ourselves to the explanation of that one thing. Now, we must keep in mind that other cycles are going on at the same time and if we want to make our story compound or complex we introduce more items exactly as an author introduces more characters into a story to make it more complex. The number of cycles, then, is just what we make it; just the numbers of processes we want described. It is just as complex as we make it, depending on how many things we wish to study simultaneously.

When the story has been told many times it becomes conventionalized. It becomes a set form so that the same terms come up again and again. As the story of your late illness, or your repeated description of an accident acquires a set form, so did the story of what mental force did in its travels, become formulated when told over and over again by the Palmers. When this story is "boiled down" to its utmost brevity and is only an outline, then we have the steps of cycles as studied in philosophy. The briefest one is the Simple Cycle.

Art. 36. The Simple Cycle.

The Simple Cycle is the briefest story from cause to effect and from effect to cause. It names six important processes:—

Efferently—Creation, Transmission, Expression.
Afferently—Impression, Transmission, Interpretation.

Notice that transmission occurs twice in it—going and coming. Also, notice that the efferent half denotes the coming out from a center; a scattering—a distribution. The afferent half denotes a drawing toward the center; a gathering in—collecting. The last word of the first series and the first word of the second series, show this very plainly. The meanings of the individual words will be given later. The student will do well to commit these steps to memory for they will be used frequently.

Art. 37. The Normal Complete Cycle.

The Normal Complete Cycle is the outline of the story of the normal functioning of Innate in the body.

In this cycle thirty-one steps are named; most of them processes. There are sixteen in the efferent half and fifteen in the afferent half. The meaning of these steps will be given later. Following is the list of the steps, numbered for convenience:

EFFERENT

1. Universal Intelligence.
2. Innate Intelligence.
3. Mental (Realm)
4. Creation.
5. Brain Cell.
6. Transformation.
7. Mental Impulse.
8. Propulsion.
9. Efferent Nerve.
10. Transmission.
11. Tissue Cell.
12. Reception.
13. Physical Personification.
14. Expression.
15. Function.
16. Coordination.

AFFERENT

1. Coordination.
2. Tissue Cell.
3. Vibration.
4. Impression (of vibrations).
5. Afferent Nerve.
6. Transmission.
7. Brain Cell.
8. Reception.
9. Mental (Realm).
10. Interpretation.
11. Sensation.
12. Ideation.
13. Innate Intelligence.
14. Intellectual Adaptation.
15. Universal Intelligence.

Art. 38. The Cycles Graphically Represented.

Fig. 1 is a cut of a "safety pin" cycle, just a simple diagram of brain cell to tissue cell. Fig. 2 is the same modified to show a little more, namely, Coordination. Fig. 3 is a still greater modification of the safety pin cycle to show, what the

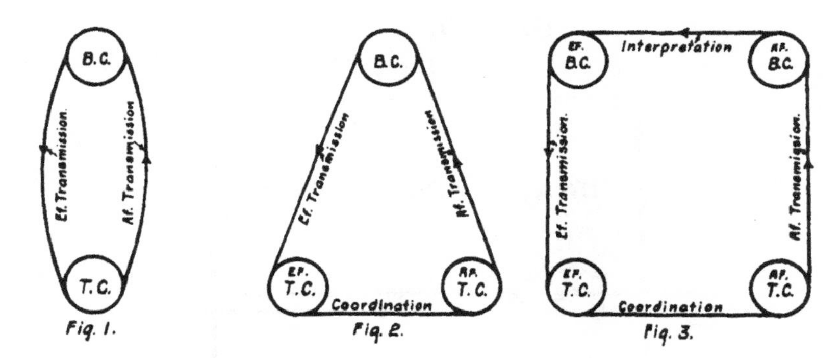

others do, but in addition, Interpretation. Fig. 4 is a cut of the "universal diagram of cycles" which is valued by B. J. most of all, as it shows, when correctly used, all the mental force cycles that are studied. We will refer to it when needed.

Art. 39. The Normal Complete Cycle Graphically Represented.

See Fig. 5 which shows a modification of the "safety pin" diagram, large enough to have all the thirty-one steps of the cycle printed on it, in their places as you follow around the circle indicated by the arrow heads and numbers.

Art. 40. Units. (78, V) (These numbers are references in Vol. V, by Palmer)

The study of the cycle is by units of force and matter.

The unit of force is the *forun.* The unit of matter is the

tissue cell or brain cell or both. The smallest unit considered in function is the tissue cell. All the steps of the cycle are the names of units of force, processes, matter, and places. As

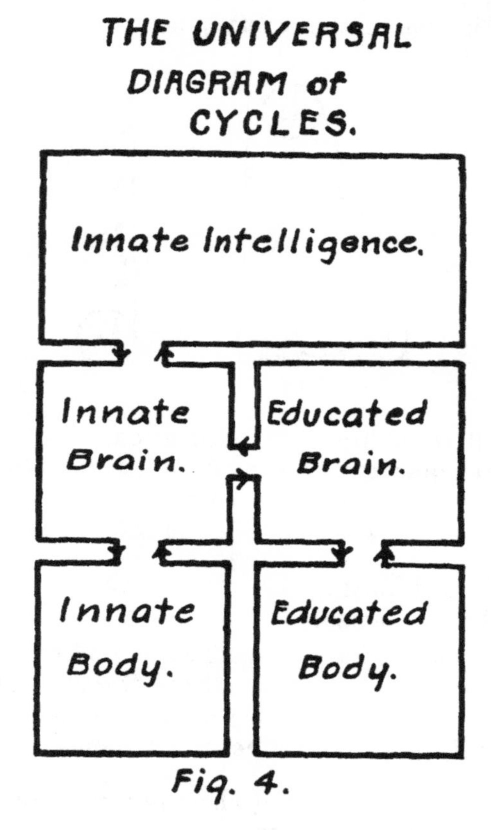

Fig. 4.

the C. G. S. system is the fundamental unit system in the study of physics and mechanics, so the forun, mental impulse, and tissue cell are fundamental units in Chiropractic.

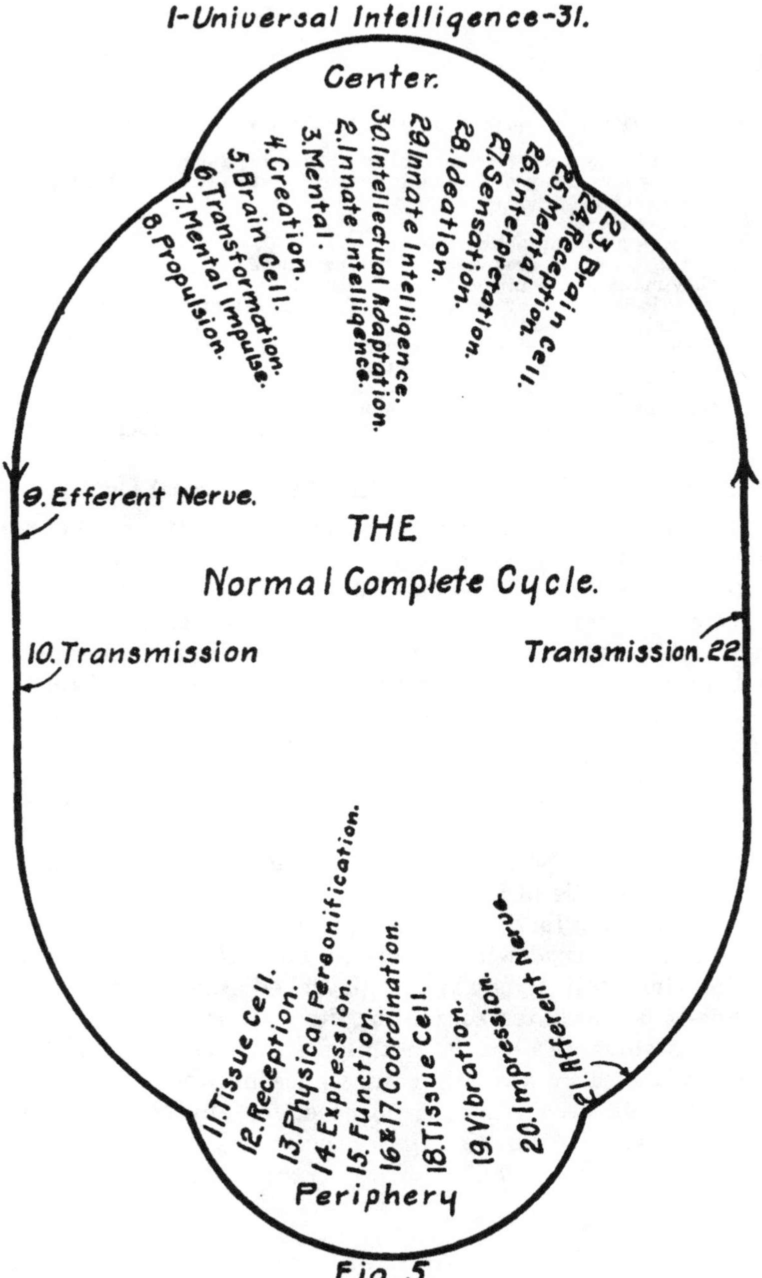

1-Universal Intelligence-31.

Center.

2. Innate Intelligence.
3. Mental.
4. Creation.
5. Brain Cell.
6. Transformation.
7. Mental Impulse.
8. Propulsion.

9. Efferent Nerve.

10. Transmission

11. Tissue Cell.
12. Reception.
13. Physical Personification.
14. Expression.
15. Function.
16 & 17. Coordination.
18. Tissue Cell.
19. Vibration.
20. Impression.
21. Afferent Nerve.

Transmission. 22.

23. Brain Cell.
24. Reception.
25. Mental.
26. Interpretation.
27. Sensation.
28. Ideation.
29. Innate Intelligence.
30. Intellectual Adaptation.

Periphery

THE
Normal Complete Cycle.

Fig. 5.

REVIEW QUESTIONS FOR ARTICLES 32 to 40, inclusive.

1. Where is the center of control in animal organisms?
2. Have we any way of knowing where Innate resides? Where does a principle reside?
3. What is a cycle?
4. What is a Chiropractic cycle?
5. In the Universe, how many cycles are there?
6. How many cycles in the human body?
7. Why is it necessary to go from the general to the specific in the study of cycles?
8. Why are the cycles of Chiropractic merely names of steps?
9. Name the steps of the Simple Cycle.
10. How many steps in the Normal Complete Cycle?
11. How many are efferent; how many are afferent?
12. What is the smallest unit of matter considered in function?
13. What is the forun?

Art. 41. THE SOURCE. (See Art. 38, Universal Diagram)

The Power that supplies the Universe with intelligence, force and matter — everything.

Another name for Universal Intelligence. (See Prin. No. 1)

We are concerned with it here as the Source of all forces and matter, as an inexhaustible supply for Innate Intelligence to draw from. Innate is not limited in her supply of forces; the only thing which prevents her from accomplishing the infinite is the limited amount of matter in the body.

Art. 42. THE SUBSOURCE. (See Universal Diagram, Art. 38)

The immediate Source of constructive forces for the collection of tissue cells in its care.

Another name for Innate Intelligence. (Prin. 20)

We are concerned with it here as an explanation of a part of the Universal Diagram. It is called Subsource because, though it is a localized source for the body it is "sub" to Universal Intelligence; but to nothing else. There is no cable of nerve tissue or any other substance between it and Universal Intelligence. There is no need, for anything universal is everywhere. **(Prin. No. 1)**

Art. 43. INNATE BRAIN. (See Universal Diagram, Art. 38)

That part of the brain used by Innate, as an organ, in which to assemble mental impulses.

It is supplied with mental impulses directly from Innate Intelligence, whose headquarters it is.

It is a vital spot and cannot be dis-eased. (317, V)

Its existence is actual, but its location is theoretical.

There is no transmission of mental impulses from Innate Intelligence to Innate brain. There is no necessity, Innate being right here. For this reason it always has 100% mental impulses. This being true it has perfect function, perfect metabolism and never has incoordination. It does not assimilate poisons from the serous stream. It is of course subject to trauma, the same as any other tissue.

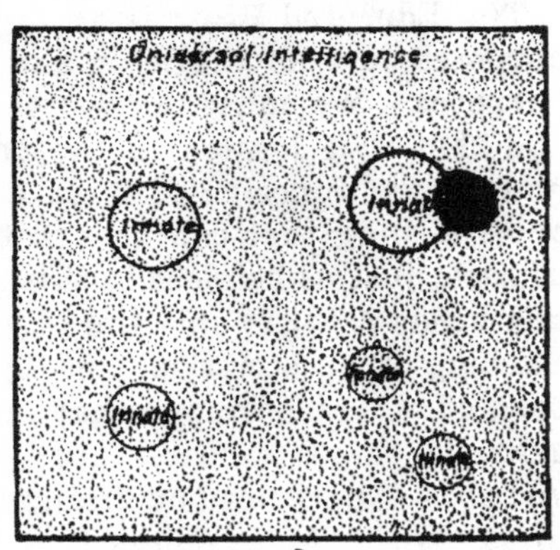

Fig. 6.

It must be supplied with nutriment and blood as any other tissue. A virulent poison *can* penetrate it. If it is injured by trauma; if it is subjected to anemia—lack of blood and nutriment; or is poisoned in spite of its resistance, then death ensues speedily, for it will not endure dis-ease or trauma. It must be remembered that although Innate's management is nothing short of miraculous, she is after all, limited in what she can do because of the limitations of matter. (Prin. 5 and 24)

Art. 44. EDUCATED BRAIN. (See Universal Diagram, Art. 38)

That part of the brain used by Innate as an organ for reason, memory, education, and the so-called voluntary functions.

The seat of Educated Mind.

It is supplied with mental impulses over nerves, as any other tissue.

It is liable to incoordination as any other tissue; it is not a vital spot.

Its existence is actual but its location is theoretical.

It is the chief organ of adaptation to environmental conditions.

The Educated Brain is an organ used by Innate for certain purposes just as the liver and stomach are used for certain purposes. We must not let the fact that it is brain tissue, and that it is located in the cranial cavity, confuse us. We must never conceive of it as a Power which create thoughts or as a thing that can govern the body. It is merely a piece of flesh, just as helpless in this matter as a steak in the butcher's window. It is only the physicists who believe that by the clashing of its atoms, physically and chemically, thoughts are born of it. Like many other organs of the body, the skin for example, it has multiple purposes. It is used by Innate, by virtue of experience and training, stored within it, as an organ to so "tincture" impulses that they are *consciously* guided—called voluntary function. *Voluntary* pertains to the will. The Educated Brain is used by Innate to receive precepts concerning the environment of the body, obtained by her able scouts, the Five Senses. The constant comparison of these precepts with former precepts and with each other, enables Innate to avoid actual or threatened dangers and to dispose of the body for its comfort and welfare. It is used by Innate to store away precepts in a manner not well understood, but about which the psychologists have plausible theories. (See Philosophy of Education in Senior Section.)

Art. 45. INNATE BODY. (See Universal Diagram, Art. 38)

Innate Body is all the tissue cells supplied with mental impulses for metabolism and the so-called involuntary functions.

The cells of Educated Body are to be considered as Innate Body so far as metabolism is concerned.

It is supplied with mental impulses through nerves from Innate Brain by the Subsource.

All the cells of the body are Innate Body. (See Fig. 7.) The classification is according to function more than anatomically. All tissues must have metabolism, even voluntary ones. The tissues which have voluntary, also have involuntary functions, at the same time.

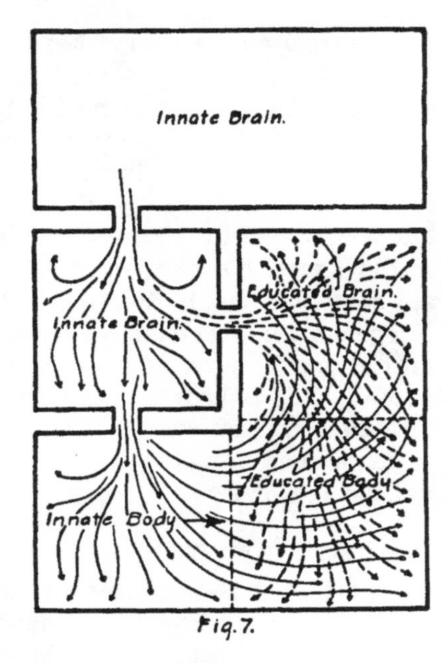

Fig. 7.

Art. 46. EDUCATED BODY. (See Universal Diagram, Art. 38)

Educated Body is all the tissue supplied with mental impulses from Innate Brain via the Educated Brain for the so-called voluntary functions.

These same cells are Innate Body so far as metabolism and the so-called involuntary functions are concerned. (See Fig. 7)

The classification is according to function; not an anatomical division. It simply has reference to those tissues, muscle predominating, which can be operated at will; voluntary or conscious movement. Educationally, we have no control over the involuntary movements that go in these tissues and while we may be conscious of some of them, we are absolutely unconscious of the metabolism that goes on in these tissues. It would certainly be a pretty poor sort of metabolism if it depended upon us to do it educationally. We, as chiropractors, believe this to be the fallacy of medicine, and of dietitians who are attempting to usurp Innate's business.

Universal means everywhere—common to every locality.

If anything is universal it is to be found everywhere you go; it is in every place, and no locality is without it. In the abstract and perfect sense this would be absolute. As *universal,* is commonly used, it is more limited. For instance, we say that buttons are universally worn. That does not mean that buttons are all over the universe, on the planets or in interstellar space, but that in most every civilized country we are apt to go, we should find buttons in use.

The universe extends everywhere; it is infinite. It has no limitations in space, distance or time; or any quality you might name. This is true of both the material and the immaterial universe. If you were to travel at any rate of speed you care to name, and any length of time you care to name, you could not get out of it.

Art. 47. Infinite.

Infinite means unlimited; no boundary; not defined.

The material universe, as mentioned in the foregoing article, is infinite; it has no boundary. The immaterial universe, meaning the intelligence which governs the universe, with all its matter, qualities, and abstractions, is likewise infinite. *Infinite* is a descriptive term applied to Universal Intelligence. therefore. (Prin. 1.)

Art. 48. Finite.

Finite means limited, or bounded.

Finite is a term applied to Innate Intelligence, because it is a finite portion of Universal Intelligence taking care of a finite portion of matter. Being finite in this sense, Innate capabilities are limited by matter. (Fig. 6.) (Prin. 5 and 24.)

Art. 49. THE FIRST STEP OF THE NORMAL COMPLETE CYCLE. (119, V.) UNIVERSAL INTELLIGENCE.

The Infinite Intelligence that is the Source of everything in the Universe.

The Infinite Intelligence pervading all space and matter, which creates and governs all things, both material and immaterial.

It occupies all space and distance. It has existed always. It is older, wiser, greater, stronger and better than anything in the Universe. It created everything and must have been first and indefinitely superior in order to do it. It must have been and is VERY intelligent. Having these virtues it must have never made a mistake and therefore is always right. Being always right is always good. Being infinitely good is God. (See Webster for definition of God.)

Being infinite, no one can define it, actually; one can get only a finite idea of it from the finite amount of manifestations we are able to perceive. This intelligence is not limited, it is we who are limited in perception. (Prin. 5, 18, and 24.) It endows "living things" with localized Power (Innate Intelligence) as a higher manifestation of its forces.

Art. 50. THE SECOND STEP OF THE NORMAL COMPLETE CYCLE. (121, V.) INNATE INTELLIGENCE.

The localized or inborn intelligence of a "living thing."

A finite portion of Universal Intelligence in a finite portion of matter, whose mission it is to keep the matter in active organization. (Prin. 21.)

Individualized Universal Intelligence.

A segment of Universal Intelligence which, though a part of it, is distinct from it. (Prin. 20.) (Fig. 6.)

While Innate Intelligence is a finite portion of Universal Intelligence, it represents the amount of attention that Universal Intelligence is giving to that amount of matter. All matter is blessed with the caretaking of the Supreme Intelligence, and if this ceases for one moment, matter would cease to exist. We do not know, of course, but it seems reasonable to believe, that the Creator's solicitude did not end when things were created; that Universal Intelligence is continuously unfolding thoughts of which everything in the universe gets its share—that amount intended for it, no more, no less. Organic things seem to be blessed with a greater amount of attention than inorganic things. So much so that Universal Intelligence has endowed the living organisms with localized or a specialized branch of itself to attend to things that must have immediate and localized decisions, in order to keep the matter organized.

Definition of *organize*: "To arrange or constitute in interdependent parts, each having a special function, act, office, or relation with respect to the whole." (Webster.)

This definition throws an interesting light upon the subject, showing that if a number of interdependent parts are to have a cooperative relation with each other, they must be grouped about a central idea, a common need or governing principle. This governing principle is Innate Intelligence.

There are various grades of "living things." Some are not much above the state of inorganic matter. (See the light circle in Fig. 6.) Yet these have 100% of intelligence, exactly proportionate to their state of organization. They have all the specialized intelligence they need; all that Universal Intelligence intended they should have. This localized intelligence is not a material thing to be measured in quarts or bushels; we speak of it in percentage, meaning that, much or little, the amount of intelligence a "living thing" has is 100%, and that is its share. Both the mouse and the elephant have 100% innates. (Prin. 7, 14, 16, 22.) That which each has is the amount required to make him what he is.

While Innate is limited as to the amount of matter she controls, which is the amount of matter in the body, she is not limited as to the amount of forces at her command. (Prin. 9.) She has the whole Universe to draw from.

Observation of manifestations seems to indicate that some Innates are deficient and that some make mistakes. A closer inspection will show that this is paradoxical. If we are acquainted with the laws of physics and chemistry, it is easy to see, that after all, Innate has not, comparatively, very much to work with. Without an infinity of matter she cannot be expected to have infinite expression. One cannot do the same work with a toothpick that he can with a crowbar. (Prin. 24.)

When Innate leaves the body, the matter in it is not destroyed but reverts to its inorganic state. It may still be called organic matter, probably because it retains the form of organic matter, as wood does, but it is no longer actively organic—not "alive." Most bodily tissues, with the exception of bone, decompose quickly, while wood or bone holds its form a long time after Innate leaves. While the localized, specialized intelligence has left and is no longer concerned with these structures, Universal Intelligence is still interested in the molecules, though not in the structures, and still gives these molecules and atoms as much care as ever. If it did not they would cease to exist at all. (Prin. 1 and 14.)

This Innate Intelligence assembles matter, for her use, adapting it so it can be used, and making it into structures pleasing to herself, but according to a Universal plan. While Universal Intelligence does not care particularly for these structures, Innate Intelligence gives them constant thought. In order to build them and keep them in repair and to function as organizations, she assembles forces from an infinite supply. Just as we educationally adapt steam, gravity, and electricity for our use and convenience, she adapts universal forces and matter for her use and convenience. After constructing the body , she continues adapting material and forces to maintain it that way through life. (Prin. 21, 23.)

Review Questions for Articles 41 to 50, inclusive.

1. What is the term *Source* synonymous with?
2. What is the term *Subsource* synonymous with, and explain the name?
3. What is Innate Brain?
4. What is the main characteristic of Innate Brain?
5. What is Educated Brain?
6. Does Educated Brain govern the body?
7. What is Innate Body?
8. What is Educated Body?
9. In what "body" are the material cells of the Educated Body?
10. What does the term *universal* mean?
11. What do the terms *finite* and *infinite* mean?
12. Explain Universal Intelligence, the first step of the cycle.
13. What is Innate Intelligence?
14. What does *organize* mean?

Art. 51. All Living Things Have Innates.

Whenever molecules and atoms have been assembled into tissues, the tissues are called organic matter; and while actively organic, have a localized intelligence, called Innate Intelligence.

Organic life extends through a wide range of development. All of them have signs of life; (Prin. 18) but some of them are organisms of such low order that the signs of life are very latent and it is very difficult to distinguish these "living things" from inorganic structures. In some organisms, some of the signs of life may be more latent than other signs of life in the same organism. If they have any organization at all, that fact is sufficient proof that an Innate Intelligence is present. (See thin line circle in Fig. 6.) High or low, through the whole gamut, man, animals, birds, fish, reptiles, insects, plants, or unicellular, they all have Innates. The higher orders have more motion of the adaptive kind than the others, which enables them to live in a wider range of environment than the others not so fortunate. Thus, we see according to

Chiropractic tenets that **life is studied generally and specifically; Universal Life and Organic Life, as contrasted phases.** Man gives to himself the highest rank, this rank being based upon his superior powers of adaptability.

Since we, as chiropractors, are interested in getting the sick well, we are naturally more interested in the Innates of our own species of organisms. From now on, when we speak of Innate Intelligence, we are referring to the human Innate Intelligence, unless otherwise stated.

Art. 52. The Third Step of the Normal Complete Cycle. Mental Realm.

The plane of Innate's activity.
The immaterial realm.
The occupation or business of Innate.

Of or pertaining to the mind." (Webster)

Mental, is strictly abstract; it is the realm of thought. Innate Intelligence, as a part of a Thinking Power, is a power which thinks. Anything which exists was first conceived in thought. **The process of thinking is creation.** Every abstract fact, every plan, every structure, every act of every part of the body, or the body as a whole, is first created in the brain by Innate Intelligence. This activity of intelligence is *mind* and is an important phase of life, not overlooked by Chiropractic. The student is cautioned to remember that **mind is not a power but the activity of power.**

Art. 53. Mind. (116 to 125, Vol. V.)

The activity of Innate Intelligence in the brain as an organ.

The introduction of thought into matter via the brain. (Prin. 3, 8, 10, 13.)

Chiropractic maintains that Innate Intelligence is the Power which governs the body; is the ego itself. You are your Innate Intelligence, your Innate Intelligence is you. If you claim that you are master of your Innate, that is a mistaken assumption of values and is the same as Innate belittling herself. Surely Innate would never do this; but when it appears that she does, it is a mis-expression. (Prin. 24, 30.)

Mind is the term applied to what Innate Intelligence does when it is at work.

Innate Mind and Educated Mind are terms used to indicate the kind of work being done.

When Innate does not work there is no mind.

Let us compare a musician to the Power; his instrument to the brain and music to mind. When the musician plays on his instrument, as an organ of expression, there is music. When the musician ceases playing there is no music expressed.

In Chiropractic, the term *mind* is considered a little differently than it is in psychology. In psychology, one mind is considered in two divisions, namely, conscious and subconscious, with no definite division between them. Psychology considers that this, the conscious mind, is the governing intellect and implies that while the subconscious mind may govern metabolism and the like, the conscious mind is the ego; is really the master. We gather from the teachings of psychology, which is based upon a materialistic view, one can willfully govern his own destinies, even to the extent of healing. Chiropractic does not use the terms, *conscious mind* and *subconscious mind* at all, for there is absolutely no application of these terms to anything Chiropractic.

Chiropractic Philosophy is not a study of psychology any more than it is of chemistry or physics. Chiropractic recognizes and honors all the findings of the psychologists as it does that of the physicists. It makes use of these findings as it does those of the physicists and agrees with psychology as long as psychology is consistent with Chiropractic. In other words, there is a Chiropractic psychology, which is the

study of the mind. (See Senior Section) All the psychology that is considered in Chiropractic, can be studied under the division called, Mental, the third step of the Normal Complete Cycle.

Art. 54. Innate Mind. (125, V)

Innate Mind is the activity of Innate Intelligence in the Innate Brain as an organ.

The product of this activity is Innate Thoughts, or Mental Force.

The act or the business of assembling forces in Innate Brain.

Even when "she" uses Educated Brain, she first uses Innate Brain. (See Universal Diagram Fig. 4) (Prin. 23.)

Art. 55. Educated Mind.

Educated Mind is the activity of Innate Intelligence in the Educated Brain as an organ.

The product of this activity is Educated Thoughts; such as, reasoning, will, memory, etc.

Innate controls the functions of the "voluntary" organs via the Educated Brain. (See Universal Diagram, Fig. 4)

Educated thoughts are mostly for adaptation to things external to the body.

Educated thoughts are never outwardly expressed until Innate does it through Innate Brain; for instance, one may have a thought but be unable to express it vocally, if Innate is unable to operate the organs of speech, owing to interference with transmission of mental impulses. In any case, we should not know how to operate the organs of speech even, though we can will them to act. The Educated thoughts may be kept within the brain and as Chiropractic says, expressed there, but which psychologists say make a physiological change in the tissue of the brain. We see no reason why we should not agree with this theory.

Art. 56. The Fourth Step of the Normal Complete Cycle. Creation. (115, 136, V)

The process of adapting Universal forces in the brain cell, so that they can be used for the maintenance and functioning of tissue cells. (Prin. 8, 23)

The assembling of forces in Brain Cell by Innate Intelligence.

Creation in the brain cell refers to the assembling of something already created, rather than the making of something out of nothing. Creation means, cause to exist, but here it means to cause to exist in a certain way. Of course there is the assembling of forces into kinds, and matter into structures, as the carpenter assembles building materials into structures and assembles forces in order to do it. We call his buildings creations but not for a moment do we think that he created them out of nothing. Innate is a creator, truly, but in the sense that she is a builder. Innate cannot change or destroy any Universal Law or matter, (Prin. 24) but can play one force against the other, adapt, use, oppose, or augment the forces at her disposal, in order to accomplish her ends. It is in this sense that he use the term *creation* in the Normal Complete Cycle. Universally, Creation is the unfolding of ideas of Universal Intelligence. Creation has not ceased, but the Supreme Intelligence is thinking about all creations constantly. This solicitude we also call creation. There are three classes of Universal creations; matter, acts, and facts. It is easy enough to grasp the first; an act must first be conceived mentally, even a natural phenomenon; a fact, something very abstract, is a creation just as much as a stone is, and it is just as indestructible. Two plus two equals four; an abstract fact. No human agency can destroy it. Therefore, it is plainly seen that in the Normal Complete Cycle, Chiropractic uses a specific meaning of creation rather than the general. An examination of the following definitions from Webster will show that Chiropractic is justified in using a specific meaning.

"Act of causing to exist, or fact of being brought into existence by a divine power or its equivalent; esp., the act of bringing the universe or this world into existence."

"Act of making, producing, fashioning, or bringing into existence, in general."

"Act of constituting or investing with a new character, title, or the like." (Webster)

Art. 57. The Fifth Step of the Normal Complete Cycle. Brain Cell. (137, V)

An organ used by Innate Intelligence for the assembling of forces.

Place where thoughts are made; place where forces are assembled.

The "clearing house" for coordination.

As the brain is an organ, so is the brain cell—a smaller unit.

The workshop of Innate Intelligence.

Metabolistically, it is a tissue cell requiring mental impulses, blood and serum.

A brain cell is a cell of nervous tissue—one of the four primary tissues. It has many of the characteristics of other tissue cells, having a body and a nucleus. Its widest difference from other cells is its branches. It has many branches; in fact it has so many of them, that a drawing or a photograph of a brain cell looks like a map of the Amazon River. The shorter body-branches are called *dendrities* and the single, long, threadlike branch, extremely long in proportion to the cell body, is called the *axis-cylinder* or *axone* or *axon*.

The body of the cell is gray, and masses of cell bodies form the gray or cortical portions of the brain. The branches are white, and bundles of them form the white or medullary portions of the brain. The white fibers pass from cell to cell, from lobe to lobe, from hemisphere to hemisphere, from brain to brain and from them to the spinal cord. They offer perfect intercommunication between all brain cells, and between brain cells and body cells. The intercommunicating parts are the axons which are believed to be the most important part of the cells, and are so long in comparison with the cell body, that if you were to imagine a cell body to be the size of a base-ball, the axon would be the size of a string and quarter of a mile long.

Very long axons pass from brain cells through the foramen magnum of the cranium. There are so many of these, that they form a cylinder about the size of a lead pencil called the spinal cord. Through this cord the axons pass to the spinal nerves, which branch and ramify to all parts of the body.

The cells of the brain are very similar in construction to the nerve cells of the spinal cord, visceral system, and peripheral organs. Nervous tissue is about the same whether in the brain or peripheral systems. The nervous tissue in the brain and spinal cord is called the *central nervous system*. anatómically. The spinal nerves and visceral system is called the *peripheral system*, in Chiropractic. Chiropractic is inclined to regard all nervous tissue outside the cranium as the peripheral system, even those portions of the cranial nerves which supply tissue cells with mental impulses.

Art. 58. The Sixth Step of the Normal Complete Cycle. Transformation. (116, 139, 233, V) (Webster)

Changing mental force to a specific unit.

Changing force from the mental realm to the material realm.

Making foruns usable in the tissue cell.

Making a force out of thought so that it can be physical enough to "get a grip" on matter.

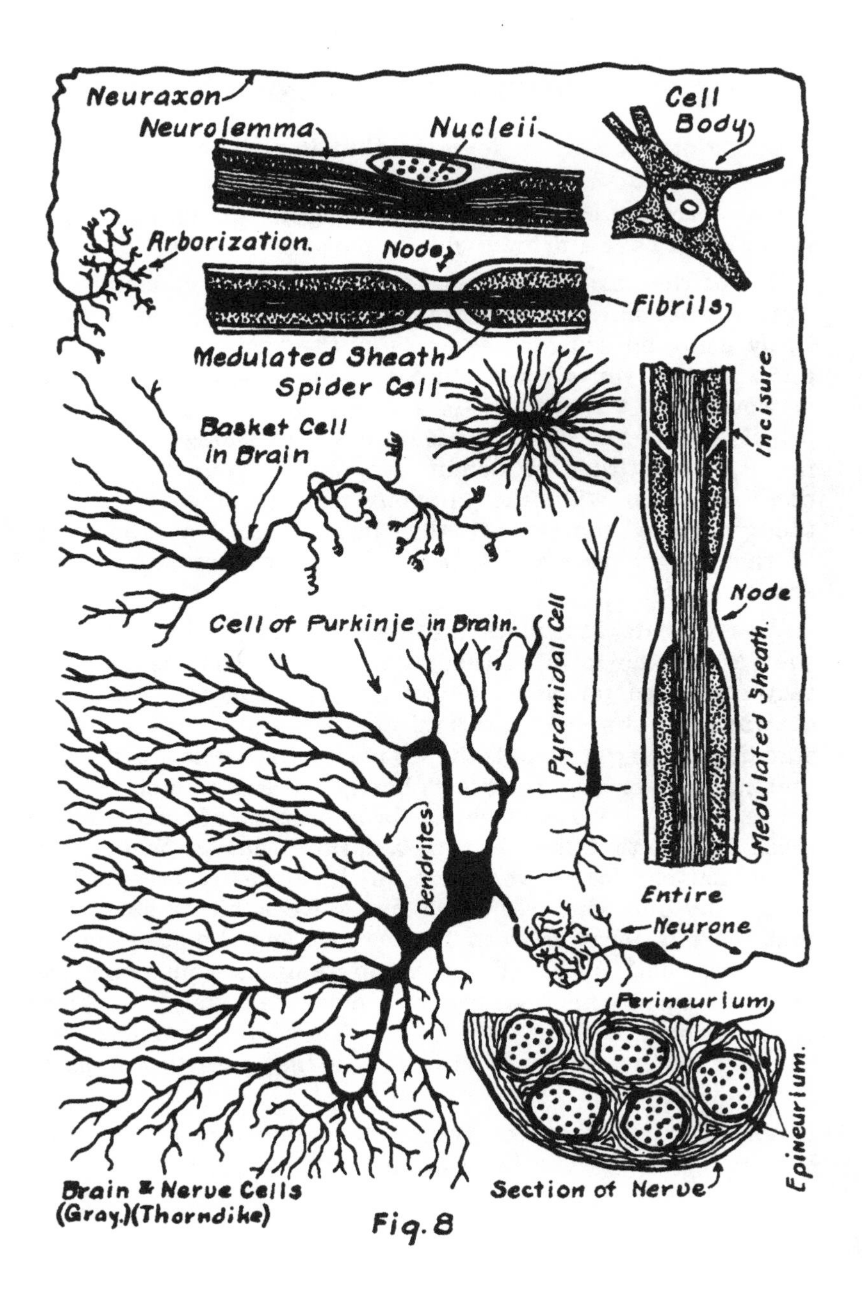
Neuraxon
Neurolemma
Nucleii
Cell Body
Arborization.
Node
Fibrils
Medulated Sheath
Spider Cell
Incisure
Basket Cell in Brain
Node
Cell of Purkinje in Brain.
Pyramidal Cell
Medulated Sheath.
Dendrites
Entire
Neurone
Perineurium
Epineurium.
Brain & Nerve Cells
(Gray.)(Thorndike)
Section of Nerve

Fig. 8

Changing thought to force so that it can be expressed in forms physical.

Concentrating or collecting mental forces into specific forms so they will have a definite aim or purpose.

One of the hardest processes of the Cycle to understand is Transformation. Perhaps we can get a slight insight into it, by using an educated example of the same thing. We all know that if you sit and stare at your pencil, wishing that it would get up and write, nothing will be done by the pencil; but if you WILL a definite set of thoughts concerning it, a multitude of definite actions in your tissues will occur and you will take up your pencil and write. Thus, thought moved matter, actually; but not until a definite set of thoughts were made specific enough to accomplish that end.

When Innate assembles universal forces in the brain cell they are in the form of thoughts. In this non-specific state they are called *foruns.* They are, as yet, thought; absolutely abstract, but the most powerful creations in nature, notwithstanding. Being abstract, they have no connection with matter; no hold on it; in this "ghostly" state, cannot grip it. (page 80, V) Transformation is a process of so changing these foruns, that they become a form of energy which does affect matter; does have a grip on it. It really becomes the link. Any one who sees a magnet move a bit of steel, sees that there is force between the magnet and the steel though they may not touch. There is no tangible connection between them, yet this invisible force moves the steel; the "lines of force" have a "grip" on matter. They are intangible, yes, but they are by no means abstract, in the sense that *hope* or *charity* is.

When foruns have been transformed they are units, called Mental Impulses. The force is now outside the mental realm and in the material realm, in which they can be reckoned a form of energy and as such, be expressed in physical forms.

Art. 59. The Seventh Step of the Normal Complete Cycle. Mental Impulse. (80, 141, 233, V)

A unit of mental force for a specific tissue cell, for a specific occasion.

A special message to a tissue cell for the present instant.

It differs from a universal force, in that it is constructive and is for a particular moment and need of coordination, while universal forces are not constructive in particular, are for all moments generally, and are too general to be coordinative. (Prin. 10, 15)

It is not fully understood what mental impulses are. This is no reflection upon Chiropractic, for, engineers and electricians do not know what electricity is. Yet they know its laws and manifestations and are so able to make practical application of this knowledge.

Chiropractors know the manifestations of mental impulses. They can make practical application of this knowledge, in getting the sick well. Whatever the force is, they know that they have named a unit of it, Mental Impulse, with as much justification as the electricians have named a unit of electrical current, *ampere.*

Each tissue cell requires specific impulses every moment. Since there are millions of cells it takes millions of impulses for them every moment. There are new ones for every adaptative change. These impulses are only good for the moment for which they are created. **They cannot be stored up or dammed back**; if this were possible the mental impulses would immediately become useless.

Art. 60. The Eighth Step of the Normal Complete Cycle. Propulsion. (117, 143, 233, V)

The sending or the starting of the mental impulse.

Dispatching the message to the right tissue cell.

The effort which causes the mental impulse to go to the tissue cell.

The term is derived from *propel,* "propel: to impel forward or onward by applied force." (Webster) Let us use the theory, here, that mental force is a form of energy. Forms of energy, as studied in physics show a decided expenditure of effort somewhere. Either given off by these energies or by something else, in giving them origin. Electric generators require the expenditure of many horsepower by their engines to propel the current. Is it not then, consistent to assume that the departure of mental impulses from brain cell, is accompanied by some kind of effort? Perhaps it is a physical movement of the cell; as, contraction.

Review Questions for Articles 51 to 60, inclusive.

1. Does a tree have an innate intelligence?
2. Which kind of "living things" can live in a wider range of environment?
3. What is Mental, the third step of the cycle?
4. What two classes of things does Innate assemble adaptatively, to build and maintain an organism?
5. What is Mind?
6. What is Innate Mind?
7. What is Educated Mind?
8. What is Creation, the fourth step of the cycle?
9. What is Brain Cell, as considered in the cycle?
10. Explain the step, Transformation.
11. What is Mental Impulse?
12. Can Mental Impulses be stored up or dammed back? Why?
13. What is Propulsion?

Art. 61. The Ninth Step of the Normal Complete Cycle. Efferent Nerve. (117, 143, 233, V)

The route of mental impulse from brain cell to tissue cell.
The nerve from brain cell to tissue cell.

The nerve-tissue cells in the brain have extremely long axons, extending to the tissue cells; or if an axon does not extend that far, it has connections of relay cells with their axons extending farther; one of these reaching the cell. While anatomy does not show any visible connections between them, the doubtful joints being called *synapses*, both laboratory and clinical findings show that there are very definite connections. In telephoning from Davenport to New York, one does not use one continuous wire with no breaks in continuity, but a relay of wires. The connections between these different wires are very definite and the route of the message continuous.

Art. 62. The Tenth Step of the Normal Complete Cycle. Transmission. (117, 144, 233,V)

The passage of the mental impulse from brain cell to tissue cell.

The conveyance of the mental force. (Prin. 23,27, 28)

The function of the nervous system is to transmit mental force to and from the tissue cell; or rather from brain cell to tissue cell and back again. The question often arises, why are nerves necessary, or why must Innate use them, "she being so infinitely wise?" A like question about electricity would be just as pertinent. Why does electricity prefer to travel through or over wires when it can travel in the radiant form? Yet a metal wire will gather to itself radiant electricity and change it to dynamic or flowing form. If this were not true, it would be impossible to have radio sets in our homes.

So far as we know, mental force may be radiated; perhaps that is the explanation of telepathy. Be that as it may, there are plenty of proofs that mental force prefers nerve tissue to travel through, and Innate adapts this natural law to her purposes, using nerve tissue to conduct mental impulses. It being a material, it has the limitations of material — hence interference is possible. (Prin. 5, 24, 27)

Art. 63. The Eleventh Step of the Normal Complete Cycle. Tissue Cell. (117, 144, 233, V) (Webster)

The smallest unit of tissue considered in function.

That unit of tissue which, with one mental impulse, will perform one unit of function.

A unit of organic matter.

It may have many functions but that one for which it is built, and which it does coordinately or cooperatively for the benefit and welfare of other tissues of the body, is the function mentioned in this cycle.

Tissue: "An aggregation of cells, fibers, and various cell products, forming a structural element." (Dorland)

Cell: "Any one of the minute protoplasmic masses which make up organized tissue, consisting of a circumscribed mass of protoplasm containing a nucleus." (Dorland)

In Chiropractic, we study the tissue cell physiologically and histologically as other sciences do. We learn in these studies that a tissue cell is the smallest unit of "living" matter; that it is organic matter and that cellular organisms have "signs of life."

Chiropractically, we consider the tissues that are actively organic. That is to say, tissues that have been built by mental force, but from which the life force has departed, leaving only the inactive structures, are not of immediate interest to Chiropractic. To put it plainer, Chiropractic is not much concerned with the laboratorical classification of "dead"

matter, though they do not underestimate its value in certain lines. Chiropractic is interested in the study of matter in the sense that it looks continually for the activity of intelligence in "live" matter. It is for a scientific purpose, not industrial, as a means to get the sick well.

Art. 64. THE SIGNS OF LIFE.

The signs of life are evidence of the intelligence of life.

The signs of life are the evidences of the "powers" of intelligence.

There are five principal signs of life.

Definition of *life*: "The quality or character which distinguishes an animal or a plant from inorganic or from dead organic bodies and which is especially manifested by metabolism, growth, reproduction and internal powers of adaptation to environment; the property by which the organs of an animal or plant, or the organism as a whole, are conceived as maintained in the performance of their functions, or the state in which all or any of the organs of a plant or animal are capable of performing all or any of their functions." (Webster)

There are other interesting definitions of life which it would be well to read in Webster's International Dictionary, for purposes of comparison. According to definitions of life as given in Webster (They are too long to quote here) life is the quality which distinguishes the matter of the vegetable and animal kingdoms from inorganic matter, or organic matter which is no longer living; "the property or capacity of adaptation to environment." According to that, then, to the physicist the signs of life mean nothing more than, signs of life; but to the chiropractor, they are signs of the attention of a localized intelligence. (Prin. 18, 19, 20)

With these Chiropractic principles in mind, let us examine the Five Signs of Life. Named in order of importance they

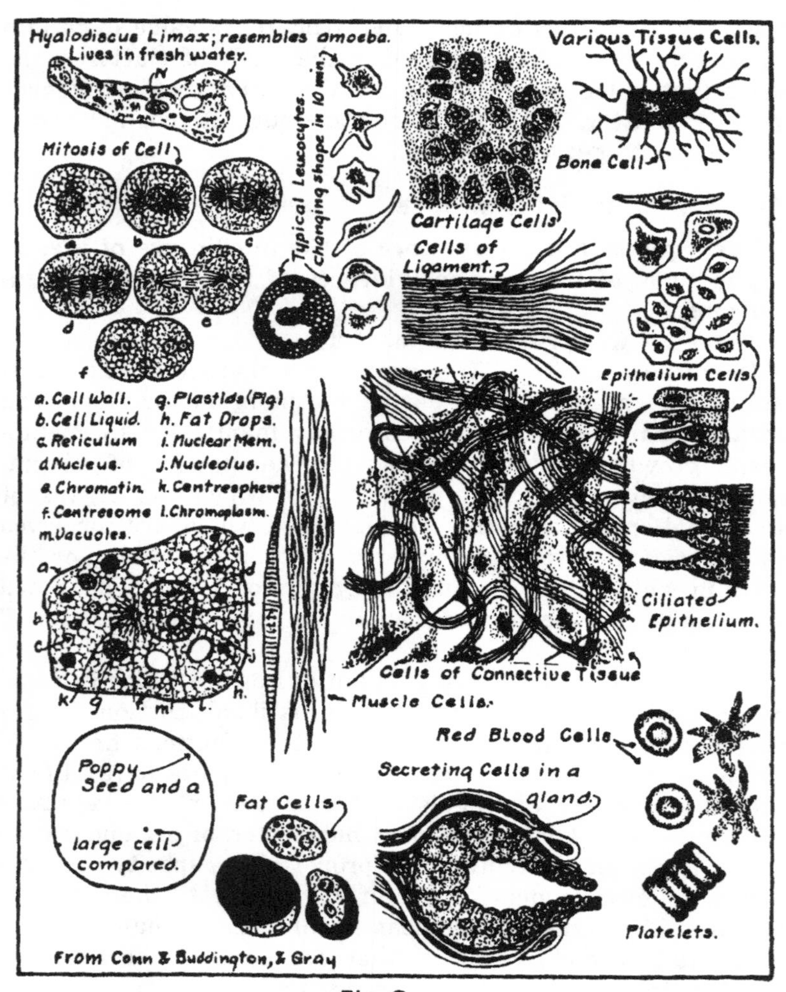
Hyalodiscus Limax; resembles amoeba.
Lives in fresh water.
N
Mitosis of Cell
a
b
c
d
e
f
Typical Leucocytes.
Changing shape in 10 min.
Various Tissue Cells.
Bone Cell
Cartilage Cells
Cells of Ligament.
Epithelium Cells
a. Cell Wall.
b. Cell Liquid.
c. Reticulum
d. Nucleus.
e. Chromatin.
f. Centresome
m. Vacuoles.
g. Plastids (Pig.)
h. Fat Drops.
i. Nuclear Mem.
j. Nucleolus.
k. Centresphere
l. Chromoplasm.
Ciliated Epithelium.
Cells of Connective Tissue
Muscle Cells.
Red Blood Cells
Poppy Seed and a large cell compared.
Fat Cells
Secreting Cells in a gland.
Platelets.
From Conn & Buddington, & Gray

Fig. 9.

are: Assimilation, Excretion, Adaptability, Growth and Reproduction. The first two are very important and the "powers" of "living things" are very latent indeed, without them.

Art. 65. ASSIMILATION. 1st Sign of Life.

The power of assimilation is the ability of an organism to take into its body food materials selectively, and make them a part of itself according to a system or intelligent plan.

Philosophically, we wish to call attention to the fact that any living thing, that is able to take food materials into its body, takes only that which it needs in its upbuilding or maintenance. It will not take anything into its body that it cannot use in that process. This indicates *selective* ability. Selection requires local and repeated judgments; judgment requires intelligence, and local judgments require a local intelligence, that is, an intelligence in the body. Besides that, to be able to take food elements and form them into the parts of a structure, (An organism is a structure) takes more than a haphazard piling-up of materials. It requires an intelligence able to plan the structure; and to build the structure according to that plan, out of the material selected. (Prin. 21)

Art. 66. EXCRETION. 2nd Sign of Life.

The power of excretion is the ability of an organism to give off waste matters selectively, which an intelligence deems are no longer of use in that structure.

Here, also, we see that intelligence is active. Non-intelligent matter is not able to judge matter; to decide which matter shall be added to matter. It requires selective ability to do this. Chiropractic has ample proof that intelligence is at work in the organism, having its welfare in mind. It takes judgment to decide which materials have served their purpose and are no longer usable. If any undesirable materials

are in the food, foreign to the uses of the organism, it requires intelligence to decide whether they are foreign materials or not; intelligence to sort them out, and an intelligently guided process to get rid of them, if they do happen to get in. Undoubtedly the forces of physics and chemistry are used in getting materials into and out of the organism, but it is plainly evident that these forces are also selected by intelligence.

Art. 67. ADAPTABILITY. 3rd Sign of Life.

Adaptability is the intellectual ability that an organism possesses of responding to all forces which come to it, whether Innate or Universal.

All the signs of life, no matter what the form, are motions of a certain kind. They must be expressed by motion of matter, else they cannot be signs. (Prin. 13)

Adaptability is the ability to adapt by virtue of having Intellectual Adaptation. The student is cautioned not to confuse *adaptability, adaptation* and *Intellectual Adaptation.*

Intellectual Adaptation is a mental process which takes place in the brain cell. It is strictly immaterial; the antithesis of physical.

Adaptation is a physical process that takes place as the expression of Intellectual Adaptation. The Physical Personification of it.

Adaptability is the ability to perform the above processes.

The definition mentions the intellectual ability to respond to forces. This implies an applied force; which would be environment. The student's attention is called, here, to the word *responding,* which indicates sensibility. If intelligence were not present the structure would receive the environmental forces passively, as a lump of clay. Organisms, however, show the presence of intelligence by the manifestations of that intelligence, in judging every circumstance of environment which may, even remotely, have something to do with the organism. This is detailed, instantaneous and specific judgment, certifying the presence of intelligence. The process of judgment and the subsequent plans of intelligence is called Intellectual Adaptation. The expression (Adaptation) of this instantaneous judgment may require some time (Prin. 6) because of the limitations of matter. (Prin. 24)

All organisms have the benefit of Intellectual Adaptation. If they did not, they could not be alive at all; (Prin. 23) but an organism having the third sign of life unusually developed, is higher in the scale of life because of its ability to make more response to environmental conditions, and thus extend its range of possible environment. Man has the most powerful organ of Intellectual Adaptation, the Educated Brain, hence a greater adaptability. He rates himself higher in the scale of life because of his higher powers of sensibility and reasoning.

Art. 68. GROWTH. 4th Sign of Life.

The power of growth is the ability to expand according to intelligent plan to mature size, and is dependent upon the power of assimilation.

That which was said about decisions in regard to assimilation and excretion will apply to intellectual actions in growth. There is plenty of evidence of intelligence shown in growth. In the first place, there must be a wonderful "know-how". Growth is always according to plan; a tissue cell or any other organism of a given kind is the same here as in India. Besides there is a control as to size and direction. Living things do not grow beyond their mature size. Who determines that size? Any moderation or variation of type must be directed by intelligence for that specific case. These decisions are the prerogative, of intelligence. (Prin. 21, 23)

Art. 69. Reproduction. 5th Sign of Life.

The power of reproduction is the ability of the unit to reproduce something of like kind; the power to perpetuate its own kind.

In this sign of life as in the others there is evidence of intelligence. It is obvious that some organisms reproduce their own kind—that shows intellectual guidance. Also, there is always a control manifested in all forms of reproduction to preserve an intelligent balance. When an organism is a unit of a race it reproduces its own kind. If this were not true, the race could not continue. Even here, we notice a control; as, in a hive of bees, all bees do not reproduce themselves, but the queen alone is allowed to do so for the whole hive.

In the body, Innate does not allow all cells to reproduce their kind *ad lib.* If they did, it would not be coordinative action to preserve the size, shape and functions of the body. When there is an uncontrolled reproduction of cells in the body, it results in pathology.

In the study of these signs of life the expression *"power of"* is mentioned frequently. It was apparently attributed to the objects of material in question; but when we say "power" we are directly referring to the intelligence in the organism, and the student is reminded that we use the word *power* and *intelligence* synonymously.

The student may wonder why motor function is not named as one of the signs of life, since the most obvious sign is motion. In answer to this, we will call attention to the fact that all five signs of life are motion, hence it is unnecessary to name motion as part of itself. (Prin. 13) The peculiarity of this motion, however, that distinguishes it from other observable motions, is that it is adaptative; it shows the guiding hand of intelligence. None of these are shown in moving inorganic matter; as, a rolling rock.

The student is cautioned not to confuse Excretion and Reproduction, the Signs of Life, with Excretion and Reproduction, the Primary Functions. There is some difference, which will be explained later.

Art. 70. REPRODUCTION OF CELLS (Webster) (Dorland) THEORY OF CELL EXPANSION. (p. 8 to 26 Incl. Vol. II)

Reproduction of cells pertains to the expansion of cells in the developmental or embryonic centers which are derived from the blastoderm.

A center is composed of cells, representing one of the forms of the four primary tissues, and there are centers of all four kinds, in order that all kinds of cells may be reproduced for growth and reparation.

Reproduction is very closely associated with growth and reparation. Considering reproduction as a function, our study can be made more exact by examining the tissue cell as a unit which is functioning. In order that the body may grow, it must have more cells, and this is accomplished by the reproduction of tissue cells; by cells whose function it is to serve that purpose.

In the body, these reproducing cells are in the reproductive centers, as, the embryonic or developmental centers derived from the blastoderm. The blastoderm is formed by the union of the spermatozoon of the male and the ovum of the female. These are in turn secreted by the glands of the reproductive organs of the parents; and this process is the result of the functioning of the expansional centers in generative organs of the parents. The purpose of these special cells is Reproductive Function, one of the Nine Primary Functions.

Under the microscope, these cells can be seen to reproduce their kind by dividing into two cells and each of these dividing into two cells, and so on. This process is called *mitosis,* commonly know as cell division. In Chiropractic the cause of it is explained by **The Theory of Cell Expansion.**

This theory states that from the time of impregnation of the ovum, the possibilities of all the cells of the body which are to be used in the development and in the maintenance of its structure are contained in that one cell.

These possibilities are expanded to full grown cells as intelligence needs them for building and repairing purposes. This action we see manifested as cell division. We can see the cell division but cannot see the unexpanded cells. This does not weaken the theory of cell expansion, however, since the theory is based upon results rather than upon what can be seen. The student should keep in mind that there is infinity in smallness as well as in magnitude; and it is not possible to see all that takes place in a tissue cell.

In the normal body, cells are not reproduced faster than they are needed for growth, reparation, or for propagation of species. If they do, through lack of Innate's control, there will be incoordination or pathology. Some cells are never allowed to reproduce; certain others are, but only at such times and in the manner that Innate desires. Example: muscle cells are reproduced from developmental centers; but at certain times, as in case of a wound, Innate will cause connective tissue to proliferate.

Reproduction as a sign of life refers to the propagation of species of the whole unit; propagation of the race.

Reproduction as a Primary Function refers to the functioning of an organ whose purpose is reproduction as a coordinative act. The fact that the expression is applied to the act of a tissue cell, does not change its meaning, for in that case, the tissue cell is considered as an organ.

Review Questions for Articles 61 to 70, inclusive.

1. What is Efferent Nerve?
2. Explain Transmission.
3. What tissue is used for Transmission?
4. What is Tissue Cell as considered in the cycle?
5. What are signs of life?
6. How many principal signs of life are there?
7. How may we know the strength of organization by the signs of life?
8. What is Assimilation?
9. What is Excretion?
10. What is Adaptability?
11. Differentiate between Adaptability, Adaptation, and Intellectual Adaptation.
12. What is Growth?
13. What is Reproduction?
14. Differentiate between Reproduction as a sign of life and Reproduction as a Primary Function?
15. What is the Theory of Cell Expansion?
16. Is the Theory of Cell Expansion opposed to the Theory of Cell Division?

Art. 71. The Spermatozoon. (Dorland) (Webster)

The spermatozoon is a single animal cell which is secreted by the testicle, an organ of the male, and consists of a body with a nucleus and a tail, which has flagellate movement.

"The motive generative element of the semen which serves to impregnate the ovum. It consists of a head, or nucleus, a middle piece, and a flagellum, or tail." (Dorland)

This animal cell is an organism with locomotion of its own, accomplished by the flagellate movement of the tail. In comparison to its size, its movement is quick and darting; unlike the movement of the amoeba. It can be kept alive for a time in artificial environment.

The spermatozoon is evidently that which carries the cell possibilities to be expanded from the race of the male, to mingle with those of the race of the female. However, this does not mean that the progenitors are depleted of something by taking away the cell possibilities, but, that they are created in the spermatozoon by the Innate Intelligence of the progenitor. This is also true of the ovum.

Art. 72. The Ovum. (Webster) (Dorland)

An ovum is a single animal cell about 1/125 of an inch in diameter, which is secreted by the ovary, an organ of the female. It is surrounded by a membrane and contains the germinal vescicle, within which is the germinal spot.

See definition in Webster's International Dictionary. It is too long to quote here.

Evidently the ovum contains all the cell possibilities to be expanded from the race of the female, which when mingled with those from the race of the male, furnish all the unexpanded cells necessary for the growth and maintenance of that individual "living thing." These mingled and combined cell possibilities represent the sum total of all the *successful* adaptations of all the progenitors in their battles with environment and their successful development. Hence it is seen that an unsuccessful attempt at adaptation which has accomplished nothing, or where the attempt has not even been made, accomplishes nothing in the progenitors' bodies and they have nothing to transmit, in those instances, to posterity. (This is the basis of the Chiropractic explanation of evolution, which is taken up later.)

Art. 73. The Pronucleus.

"Either of the two nuclei of a fertilized egg cell after maturation but before segmentation—the female pronucleus, formed from the chromosomes left in the egg after forming the polar bodies, and male pronucleus, formed by the nucleus or head of the spermatozoon." (Webster)

Nucleus: "An organ present in the protoplasm of most plant and animal cells, except in certain forms of low organization, and regarded as an essential factor in their constructive metabolism, growth, and reproduction and in the hereditary transmission of characters. . . ." (Webster)

The ovum is a single cell, which when impregnated, contains chromatin from both parents, by means of which the characteristics of both male and female are transmitted to the offspring. In the process of fertilization, the head of the spermatozoon penetrates the ovum, leaving its tail to drop off and be absorbed. The ovum then has two nuclei; one of its own and one that came with the spermatozoon. These two centrosomes then act as a basis for the first cleavage or cell division. This single cell or ovum, with its two nuclei is then ready for immediate development.

Art. 74. Mulberry Mass or Morula.

"The segmented ovum in the mulberry stage, forming a solid mass of cells." (Dorland)

Morula: "The globular mass of cells (blastomeres) formed by clevage of the egg of many animals in its early development. A typical morula differs from a typical blastula (which in many animals it precedes) by having no central cavity." (Webster)

In a few hours after the impregnation of the ovum, the cell has divided into many other cells by mitosis, forming a solid mass of cells resembling a bunch of grapes or a mulberry with its little globules. It then becomes stationary in the uterus, upon a spot of the surface which has been prepared for it by menstruation.

Art. 75. The Primitive Streak or Trace.

"An opaque band which appears in the vertebrate blastoderm in the axial line of the future embryo, but somewhat behind the place where the embryo proper begins to develop. In it the epiblast and hypoblast are not distinguishable as distinct layers; along each side of the mesoblast begins to differentiate." (Webster)

In the course of a very short time a dark line appears on the surface of the mulberry mass; it has a knob on the anterior end. This dark streak with the knob, is the spinal cord and brain—the first recognizable structure to appear. It stays on the surface for a short time and then sinks slowly into the mulberry mass as the layers are formed.

It would seem that the inborn intelligence is a contractor and builder and has brought on the grounds the contractor's shack and tools.

Art. 76. The Blastoderm.

"A membrane formed by the repeated segmentation of the blastomeres; specif., that formed by the actively segmenting part of the eggs of most vertebrates in their early stages. It soon becomes differentiated into the germ layers, and from it the embryo forms." (Webster)

"The delicate membrane which lines the zona pellucida of the impregnated ovum. The blastoderm is formed by the cells (blastomeres) which result from the splitting up of the ovum after impregnation, and have been pushed from the center of the accumulation of the blastochyle. The blastoderm forms a hollow sphere (blastodermic vesicle). Trilaminar blastoderm, the state of development in which the embryo is represented by the three primary layers; the ectoderm, the mesoderm and the entoderm" (Dorland)

In the blastoderm the cells are arranged in three layers. These three layers are the germinal cells from which the tissues of the body are developed. They are named epiblast, mesoblast and hypoblast; or ectoderm, mesoderm and entoderm.

Art. 77. THE THREE LAYERS OF THE BLASTODERM.

From the outer layer, the epiblast, the skin and nervous tissues are developed.

From the middle layer, the mesoblast, is derived the tissues that make up the bulk of the body.

From the inner layer, the hypoblast, is derived the tissues that make up the mucous linings of the inner organs of the body.

From these three layers, the four primary tissues of the body are derived.

As the blastoderm becomes the body, the germinal cells of its three layers become the expansive centers of the body; in which cells are expanded for the purpose of growth and reparation. These germinal cells are actually maintained as a clan, throughout, whose purpose it is to reproduce cells; not only their own kind, but there are germs that reproduce cells that are race vehicles to carry forth cell possibilities to the next generation. The purpose of the latter germinal cells is a Primary Function, called Reproductive Function, for their work is to benefit the body as a whole.

Art. 78. THE FOUR PRIMARY TISSUES.

The four primary tissues derived from the three layers of the germinal cells of the blastoderm are: Epithelium, Muscular, Connective, and Nervous.

Our purpose in introducing the study of these tissues is so the student will not fail to notice the structure and capabilities of each form of these primary tissues. Be sure to note the characteristic structure according to the purpose which accounts for its presence in the body; as, when Innate wants motor function, she uses a soft, elongated elastic cell with a movable protoplasm. Its function is active, not passive. When she wants a framework to support the body, she uses some hard, rock-like cells, capable of passive resistance. Innate needs a variety of tools, just as the carpenter does. As the structure of the carpenter's tools are characteristic of the functions they perform, so are the tools which Innate uses. You could not expect the carpenter to saw with his plane; neither can you expect Innate to produce motor function with a bone cell; she has muscle cells for that purpose.

Art. 79. The Twelfth Step of the Normal Complete Cycle. Reception.

The arrival of the mental impulse at the tissue cell.

The receipt of Innate's message.

When a tissue cell is healthy; in a good state of construction, strong and ready, it can receive normally and immediately act adaptatively to the mental impulses. (See Signs of Life). We say it is able to obey Innate readily and normally and has "good resistance." On the other hand, if the tissue cell is sick or injured or poisoned it cannot receive normally or act efficiently. When the tissue cell is not at its best, it is not in as high a state of organization as it should be and it is easy to see that its adaptative action will always be proportionate to its state of organization. Even after perfect transmission has been restored it will require some time for the cell to be brought back to its proper state, therefore the element of time enters. (Prin. 6.) Also, we can see how Innate is hindered by the limitations of matter for awhile, even after transmission is restored. (Prin. 5, 24)

Art. 80. The Thirteenth Step of the Normal Complete Cycle. Physical Personification.

The immaterial expressed in material.

The physical representation of a mental creation.

A material form of a mental conception.

Innate's plans "coming true."

When Intelligence creates, the creations are entirely mental, but none the less real, for that. As evidence to our educated minds, they must be expressed. All forces, mental or physical, must be expressed by matter. (Prin. 10, 15.) We could not be aware of motion unless we perceive matter moving. When we perceive matter moving, we must know, if we reason, that either Universal Intelligence or Innate Intelligence or both, created the forces that set the matter in motion. We know that intelligence created these forces, because the motions are always according to law; either precise unchangeable laws or the laws of precise change—adaptation. Present motion, then, is the physical expression of the mental "plane" of intelligence, and structures of matter are monuments—physical personifications of motions that have been.

An architect plans his great bridge or building. To him the building is real. He can visualize the mental edifice but it will exist only to him and not to any one else until the finished edifice portrays to every one what the creator had in mind.

A planned event, as a party, is but a mental conception, but when it is taking place it is a physical expression (personification) of the mental plans.

How would any one ever know your thoughts if you did not express them through media of material — by speaking, writing, gestures, facial expression, etc., etc.? In the same manner the more profound thoughts (creations) of Innate Intelligence are expressed through the material of every tissue cell.

REVIEW QUESTIONS FOR ARTICLES 71 to 80, inclusive.

1. Describe the spermatozoon.
2. Describe an ovum.
3. Describe the pronucleus and how it develops.
4. What is the mulberry mass?
5. What is the primitive streak?
6. What important significance has the primitive streak?

7. What is a blastoderm?
8. Describe the layers of the blastoderm.
9. Name the Four Primary Tissues and give their origins.
10. What is Reception, the 12th step of the cycle?
11. Explain Physical Personification.

Art. 81. The Fourteenth Step of the Normal Complete Cycle. Expression. (118, 146, 233 V)

The activity of matter which reveals the presence of Innate Intelligence. (Prin. 15, 18)

A "showing" of intelligence—manifestation.

This term is used to indicate Innate's function which is intellectual adaptation.

Expression means just what the word indicates — pushing outward. It is the coming out of something; something becoming evident. This something is the force of Innate Intelligence—mental impulses. The manner of its coming out is very important and significant, for the quantity and direction of these forces are predetermined by the intelligence behind them and the quality is determined by the vehicle of expression; by the character of the structure, or instrument (organ) which Innate uses for that particular purpose. The study of the purposes of these vehicles of expression is the study of *Function.* (Prin. 18, 23).

Art. 82. The Fifteenth Step of the Normal Complete Cycle. Function (118, 146, 233, V)

The purpose or action of a tissue cell, as used by Innate as an organ.

It has reference to the purpose of a unit of matter; the smallest possible organ; the tissue cell.

As expression refers to what Innate does, so function refers to what a tissue cell does.

The function of a tissue cell is always according to its characteristic build, and is the coordinative service it renders the whole body. (Prin. 13)

Function is the fulfilling of a purpose — the purpose being the reason for the existence of anything. Everything in existence has reason for existing; one or more purposes in the scheme of things. The fulfillment of that purpose, whether active or passive, is function. The student should bear in mind that the term *passive* is comparative, for everything in the Universe is in action and also *fulfillment* is action. Hence everything has function; the function of a pen is to be used for writing; an inkwell to hold ink; an envelope to envelope a letter; a steamship's function is to cross the ocean. The fact that these things are sometimes at rest does not change their function in the least. They may not always be *functioning*. The function of an empty inkwell is still to contain ink; and though the steamship is at the dock, its function is to cross the ocean. When they are being used, they are expressing the intelligence of their users. Though intelligence determines the quantity, timeliness, and direction of these functions, the quality of the function depends upon the structural characteristics of the instrument. Thus, the envelope could not conveniently be used for writing, or the pen for enveloping a letter; and the steamship would not make a serviceable inkwell. While this latter is sublimely ridiculous, yet it strongly points out that everything has its own functions and those functions, are what a thing is built to do and accounts for its existence.

A thing may have more than one function or a different function at a different time. Some things have dual, triple or multiple functions. Thus, a chair may be used for sitting, as a footstool, standing upon, as an improvised table or a door prop. Again, we point out that the user expresses himself through these structures as instruments or organs.

Art. 83. PRIMARY FUNCTION. (46, M & M) (332, V) (600, II)

The purpose or action of a tissue cell or organ for coordination.

The cooperative service rendered to the body by a tissue cell or organ.

The characteristic structure of a cell is always in accordance with its primary function.

A tissue cell may have many movements but only those for coordination are primary; it may fulfill its office with no movement; as, a bone cell.

In the foregoing article it was pointed out that a chair might be used for a number of things; but it is obvious that the Primary Function of the chair is to be used for sitting. While it might be used for other things, its harmonious use in the household is strictly its primary function.

Most organs of the body have more than one purpose; as, the skin serves as a covering for the body, secretion, excretion, respiration, radiation, and sensation; and all these are primary functions. In the Normal Complete Cycle, however, following our deductive system, we have narrowed our study down to the ultimate unit organ—the tissue cell. As we go from the general to the specific, it is evident that the study of function will be the primary purpose of *one* tissue cell.

There are four primary tissues in the body, and these four classes are subdivided into other kinds; and these kinds are built into a great variety of structures. Yet there is a reason for so many different kinds of structures, for Innate requires a great many kinds of things to be done.

An examination of the outstanding of these, shows us that; muscle cells are made to produce movement for the benefit of the whole body, bone cells to offer framework, ligaments to serve as guys, epithelial cells to serve as lining and covering, nerve cells to conduct, and glandular cells to secrete.

While all of these cells have other movements and purposes than those named, these other movements are for the cell itself — its private affairs; as, the Signs of Life of the cell. Certain classes of these cells are so important in the body scheme, that when they go wrong they cause more trouble than others. Perhaps some more are susceptible to trouble than others, when there is interference with transmission. At any rate, there are some functions that are more noticeable than others, and clinical findings prove that the functions, that are notorious for going wrong, are about nine in number. These are known in Chiropractic as "The Nine Primary Functions." Not that these are all the primary functions, but they are the nine cardinal trouble makers when there is incoordination.

Art. 84. The Nine Primary Functions. (46, M & M) (332, V) (600, II)

The primary functions which are most commonly involved in incoordinations are approximately nine in number.

This is an arbitrary number, because nine were selected and named.

List of The Nine Primary Functions:

- **Motor Function.**
- **Calorific Function.**
- **Sensory Function.**
- **Secretory Function.**
- **Excretory Function.**
- **Nutritive Function.**
- **Reparatory Function.**
- **Expansive Function.**
- **Reproductive Function.**

The student is advised to learn the names of the Nine Primary Functions.

The subject of function will be taken up in detail in the Junior Section.

Art. 85. The Sixteenth Step of the Normal Complete Cycle. Coordination. (118, 147, V)

The harmonious cooperative action of the tissue cells, controlled and synchronized by Innate Intelligence.

The perfectly coordinated mutual functioning of all the structural elements of the body.

Harmony of primary functions.

Perfect relation of functional activities for the welfare of the whole body as a unit.

Good "team work" by the tissue cells. (Prin. 23, 32)

The principle of Coordination is one of the most fundamental principles of Chiropractic. The fact, that a cell is in the body at all, is ample proof that Innate requires it to serve a purpose. Any tissue cell in the body that Innate has no need for is an abnormality and is known in Chiropractic as a *tumor.* Innate has no excess property—she keeps a close inventory and possesses no tools that are not used. Therefore, each tissue cell is an organism and therefore, there is intelligence in it. It is absolutely essential that the units comprising the body be of this nature, else Innate could not control them. If it were not necessary for these units to have some intelligence, Innate could just as conveniently use a bit of inorganic matter such as stone, metals, etc. Obviously this is not possible; Innate must have units with adaptability that respond to her urge; the law of demand and supply.

Art. 86. The First Afferent Step of the Normal Complete Cycle. Coordination.

The same as Coordination in the Efferent Half of the Normal Complete Cycle but with the afferent aspect, and consideration.

Art. 87. The Second Afferent Step of the Cycle. Tissue Cell.

The tissue cell that received the mental impulse and responded.

The material that is obeying the mental impulse.

The material that is responding to environment, by its adaptability.

The tissue cell must be sound in order to obey Innate perfectly. (Prin. 5)

In Chiropractic the tissue cell is the unit of material, considered as the smallest organ, which with one unit of force expresses one unit of function. It responds to environmental forces; to the influence of its neighbors, and the urge of Innate. All of these factors enter into what it does. If normal and sane (sound) it will do exactly what Innate wants it to do coordinately; within its limitations, of course. (Prin. 5, 24)

Art. 88. The Third Afferent Step of the Cycle. Vibration.

The motion of a tissue cell in performing its function.

Tissue cells may be said to have three kinds of motion; namely, functional, metabolistic, and physical. The functional is its movement in coordinating—its primary function. The metabolistic, its movement in expressing its signs of life; living for itself. Physical, molecular movement which all matter has, whether it is in the body of a living thing or in common matter outside of the body.

The functional and metabolistic movements have the characteristic of being managed by intelligence.

In order to have perfect functional and metabolistic vibrations, the structure must be sound. (Prin. 5, 24)

Since all matter has physical vibration, it is clear that Innate cannot break this universal law, (Prin. 24) yet she can adapt it to her uses. This is mentioned, since, bone, a hard rock-like material, does not move its cells when it functions, as does muscle. Yet, its function, which is support, depends upon its hardness and resistive strength. Hardness and resistance are physical "properties" of matter, as the result of cohesion, valency etc. Innate, of course, wants this substance to be hard and resistive and she is the cause of it being that way, by determining the amount of cohesion and managing the valency. Thus, we know that the function of bone depends upon "managed" physical "properties" and that these are given to matter by intelligence. (Prin. 1.) Valency and cohesion etc. are forces expressed by molecules and atoms, hence motion exists there. Therefore, a material of the body which seemingly has a passive function is really dependent upon functional impulses as well as metabolistic. A little further thought along this line will show that the functioning of *any* tissue of the body is the result of "managed" natural forces of the universe.

Art. 89. The Fourth Afferent Step of the Cycle. Impressions of Vibrations. (109, 171 V)

The message from the tissue cell to Innate Intelligence concerning its welfare and doings.

The effect of vibrations of tissue cell upon the afferent nerve.

In the Normal Complete Cycle this refers to the afferent current from any and every tissue cell and does not refer to special sense impressions. (See Art. 109, Special Sense Cycle.)

The vibrations are not transmitted over the afferent nerve, but the vibrations are impressed and the impressions are transmitted.

An analogy may help to make this clear. When a person steps into a telephone booth and takes down the receiver, he at once makes a complete electrical circuit which is unvariable and smooth. It makes no sound for the unvariable current does not change the strength of the magnets in the telephone mechanism, and the diaphragms do not vibrate, hence there is no sound. Then the person begins to speak. His voice vibrates the diaphragm in the transmitter which "makes and breaks" the electrical current, which, then, is no longer smooth and travels in fluctuating strength. This fluctuating current changes the strength of the magnet in the receiver at the listener's end of the cycle, which causes the diaphragm in his receiver to vibrate, thus new sound is created which is a replica of the original sound at the transmitter. At no time do the vibrations of the speaker's voice leave the telephone booth, or travel over the wire, as is popularly supposed by many persons who do not have much knowledge of electricity. The voice that the listener hears is re-created by *his* telephone in *his* booth, perhaps a thousand miles away from the speaker.

Art. 90. The Fifth Afferent Step of the Normal Complete Cycle. Afferent Nerve.

The route from tissue cell to brain cell.

The nerve from tissue cell to brain cell.

In the Normal Complete Cycle, this does not refer to the Special Sense Nerves, but to the communication that each and every tissue cell has with Innate Intelligence. (See Junior Section for General Sense.)

The route of the Afferent part of the Normal Complete Cycle has long been a debated question. While the Afferent route is not definitely known; it is definitely known that there is an Afferent route. As Chiropractic grows older and people's knowledge of nerve physiology increases, more is known about the afferent nerves, and year by year the findings of the anatomist support the Chiropractic theories along this line. Afferent nerve cells are visible enough and easily distinguishable from efferent nerve cells, but it is not clear, in every case, which are special sense nerves and which are merely general sense nerves. It is clear that some special sense nerves, as the optic, are not common general sense nerves, but are highly specialized organs of nerve tissue, which besides their afferent report of vibrations of light, may or may not report general functional metabolistic conditions. (See Fig. 8)

After several years of study based upon clinical findings, study of the nervous system—its anatomy and physiology—linked up with the fundamentals of Chiropractic, the writer offers the following explanation.

Every tissue cell has communication with Innate Intelligence in the brain by means of afferent nerves. By infinitely gradual differences, some of these cells are able to do more communicating than others. Because of this fact it is difficult to make any hard and fast demarcation into classes and any classification must be more or less arbitrary. When this ability of a tissue cell becomes so great that a scientist can observe it, then it can be placed in the rank of special sense, and it is also very evident that such a cell, having so much ability of this kind, can do very little else, and clearly, is a special sense organ. If a cell is so specially built, that reporting to Innate is its specialty, its special purpose; then its function is Sensory Function, one of the nine primary functions. As all cells receive functional impulses in order to act coordinately, so the special sense cell must receive its functional impulses over efferent nerves, in order to act coordinately. Such a cell is able to send to Innate impressions of both kinds of senses; viz., special and general; those concerning environment and those concerning itself; (See Fig. 27) while less sensitive cells can only communicate about themselves. The student can see that the only possible line of demarcation between these two kinds of senses is arbitrarily determined by objective manifestations.

Review Questions for Articles 81 to 90, inclusive.

1. What is Expression?
2. What is Function as considered in the cycle?

3. What is Primary Function?
4. Name The Nine Primary Functions.
5. What is Coordination?
6. What is Vibration as considered in the cycle?
7. What are Impressions of Vibrations?
8. Which are transmitted to the brain, Vibrations or the Impressions of them?
9. What is the Afferent Nerve?
10. Can we anatomically point out the Afferent Nerves of the Normal Complete Cycle?

Art. 91. The Sixth Afferent Step of the Normal Complete Cycle. Transmission.

The carrying of impressions of vibrations to the brain.

The afferent message being conveyed to Innate Intelligence.

It is not a mechanical trembling of the nerve.

Transmission is just the same in Afferent nerves as in Efferent nerves. Impressions of vibrations are mental force just as much as mental impulses are; and their transmission is accomplished in the same way. The student is cautioned not to fall into the error of believing that impressions are a mechanical thrust or punch on nerve ends which "jiggle" their way to the brain, where they violently shake the brain and alarm Innate. An impression is the intellectual personification of the adaptability of the tissue cell, (Prin. 7, 18) and this intellectual force is transmitted, not as vibrations, but as representing the intellectuality behind the vibrations.

Art. 92. The Seventh Afferent Step of the Normal Complete Cycle. Brain Cell.

The place where Innate interprets the impression of vibration.

The place where the impression is changed to enter the mental realm.

It is the receiving department of Innate's workshop.

The same kind of brain cell as efferent and perhaps in some cases the same one.

Art. 93. THE EIGHTH AFFERENT STEP OF THE NORMAL COMPLETE CYCLE. RECEPTION.

Impressions arriving at the mental establishment.

Receipt of the afferent messages.

Brain cell is a tissue cell and receives the same way as any tissue cell.

The receipt is in Innate Brain.

Art. 94. THE NINTH AFFERENT STEP OF THE NORMAL COMPLETE CYCLE. MENTAL.

The same mental establishment as studied in the efferent half of the cycle.

Art. 95. THE TENTH AFFERENT STEP OF THE NORMAL COMPLETE CYCLE. INTERPRETATION.

Analysis of the impression by Innate Intelligence.

Judging the impression.

Transforming the impression into thought.

Changing from the material realm to the immaterial realm.

When the unit of information, the impression, reaches the brain cell it is judged by Innate. This judgment is a thought and therefore in the mental realm. The process is just the reverse to that of transformation, in the efferent half of the cycle. When it is thus changed Innate knows the character of the vibration; whether it is normal or abnormal, good or bad for the body. This knowledge is named in the next step.

Art. 96. THE ELEVENTH STEP OF THE NORMAL COMPLETE CYCLE. SENSATION (152 V).

What Innate knows about one impression.

A unit of knowledge, from a unit of interpretation, of a unit message, concerning a unit of condition, of a unit of matter doing a unit of function, impelled by a unit of mental force, in a unit of time.

The product of interpretation.

A form of energy, that has been transformed back into thought by Innate.

Innate now knows what it is and whether or not, it is good for the body.

Sensation is strictly a mental process or the product of a mental process. It is never abnormal. It may be knowledge of something abnormal but it is never abnormal itself. Sensation is always in the brain. In case of sensation from special sense, the popular belief is that it is in the periphery, but such is not the case. For instance, when you touch an object it seems to you that the sensation, of the object felt, is in the fingers. The object *is at* the fingers but the sensation is *in* the brain. The cells of the fingers could report in vain, if there were not this mental process.

Art. 97. The Twelfth Afferent Step of the Normal Complete Cycle. (152, V)

The sum total of sensations.

The ultimate conclusion of Innate, based upon the total news received.

The completed mental picture.

The opinion which Innate has formed about the periphery, based upon the total of sensations.

Sensation is merely one unit; it is not enough to give complete information. Let us use an analogy. We read the headlines of a newspaper stating that there has been a bad train wreck. The information conveys but little at first and it is not until we read further particulars that we are able to begin to visualize it. When we have read several subsequent newspapers we are able to picture the wreck quite clearly.

Art. 98. The Thirteenth Afferent Step of the Normal Complete Cycle. Innate Intelligence.

The judge of impressions.

The intellect that has the ideation.

The same Innate as studied in the efferent half.

Art. 99. The Fourteenth Afferent Step of the Normal Complete Cycle. Intellectual Adaptation. (155, V)

The plans of Innate to meet circumstances.

The planning of ways and means to overcome or utilize universal forces and matter.

Innate's only function.

It differs from adaptation in that intellectual adaptation is a mental process, and adaptation is the physical personification of intellectual adaptation; mental and physical contrast.

It differs from adaptability in that intellectual adaptation is the action of intelligence, while adaptability indicates the possession of said intellect; contrast between the ability of the actor and the action of the actor.

When Innate receives the impressions from the tissue cell, the material conditions of the cell and the forces existent there, through ideation, become known to Innate, in quantity, quality and intensity. Upon these then, are based the response. In order to maintain harmony, the response will have to be of such quantity, quality and intensity as to give a balance for that moment. The next moment will bring forth a new set of affairs. Thus we see that instead of a steady flow of force from brain cell to tissue cell, there is a continual change. (See Fig. 10) The amount of attention from Innate Intelligence, for any given moment, is always one hundred per cent, although this may be more or less than at the moment before. It is a very fine working of the law of systematic change.

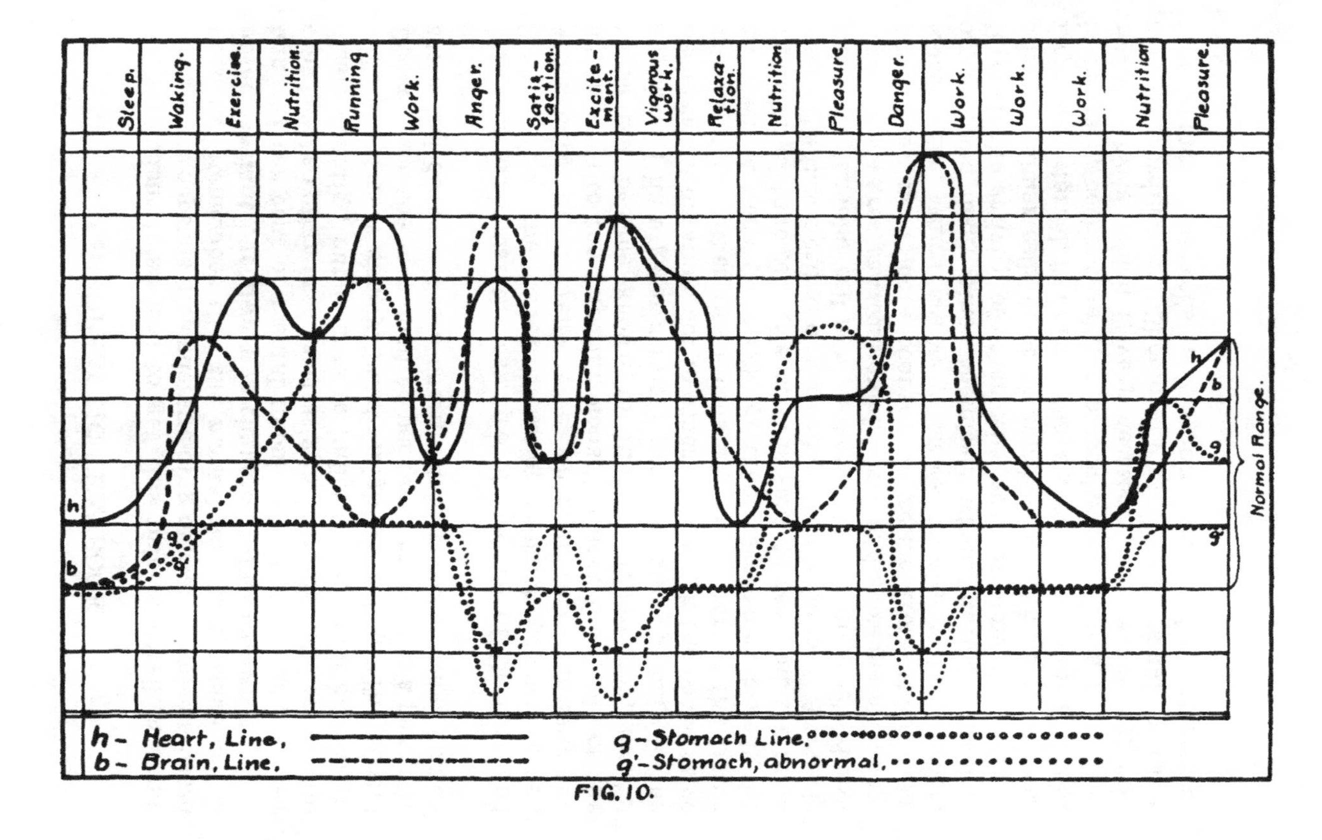
Sleep.
Waking.
Exercise.
Nutrition.
Running
Work.
Anger.
Satis-faction.
Excite-ment.
Vigorous work.
Relaxa-tion.
Nutrition
Pleasure.
Danger.
Work.
Work.
Work.
Nutrition
Pleasure.
Normal Range.
h- Heart, Line,
b- Brain, Line,
g- Stomach Line,
g'- Stomach, abnormal,

FIG. 10.

The student is advised to get this principle well in mind, for upon it depends his understanding of many subjects based upon it. Remember that **the mental flow to a tissue cell is never constant but always is changing.** The expression "one hundred per cent of mental impulses," or "one hundred per cent flow" so often used carelessly in Chiropractic, does not indicate quantity, but is used to indicate *perfection of change.*

To put it very simply, Innate might be called "The Artful Dodger" and the "one hundred per cent" represents a perfectly successful dodge. It is a one hundred per cent manipulation of forces.

Let us again use the example of the law of Demand and Supply. From the tissue cell's actions emanate physical forces, which affect the afferent nerve, which in turn transmits the impressions to the "clearing house", where the needs of the tissue cell become known to Innate. Whereupon, mental impulses, (the urge of service) are sent out, not only to the tissue cell in question, but to others. Through the cooperative actions of the other tissue cells and the action of the tissue cell itself, actions (functioning) take place which benefit the condition of that cell. Hence it is easy to see that the more active the tissue cell, the more adaptation it needs. A muscle cell or a glandular cell is more active than a bone cell, therefore needs a greater variation of forces and more material supply. They need more cooperative action from other cells. Muscle cells, which are very active, require water, carbon, oxygen, and many other chemicals which must be supplied through the activity of other cells, such as glandular. These other glandular cells must be supplied with these substances from the external, in order to have them to prepare; and that is the task, perhaps, of this muscular cell. Thus there is a round, a cycle, which is very necessary, and when perfectly done is coordination. Should any of these cells fail in their functioning, some cells, somewhere, will suffer. Imperfections in the working of the law of Demand and Supply, any where, will cause neglect, inconvenience or suffering.

Art. 100. THE FIFTEENTH AFFERENT STEP OF THE NORMAL COMPLETE CYCLE. UNIVERSAL INTELLIGENCE.

The source of the energy which performs all the foregoing miracles. It being infinite, cannot fully be described, and cannot be defined at all. The beginning and ending of the Normal Complete Cycle.

Art. 101. RESUME OF THE NORMAL COMPLETE CYCLE.

The Normal Complete Cycle is the story of what happens between cause and effect and effect and cause.

The list of thirty-one steps is the conventional outline of the story.

The Story.

Universal Intelligence is in all matter and continually gives to it all the properties and actions. The expression of this intelligence through matter is the Chiropractic meaning of life; therefore life is necessarily the union of intelligence and matter. Force unites intelligence and matter. Universal Intelligence gives force to both inorganic and organic matter. That force which Universal gives to organic matter as a higher order of its manifestations, is called **Innate Intelligence.** The mission of Innate Intelligence is to maintain the material of the body of the organic unit in active organization. It does this by adapting the forces of universal, (which as physical laws are unswerving and unadapted and have no solicitude for matter) so they can be used in the body; so that all parts will have co-ordinated action, thus every part has mutual benefit. This work of Innate is entirely **Mental.** For this reason the forces of Innate never injure or destroy the tissues. The forces of Innate are mental for they are far superior to physical forces, because they control physical forces. This assembling of universal forces is called **Creation,** for they have definite form and purpose, eventually. The headquarters of Innate's control, in the body, is the brain, and the definite unit of this is called **Brain Cell.** From the brain cell as a unit, Innate controls a unit of matter. In the brain cell as a physical workshop of material, Innate **Transforms** the mental force into a definite unit, for a given tissue cell, for a given moment. This specific force, when transformed, is a force which is either a physical energy or a form that controls or sets into action, physical energies. It is called **Mental Impulse.** The departure of the mental impulse from the brain cell is called **Propulsion.** If it is like a physical energy it requires effort. The forces of Innate Intelligence operate through or over the nervous system. That which has efferent direction and which conducts the mental impulse is called **Efferent Nerve.** Since the physical energies can suffer interruption in their transmission, in a like manner, the forces of Innate can suffer interference with transmission; and that is the basis for the existence of Chiropractic. This comparison, also, is the basis of some theories, which contend that the mental impulse is a physical force and therefore subject to the same laws as any other physical force; but it should always be remembered that these physical energies are in the *adapted form* (if this theory is used) and therefore not injurious to tissue as electricity would be.

The conveyance of the mental impulse over the efferent nerve is **Transmission.** Over this route of specialized material the mental impulse travels to **Tissue Cell** where it is **Received,** whereupon the mental conception of Innate, as to what that cell should be or how it should act, comes to pass. That which was only mental, now becomes a physical fact. It shows by its very character that an intelligence planned the form or the action, and this evidence of intelligence is called **Expression;** meaning the coming forth through matter; the showing of intelligence. Things which show this are said to be alive and such expression is called *life.* The character of this action is determined by the character of the tool used by Innate to express herself, therefore the purpose or the action of this tool which is the tissue cell, is **Function.** The function of matter is to express force. In the tissue cell, which is a specific kind of matter, the specific forces of Innate are expressed in a specific manner by an instrument built for the particular kind of expression. The prompt and correct action of that tissue cell, being actuated by Innate's specific force in harmony with all other cells, is called **Coordination.** In this, we see the working of the law of cause and effect, and that every process requires time. In order to perform its function, the tissue cell has motion, both molecular and as a whole cell. This movement is called **Vibration.** These vibrations give off physical forces which are impressed upon the afferent nerve as a form of force called **Impression.** These impressions are transmitted over the **Afferent Nerve.** This **Transmission** is similar to transmission in the efferent half of the cycle, for the forces are similar. When it reaches the afferent **Brain Cell,** it is **Received** much in the same manner as the tissue cell receives, for brain cell is a tissue cell, after all. When this force has reached brain cell, it is immediately admitted into the **Mental** realm by **Mental Interpretation.** The product of this act of interpretation by Innate is a **Sensation.** When Innate has a number of sensations, she has a correct image of the condition of the tissue cell and this is named **Ideation.** Ideation can be the possession of nothing but intelligence. The intelligence in the body, of course, is **Innate Intelligence.** When Innate Intelligence knows what the tissue cell needs, she plans ways and means to make it adapt to its environmental conditions and the mental process of doing this is **Intellectual Adaptation.** The great source of supply from which Innate draws her forces is **UNIVERSAL INTELLIGENCE.**

REVIEW QUESTIONS FOR ARTICLES 91 to 101, inclusive.

1. What is afferent Transmission?
2. What is afferent Brain Cell?
3. What is afferent Reception?
4. In which brain is afferent Reception, as considered in the Normal Complete Cycle?
5. What is Interpretation?
6. What is Sensation?
7. Where is Sensation as considered in the Normal Complete Cycle?
8. What is Ideation?
9. What is Intellectual Adaptation and where does it take place?
10. Is the flow of mental impulses constant or changing?
11. What expression means the same as the Law of Systematic Change?
12. Be able to give a complete resume of the Normal Complete Cycle.

Art. 102. REVIEW OF PRINCIPLES.

As a conclusion to the Freshman Section, the student should turn back to the Introduction and study carefully the principles of Chiropractic. He should learn to give, verbatim, the thirty-three principles. Review Article 22, Art. 23, and Art. 24 and be able to answer the review questions on those three articles. Having done this, as well as a review of the whole Introduction, the student is ready for the study of the Sophomore Section.

Sophomore Text

The Sophomore Section is the study of cycles and the condition of matter. These itemized are: cycles, normal, abnormal, subluxation, restoration, practical, special sense, interbrain, universal, serous cycle, poison, fever, evolution, etc. The Article numbers are continued and the method is the same as in Freshman.

Art. 103. Chiropractic Cycles.

The explanation of the successive steps from cause to effect and back again to the cause.

Sophomore work teaches a broader idea of cycles than was given in the Freshman work. In the Freshman work the Simple and the Normal Complete Cycles were given, and their stories pertained to what happens when Innate Intelligence functions in the human body. Whereas, Chiropractic Cycles really take in a much broader field than that. They pertain to the stories of cause and effect about anything, anywhere, in the Universe, from the Chiropractic standpoint of reasoning; and particularly to the events resulting from the Cause of Dis-ease.

Art. 104. How to Tell the Story.

The story that is the explanation of the cyclic steps may be reversed; that is, going from the effect to the cause and from cause back to effect.

The place to start reasoning is always at the cause or at the effect.

In the Normal Complete Cycle, the cause is in the brain, and is Innate Intelligence.

In the Normal Special Sense Cycles, the cause is environmental or in the periphery.

In the Abnormal Cycle, the cause is the subluxation.

In the restoration Cycle, the cause is the adjustment.

In general, Universal Intelligence is the cause, and that is why most cycles begin naming steps with "Universal."

Art. 105. Physiological Cycles of the Body.

The Serous Cycle; the circulation of the fluids of the body.

The Blood Cycle; circulation of the blood in a cyclic course.

Respiration Cycle; the course of the air into and out of the lungs; and the course of the oxygen to the periphery and back again to environment.

Nutrition Cycle: the course of food from environment to digestive tract, thence to the periphery and back again to environment.

Heat Cycle: the generation, distribution, and dissipation of heat.

Nerve Cycle: the cyclic arrangement of nerve tissue from brain to periphery and back again to brain.

The study of these cycles is found in, and forms the basis for Chiropractic Physiology.

Art. 106. Normal Cycles.

Normal Cycles are those in which the orderly and normal sequence of their steps is unbroken; all of the steps being in perfect harmony.

The cause in Normal Cycles is in the brain; or in environment or periphery.

The Simple Cycle and the Normal Complete Cycle are the ones most studied in Chiropractic.

Normal Cycles are the study of normality. The question of abnormality does not enter, except for comparison. All the work in Freshman was the study of normality. When abnormality was mentioned or described, it was for comparison or for further explanation of the normal. *Normal* means running true to form—nothing going wrong. It is necessary for us to **understand normality before we can understand abnormality.**

Art. 107. ABNORMAL CYCLES.

Abnormal Cycles are those in which the orderly, normal sequence of steps of the Normal Cycles is broken.

The cause, in Abnormal Cycles, is the cause of the disorder; as in the body, interference with transmission (subluxation).

Art. 108. COMPOUND OR COMPLEX CYCLES.

A Compound Cycle is the combination of two cycles working together simultaneously and dependent upon each other.

A Complex Cycle is two or more cycles combined, working together simultaneously and dependent upon each other.

Compound and Complex Cycles must have harmony within themselves in order to have normality and coordination.

We should train ourselves to think of, or to visualize, more than one cycle at work at the same time.

Art. 109. SPECIAL SENSE CYCLES.

A Special Sense Cycle is the story of what happens between the special sense organ and brain cell and back again to periphery.

In each, the cause is in the periphery or in the environment (depending upon where you begin).

The names of these are: sight, sound, smell, taste, and touch.

When the normalcy of a Special Sense Cycle is distributed by a cause, it becomes an Abnormal Cycle.

The subject of special sense is taken up in detail in Senior work, and for that reason only two Special Sense Cycles will be given in Sophomore work, as examples.

The student should know early in the course that general sense, as described in the Normal Complete Cycle, is not the same as the sense studied in the Special Sense Cycles; the latter pertain to Sensory Function.

Art. 110. The Cycle of Sight.

The explanation of the process of sight from the organ of sight to brain cell and back again to periphery.

The organs of sight have specialized nerve cells, whose special function is Sensory; to register the subtle vibrations of light.

The cycle given here starts with the origin of light in the environment.

The steps of this cycle are given in the scheme in Fig. 11.

The steps are self-explanatory with the exception of a few.

The student should bear in mind that a single cycle is given here, though it is really a Compound Cycle.

Light is given off from an origin and travels through space and when it reaches the eye, it is refracted through the lens there and falls upon the retina. In the retina are the specially constructed nerve cells that are able to register vibrations of this kind. These nerve axons begin in structures of nerve tissue called rods and cones. From there, the impressions of vibrations are transmitted over the afferent nerve (optic nerve) to the brain cell, where they are received and admitted into the mental realm by the process of interpretation. Then from one unit of impression Innate derives one unit of sensation. This is the sensation of light. From the sensation of light, Innate has knowledge of the character of the light, and if it is from the secondary rays, which come from an object, Innate gets an ideation of the character of that object and knows what relation the object may have to the body, which "she" is guarding. In order to make response to this element of environment, Innate assembles forces from Universal, from which she can get an inexhaustible supply. The mental process of planning the response is Intellectual Adaptation; and the process of accurately assembling the forces is Creation. This, however, is *thought,* and from the study of brain con-

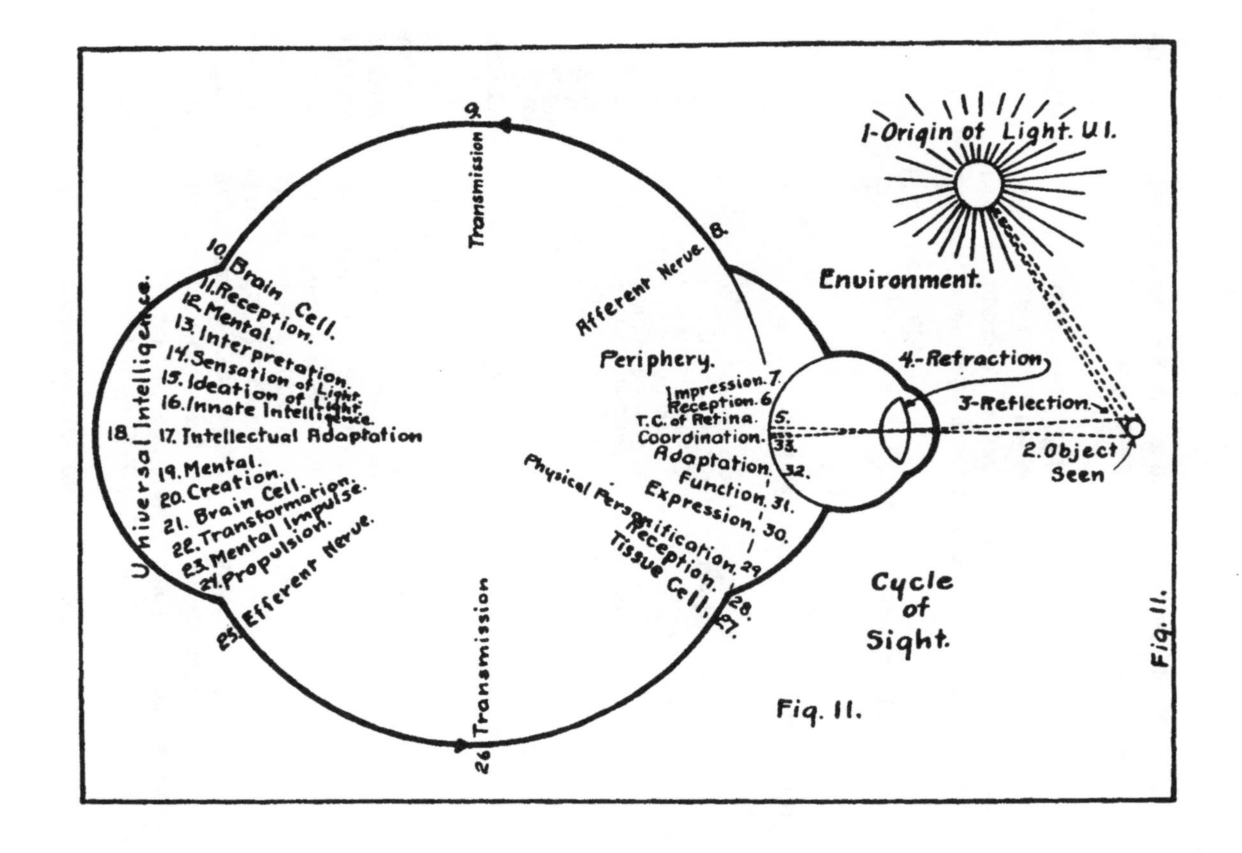
1-Origin of Light. U.I.
Environment.
4.-Refraction.
3-Reflection.
2. Object Seen
Cycle of Sight.
9
Transmission
8.
Afferent Nerve.
Periphery.
Impression. 7.
Reception. 6
T.C. of Retina. 5.
Coordination. 33.
Adaptation. 32.
Function. 31.
Expression. 30.
Physical Personification. 29
Reception. 28.
Tissue Cell. 27.
10. Brain Cell.
11. Reception.
12. Mental.
13. Interpretation.
14. Sensation of Light.
15. Ideation of Light.
16. Innate Intelligence.
18. Universal Intelligence.
17. Intellectual Adaptation
19. Mental.
20. Creation.
21. Brain Cell.
22. Transformation.
23. Mental Impulse.
24. Propulsion.
25. Efferent Nerve.
26 Transmission
Fig. 11.

Fig. 11.

struction is thought to be another brain cell, called "efferent brain cell." In this brain cell, the creation is transformed into a mental impulse which is then propelled on its way, and conducted by the efferent nerve. This nerve is not the optic nerve, for the optic nerve has the typical afferent nerve construction. (See Fig. 33) When the impulse reaches the tissue cell which is functioning (to send impressions of light to the brain), the said tissue cell receives it, and what Innate planned becomes a physical fact (physical personification); and Innate's wishes are expressed by the further functioning of the tissue cell, for the sake of coordination.

Review Questions for Articles 103 to 110, inclusive.

1. What is a Chiropractic Cycle?
2. What is a Compound Cycle?
3. What is a Complex Cycle?
4. Where should we always start reasoning in a Chiropractic Cycle?
5. What is the Cause in the Normal Complete Cycle?
6. What is the Cause in the Normal Special Sense Cycle?
7. What is the Cause in all Abnormal Cycles?
8. What is the Cause in Restoration Cycles?
9. What is the General Cause of all things in the Universe?
10. Name the physiological cycles in the body.
11. What is a Normal Cycle?
12. What is an Abnormal Cycle?
13. When the normalcy of the Special Sense Cycle is distributed, what does it become?
14. What is the Cause in the Cycle of Sight?

Art. 111. Special Sense and Normal Complete Cycles, Compounded.

A special Sense Cycle can be made abnormal by impingement on sensory nerves, especially if nerves of feeling are involved.

A special Sense Cycle can be made abnormal by impingement on efferent functional nerves. This is the most common possibility.

A Special Sense Cycle can be made abnormal by interference with transmission affecting the condition of the special sense

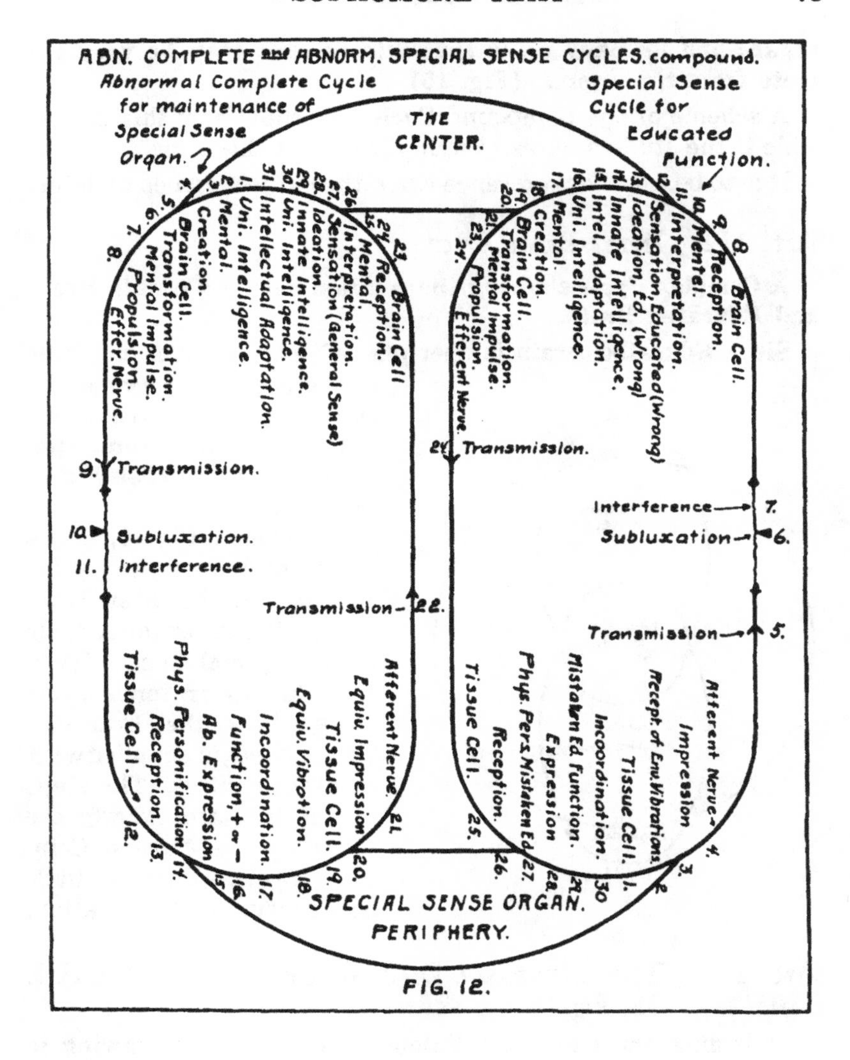
ABN. COMPLETE and ABNORM. SPECIAL SENSE CYCLES. compound.
Abnormal Complete Cycle for maintenance of Special Sense Organ.
Special Sense Cycle for Educated Function.
THE CENTER.
1. Uni. Intelligence.
2. Mental.
3. Creation.
4. Brain Cell.
5. Transformation.
6. Mental Impulse.
7. Propulsion.
8. Effer. Nerve.
9. Transmission.
10. Subluxation.
11. Interference.
12. Tissue Cell.
13. Reception.
14. Phys. Personification
15. Ab. Expression
16. Function, + or −
17. Incoordination.
18. Equiv. Vibration.
19. Tissue Cell.
20. Equiv. Impression
21. Afferent Nerve.
22. Transmission
23. Brain Cell
24. Reception.
25. Mental.
26. Interpretation.
27. Sensation (General Sense)
28. Ideation.
29. Innate Intelligence.
30. Uni. Intelligence.
31. Intellectual Adaptation.
1. Tissue Cell.
2. Recept. of Env. Vibrations.
3. Impression
4. Afferent Nerve
5. Transmission
6. Subluxation
7. Interference
8. Brain Cell.
9. Reception.
10. Mental.
11. Interpretation.
12. Sensation, Educated (Wrong)
13. Ideation, Ed. (Wrong)
14. Innate Intelligence.
15. Intel. Adaptation.
16. Uni. Intelligence.
17. Mental.
18. Creation.
19. Brain Cell.
20. Transformation.
21. Mental Impulse.
22. Propulsion.
23. Efferent Nerve.
24. Transmission.
25. Tissue Cell.
26. Reception.
27. Phys. Pers. Mistaken Ed.
28. Expression
29. Mistaken Ed. Function.
30. Incoordination.
SPECIAL SENSE ORGAN.
PERIPHERY.

FIG. 12.

organ; and in many cases that interference may be very remote from the organ. (Fig. 15)

A scheme of the Compound Cycle will show how this is possible if the student cares to study it out, at this time.

It is to be used for reference when the subject comes up later.

Art. 112. Inter-Brain Cycle.

A Complex Cycle showing the relation between Innate Brain and Educated Brain.

Since Educated Brain is "periphery," because it is made of tissue cells (of nervous tissue), it requires mental impulses, blood, serum, etc. (See Art. 44.) (See Fig. 4 in Art. 38.)

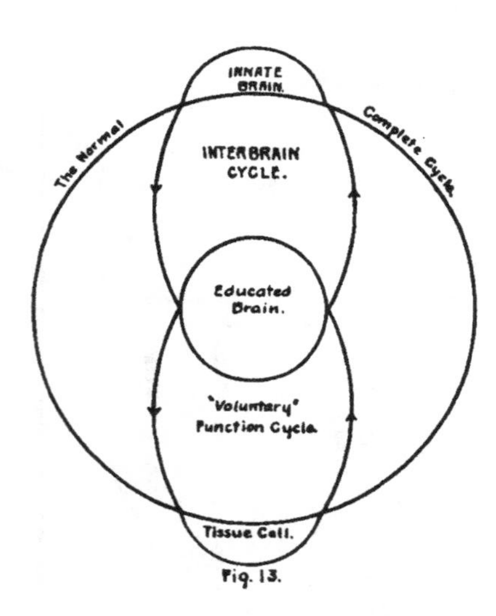

Fig. 13.

The scheme, Fig. 13, shows the relations of the cycles constituting the Inter-Brain Cycle; the lower inner cycle is the Special Sense Cycle, and the upper inner cycle shows how the Educated Brain, itself, is supplied with mental impulses. The steps of the last are exactly the same as the Normal Complete Cycle. There is little need for further explanation.

Art. 113. The Universal Diagram of Cycles. (See Art. 38, Fig.4)

This diagram, which Dr. Palmer calls "the best drawing in the world," shows all the relationships of all cycles.

The course of mental force is followed around the border line of the diagram, as shown by the arrows in the scheme in Fig. 4. Following these arrows from Innate Intelligence, we see that Innate Brain is supplied first. It is really the place from which Innate works. Next, we notice that Innate Body gets its impulses from Innate Brain. Of course this must be, since all the tissues of the body are "innate body," with the exception of Innate Brain; therefore, Educated Brain and Educated Body are Innate Body, so far as metabolism and "involuntary" functions are concerned. From Innate Body, we follow the course back to Innate Brain. Immediately, the arrows lead us from Innate Brain to Educated Brain. This shows us that Innate, if she so chooses, records what has taken place in Innate Body (Pain is a good example of this) so that Educated Mind is conscious of what has been done. Next, we follow the Innate Force through the Educated Brain, where it becomes "tinctured" with whatever quality Educated Mind can give it; thence to Educated Body, where "voluntary" functions take place. Thus, we see that Educated Brain "controls" nothing, but the mental impulses pass through it and further assembling is done there (by Innate), so that there can be conscious action. The arrows lead back to Educated Brain, showing us that there is awareness, educationally, of the action of Educated Body. From Educated Brain, we trace back to Innate Brain, the "cab" from which Innate controls the whole engine. (See Fig. 7.)

This diagram, if the student will take the trouble to use it, can be applied to many kinds of cycles, simple, compound, and complex.

Art. 114. A Written Diagram Showing Innate and Educated Realms.

(See Fig. 7) Innate's possessions	function	voluntary	Educated Brain and Educated Body
		involuntary	Innate Body
	matter	all of body and brain	

Art. 115. The Normal Vertemere Cycle. (Also see Senior Section.)

The Vertemere Cycle is the cycle from Innate Brain to the tissues, holding in situ the vertebra in question.

A subluxation impinging a nerve from brain to organ, also impinges the nerves supplying its own tissues; and that is why it exists as a subluxation. (See this subject in Senior Section.)

In the scheme in Fig. 14, the outer cycle represents the Normal Complete Cycle from brain to the organ in question; and the inner cycle represents a Normal Complete Cycle from Brain Cell to "tissue cell" in the region of the vertebra itself. This makes a Compound Cycle for study. This is one of the most important cycles in the study of Chiropractic, and the student should make himself well acquainted with it. It is the only cycle with immediate practical application, and is the basis for the Art or Technic of Chiropractic.

Art. 116. Universal Forces.

Synonyms: External Forces, Environmental Forces, Physical or Chemical Forces.

Universal Forces are the generalized forces of the Universe, which obey Universal (physical) laws, and are not adapted for constructive purposes.. (Prin. 11.)

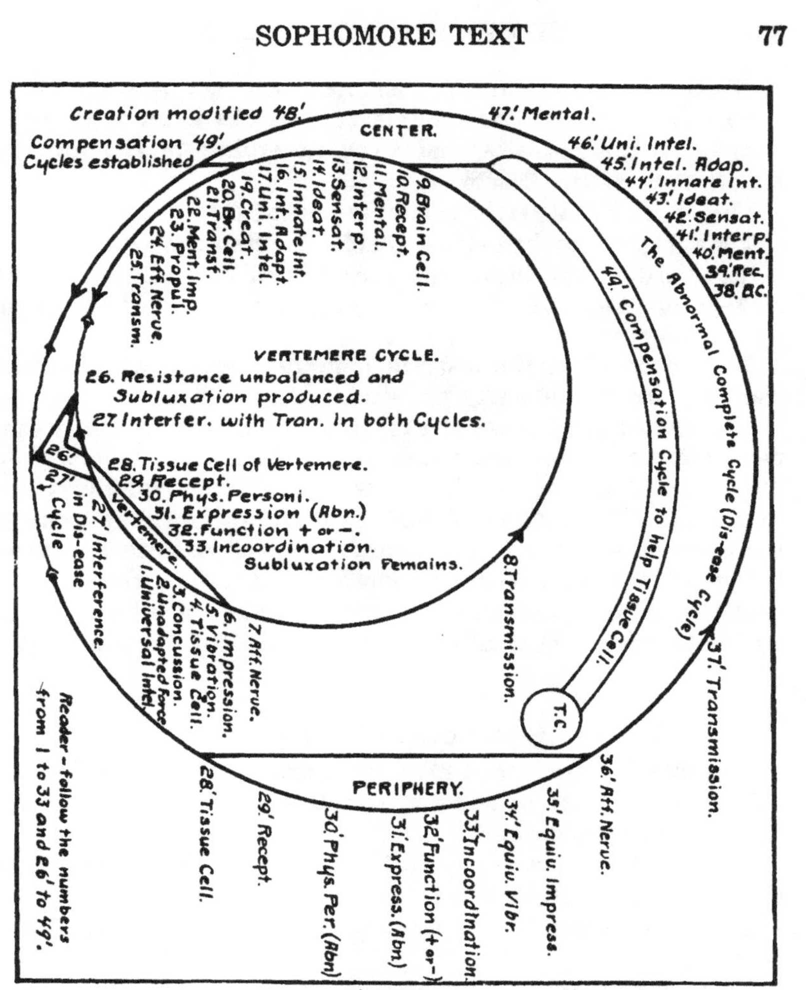
Creation modified 48.'
47.' Mental.
CENTER.
Compensation 49.'
Cycles established
46.' Uni. Intel.
45.' Intel. Adap.
44.' Innate Int.
43.' Ideat.
42.' Sensat.
41.' Interp.
40.' Ment.
39.' Rec.
38.' B.C.
9. Brain Cell.
10. Recept.
11. Mental.
12. Interp.
13. Sensat.
14. Ideat.
15. Innate Int.
16. Int. Adapt.
17. Uni. Intel.
19. Creat.
20. Br. Cell.
21. Transf.
22. Ment. Imp.
23. Propul.
24. Eff. Nerve.
25. Transm.
The Abnormal Complete Cycle (Dis-ease Cycle)
49.' Compensation Cycle to help Tissue Cell.
VERTEMERE CYCLE.
26. Resistance unbalanced and Subluxation produced.
27. Interfer. with Tran. in both Cycles.
26'
27'
Cycle
in Dis-ease
28. Tissue Cell of Vertemere.
29. Recept.
30. Phys. Personi.
31. Expression (Abn.)
32. Function + or −.
33. Incoordination.
Subluxation Remains.
Vertemere.
27.' Interference.
1. Universal Intel.
2. Unadapted Force.
3. Concussion.
4. Tissue Cell.
5. Vibration.
6. Impression.
7. Aff. Nerve.
8. Transmission.
T.C.
37.' Transmission.
Reader - follow the numbers from 1 to 33 and 26' to 49'.
PERIPHERY.
28.' Tissue Cell.
29.' Recept.
30.' Phys. Per. (Abn)
31.' Express. (Abn)
32.' Function (+ or −)
33.' Incoordination.
34.' Equiv. Vibr.
35.' Equiv. Impress.
36.' Aff. Nerve.

Fig. 14.

While Universal Forces, absolutely are not adapted, they can be adapted, and when they are, their character is changed exactly to the opposite, and work according to the laws of adaptation. (Prin. 25, 26)

They may be either beneficial or harmful to the body.

They may be applied either inside or outside of the body.

Some are always inside the body (Prin. 1, 16), they cannot be kept out; but if the body is normal, they are always adapted, when inside.

They may affect the body in numerous ways; as, physical, chemical, or mechanically physical.

Universal Forces have already been described in the Freshman Section. They are necessary to the body, to maintain universal balance, so that Innate will have some dynamic forces to manage. The student should understand that they come to the body in necessary circumstances as well as possible harmful ones. We know them as incidents, weather, food, drink, sunlight—myriads of ways. Sometimes they are harmful, as accidents, inclement weather, poison, unhealthful environment, etc.

Art. 117. Invasive Forces. (Penetrative Forces.)

Invasive Forces are Universal Forces which force their effects upon tissue in spite of Innate's resistance; or in case the resistance is lowered.

Invasive Forces are physical or chemical forces which, in spite of Innate's objection, act in an unadapted way.

They are in numerous forms: as, mechanical (physical) and chemical.

These forces are well known. We fail to acknowledge some of them because they are insidious. They may enter the body as chemical forces and begin their destructive work by corrosion; or they may call for very violent adaptation. The forces of weather, or heat, or cold, etc., call upon the material

resources and Innate of the body for very severe adaptation, and, if the resisting powers are low, do harm. However, all the Invasive Forces do not provoke violent resistance—some are more subtle.

Art. 118. Innate Forces.

Forces arranged by Innate for use in the body.

They are Universal Forces assembled or adapted for dynamic functional power; to cause tissue cells to function; or to offer resistance to environment.

Innate Forces may be for adaptation to other Universal Forces, which have not been adapted; to balance, annul, check, augment, or otherwise adapt them.

Art. 119. Resistive Forces.

Resistive Forces are Innate Forces called into being to oppose Invasive Forces. They are not called Resistive Forces unless they are of that character.

They may be in many forms; as, mechanical (physical) or chemical. Examples of physical form; movement of tissue cells; chemical, antidotes, oxidations, etc.; mechanical, as "bucking" when a patient is being adjusted, sometimes; or as educated adaptations; will, reasoning, etc.

When ill-timed or unbalanced they may produce strains, torn tissues, fractures, luxations, or subluxations. (destructive jujitsu)

When ill-timed or unbalanced it is not the fault of Innate, but the limitations of matter. (Prin. 24)

They may oppose or join some Invasive Forces as determined by Innate.

In adjusting, Innate approves a correct move, but will oppose a wrong move.

The body (Innate managing), will always oppose an Invading Force if it is not beyond the limits of adaptation of the tissues.

Art. 120. Trauma.

Trauma is injury to tissue cells, due to accident or poisoning.

In Trauma, the tissue cells are not sick, necessarily, when injured. The tissues are not incoordinating and if transmission remains normal, healing will quickly ensue.

In the sense that tissue cells will "not be at ease" when injured, a traumatic condition might be called dis-ease, but never incoordination, unless there is interference with transmission.

A distinction might be made in this way; in Trauma the tissue cells are clean and in incoordination they are not.

Trauma is in the field of surgery, and a chiropractor would have no work to do, in this case, unless there are subluxations causing interferences with transmission of mental impulses.

"Trauma, pl. Traumata — A wound or injury. Physic Trauma—an emotional shock that makes a lasting impression on the mind, especially the subconscious mind." (Dorland's Medical Dictionary.)

Art. 121. Disease and Dis-ease. (55, M & M)

Disease is a term used by physicians for sickness. To them it is an entity that one can have and is worthy of a name, hence diagnosis.

Dis-ease is a term used in Chiropractic, meaning not having ease. It is the condition of matter when it does not have ease. In Chiropractic, ease is the entity, and dis-ease is the lack of it.

Dis-ease, in Chiropractic, is indicative of the body being minus something that should be restored, in order to make it normal; that is, in various modes of expression the body lacks ease, health, coordination, transmission, adaptation, well being, 100% quality, soundness, sanity, etc., which must be brought

up to 100%, or RESTORED. That is what Chiropractic aims to do; remember it, RESTORATION.

In Trauma the tissues are not degenerated or depleted. They are just injured; and this is proven by the fact that a wound will heal readily and healthily if the region of injury, or the body is not suffering incoordination.

Dis-ease is the condition of tissue cells when there is incoordination. It is the result of incoordination when the tissue cells do not do their duties coordinately. The tissue cells that fail to function are not always where the symptoms of trouble are; example, gas and tympanites when the liver is not functioning coordinately. When there is incoordination tissue cells are sick; not clean as they are in Trauma. When there is coordination there is a good supply of things, to make a tissue cell healthy. If it is healthy, it is sound. If tissue cells are not coordinating, some tissue cells will be made unsound; therefore, they are sick and not at ease.

So many terms, namely, dis-ease, incoordination, paralysis, physical insanity, used almost synonymously, are confusing to the student. To simplify matters, the writer suggests that the terms dis-ease be used, with the understanding that it indicates *unsound tissue* (physical insanity); tissue which is not clean as healthy tissue is, and that will clearly differentiate it from traumatically injured tissue. (See Paralysis, Art. 264, Jr.)

Unsound tissue can be restored to soundness only by something from within; something from Innate. Dis-ease is the result of the prevention of something from within, coming to the outside. A tissue cell is happy and at ease when it gets it. To restore ease to a tissue cell, that something from within must be restored to it from within; hence the "cure" of dis-ease is from within, and never from without. No treatments or medicines (from without) can give soundness to the tissue cell. It must come from Innate.

Review Questions for Articles 111 to 121, inclusive.

1. Give three ways in which Special Sense can be made abnormal.
2. In the Inter Brain Cycle, what tissue is "periphery"?
3. What Cycle has the most practical application?
4. Why does a misplaced vertebra which is subluxated remain a subluxation?
5. Where is "periphery" in the Vertemere Cycle?
6. What is the character of Universal Forces?
7. Are Universal Forces applied inside or outside the body?
8. What are Invasive Forces?
9. Are Invasive Forces synonymous with Universal Forces, or are they a specific class of Universal Forces?
10. What are Innate Forces?
11. What are Resistive Forces?
12. Are Resistive Forces synonymous with Innate Forces, or are they a specific class of Innate Forces?
13. When Resistive Forces are ill-timed or unbalanced, what are they apt to produce?
14. When Resistive Forces are ill-timed or unbalanced, whose fault is it?
15. What is Trauma?
16. What is Disease?
17. What is Dis-ease?
18. What is the difference between Trauma and Incoordination?
19. In regard to dis-ease what is the sole aim of Chiropractic?

Art. 122. The Cause of Dis-ease.

The cause of Dis-ease is interference with transmission of mental impulses.

The subluxation is the physical representation of the Cause.

Art. 123. How the Cause, Causes Dis-ease.

Interference with transmission causes Dis-ease by preventing Innate from producing adaptation in the tissue cell; hence it becomes unsound and not at ease.

If there is interference with Innate's forces, there is lack of adaptation; lack of adaptation means that Universal Forces will work uncontrolled. Uncontrolled Universal Forces injure tissue cells or make them act incoordinately. Incoordination results in unsound tissue—hence dis-ease.

Art. 124. THE ABNORMAL COMPLETE CYCLE. (185 V)

The Abnormal Complete Cycle is a Compound Cycle consisting of the Abnormal Cycle from brain to organ, combined with the Abnormal Cycle from brain to vertemere.

The orderly sequence of steps has been broken simultaneously in both cycles.

The table of steps is given in Fig. 14. The student is not required to commit to memory the steps of all these cycles, but to be able to reason with the steps as guides. Follow the steps from 1 up to 33 and from 26' to 49'.

From step 26' the nerve no longer functions quietly, in carrying the "scrambled" mental impulse. There is an abnormal molecular activity along the course of the neuromere, giving off heat. When it reaches the tissue cell, it is received by a *normal* tissue cell reluctantly, as something "off color," if not obnoxious, depending on how much the impulse has been tampered with. No longer a perfectly assembled force of Innate's, it now is practically a common universal force. It is not what Innate intended when she made intellectual adaptation; hence there will be abnormal physical personification. Since Innate's intentions did not reach the tissue cell in completeness, it (the tissue cell) will abnormally express Innate. Since the tissue cell has adaptability (Prin. 18, 19) it will react exactly according to the forces it receives; coordinately for the innate part of it, and incoordinately for the universal part of it. Of course, the tissue cell suffers under such ministrations and indirectly causes other tissue cells to suffer. It takes on a degree of unsoundness and its non-cooperative action will make other tissue cells unsound.

This *now* abnormal Tissue Cell, acting (functioning) gives off forces exactly corresponding to its character, which are called **Equivalent Vibrations.** These composite forces are collected (a representative amount) by the afferent nerve, and normally **Transmitted** by the **Afferent Nerve** as **Equivalent Impressions.** Reaching the **Brain Cell,** it is **Received** into the **Mental** establishment by **Interpretation,** giving **Innate Intelligence, Equivalent Sensation.** By this, she knows the exact percentage of normality and abnormality in the cell; especially when enough sensations give her an **Equivalent Ideation.** Innate Intelligence then knows what to do next, to make the best of a bad business. A student will always do well to emulate Innate as a "good loser," a "one hundred per cent sportsman." She plans ways and means, "cashes" some more forces from **Universal Intelligence** and proceeds to make **Compensation** (as shown in Fig. 14).

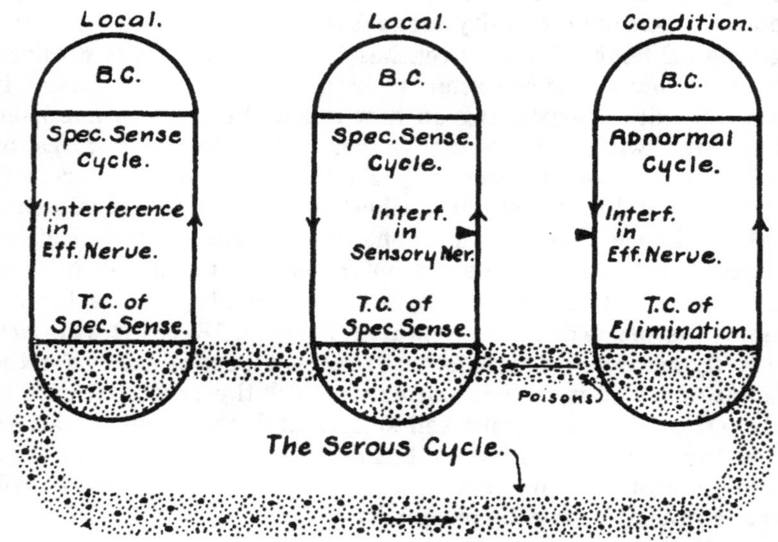

Scheme showing interference in Special Sense Cycle in the Efferent Half, the Afferent Half, and how the conditions are further aggravated

Fig. 15.

Art. 125. The Abnormal Sense Cycle. (Direct and Indirect)

An Abnormal Sense Cycle is a Normal Sense Cycle made abnormal by direct interference with transmission on the afferent sensory nerve; or indirectly by interference on the efferent nerve supplying the special sense organs; or another kind of indirect effect through the Serous Circulation.

NOTE: Any and all tissue cells, except Innate brain may be made more unsound (hence, incoordinating) by an abnormal Serous Circulation—see Serous Circulation articles.

The cycles are shown in Fig. 12 and Fig. 15. They are combined with the Vertemere Cycles. The drawings are self-explanatory, if the student has studied the preceding.

Art. 126. How to Apply the Normal Cycle to Any Function.

Take, for example, the stomach as an organ.

To deal with introduced external forces and matter.

The function considered is digestion, one of the nutritional group.

The cycle is given in Fig. 16, and is self-explanatory. Follow the step numbers from 1 to 57, in the diagram.

Art. 127. Special Sense Adaptation. (Two phases)

Special Sense Adaptation Cycles explain the process resulting from the news received from environment through the special senses.

The lists of steps given below will explain:

IN THE SPECIAL SENSE CYCLE	IN THE NORMAL COMPLETE CYCLE
1. Fire.	1. Fire.
2. Tissue cell of finger.	2. Tissue cell of finger.
3. Penetrative forces.	3. Penetrative forces.
4. Dangerous vibrations.	4. Traumatic vibrations.
5. Impressions.	5. Equivalent impressions.
6. Afferent nerve.	6. Afferent nerve.

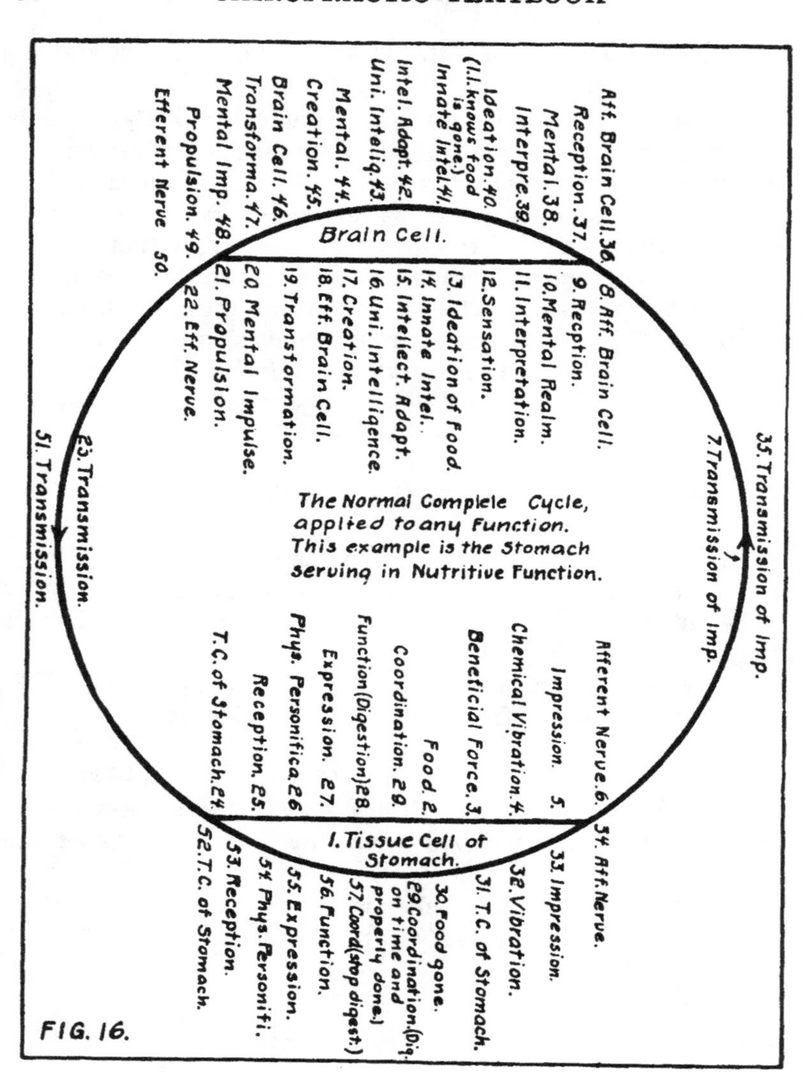
35. Transmission of Imp.
7. Transmission of Imp.
Aff. Brain Cell. 36.
Reception. 37.
Mental. 38.
Interpre. 39.
Ideation. 40.
(I.I. knows food is gone.)
Innate Intel. 41.
Intel. Adapt. 42.
Uni. Inteliq. 43.
Mental. 44.
Creation. 45.
Brain Cell. 46.
Transforma. 47.
Mental Imp. 48.
Propulsion. 49.
Efferent Nerve 50.
Brain Cell.
8. Aff. Brain Cell.
9. Recption.
10. Mental Realm.
11. Interpretation.
12. Sensation.
13. Ideation of Food.
14. Innate Intel.
15. Intellect. Adapt.
16. Uni. Intelligence.
17. Creation.
18. Eff. Brain Cell.
19. Transformation.
20. Mental Impulse.
21. Propulsion.
22. Eff. Nerve.
The Normal Complete Cycle, applied to any Function. This example is the Stomach serving in Nutritive Function.
Afferent Nerve. 6.
Impression. 5.
Chemical Vibration. 4.
Beneficial Force. 3.
Food. 2.
Coordination. 29.
Function (Digestion) 28.
Expression. 27.
Phys. Personifica. 26
Reception. 25.
T.C. of Stomach. 24.
1. Tissue Cell of Stomach.
34. Aff. Nerve.
33. Impression.
32. Vibration.
31. T.C. of Stomach.
30. Food gone.
29. Coordination. (Dig. on time and properly done.)
57. Coord (stop digest.)
56. Function.
55. Expression.
54. Phys. Personifi.
53. Reception.
52. T.C. of Stomach.
23. Transmission.
51. Transmission.
FIG. 16.

IN THE SPECIAL SENSE CYCLE (Continued)	IN THE NORMAL COMPLETE CYCLE (Continued)
7. Transmission of impressions.	7. Transmission of equivalent impressions.
8. Aff. brain cell.	8. Aff. brain cell.
9. Reception of impressions.	9. Reception of impressions.
10. Mental Realm.	10. Mental realm.
11. Mental interpretation.	11. Mental interpretation.
12. Sensation of danger.	12. Sensation of injury and pain.
13. Ideation of danger.	13. Ideation of damage.
14. Innate Intelligence.	14. Innate Intelligence.
15. Intellectual adaptation.	15. Intellectual adaptation.
16. Universal Intelligence.	16. Universal Intelligence.
17. Creation.	17. Creation.
18. Eff. brain cell.	18. Eff. brain cell.
19. Transformation.	19. Transformation.
20. Mental impulses.	20. Mental Impulses.
21. Propulsion.	21. Propulsion.
22. Eff. nerve.	22. Eff. nerve.
23. Transmission.	23. Transmission.
24. Muscle tissue cells of arm and fingers, etc.	24. Tissue cells of burnt fingers—reception may be difficult.
25. Reception of mental impulses.	25. Reception of mental impulses.
26. Physical personification of action.	26. Physical personification of reparatory design and plan.
27. Expression.	27. Expression.
28. Functioning—movement.	28. Function—reparation.
29. Coordination—saved.	29. Coordination—finger getting repaired.

Art. 128. How to Apply the Abnormal Cycle to Any Dis-ease in Symptomatology.

Example: coryza with chronic subluxations in C. P.; K. P., and an acute subluxation (newly made) in Mid. Cer. P.

Steps in bold faced type are steps in the Vertemere Cycle.

FUNCTIONS INVOLVED: CALORIFIC AND SECRETORY Direct	FUNCTIONS INVOLVED: CALORIFIC AND EXCRETORY Indirect
1. **v. Draft.**	1. Draft.
2. **v. Shock.**	2. Sudden closing of pores.
3. **v. Concussion of forces.**	3. Accumulation of poisons.
4. **v. New Subluxation at 4th Cerv.**	4. Serum poisoned.

FUNCTIONS INVOLVED:
CALORIFIC AND SECRETORY
Direct (Continued)

5. Interference with transmission.
6. Tissue cells of nasal pharynx.
7. Reception.
8. Abnormal personification.
9. Abnormal expression.
10. Abnormal function.
11. Incoordination.
12. Tissue cells of nasal pharynx.
13. Tissue cell incoordinated and unsound.
14. Equivalent vibrations.
15. Equivalent impressions.
16. Afferent nerve.
17. Transmission of equiv impress.
18. Afferent brain cell.
19. Reception.
20. Mental.
21. Mental interpretation.
22. Equivalent sensation.
23. Equivalent ideation.
24. Innate Intelligence.
25. Intellectual Adaptation.
26. Universal Intelligence.
27. Creation of extra adaptative forces.
28. Skip several regular steps.
29. Decreased carrying capacity.
30. Interference with transmission.
31. Hot box.

"local"

FUNCTIONS INVOLVED:
CALORIFIC AND EXCRETORY
Indirect (Continued)

5. Existing C. P. and K. P. subluxations.
6. Failure of compensatory elimination.
7. Efferent nerves.
8. Tissue cells all over the body.
9. Poisoned tissue cells.
10. Equivalent vibrations.
11. Equivalent impressions.
12. Afferent nerve.
13. Transmission of impressions.
14. Afferent brain cell.
15. Reception.
16. Mental realm.
17. Mental interpretation.
18. Equivalent sensation.
19. Equivalent ideation.
20. Innate Intelligence.
21. Intellectual adaptation.
22. Efferent brain cell.
23. Transformation.
24. Mental Impulses
25. Propulsion.
26. Efferent nerves to calorific organs.
27. 5th dor. impingement on them.
28. Abnormal transmission.
29. Skip several regular steps.
30. Calorific function, burning poison.
31. Calorific out of control.
32. Fever.

"condition"

Art. 129. The Complete Dis-Ease Cycle.

The Dis-ease Cycle is a Complex Cycle, combining the Abnormal, the Vertemere, and various compensating cycles.

The compensating cycles are the functional cycles of adaptation to various organs to compensate as far as possible by the work of other organs; to do the work that the organ in question fails to do. Thus, if the liver fails to secrete the proper kind or amount of bile, Innate causes the pancreas

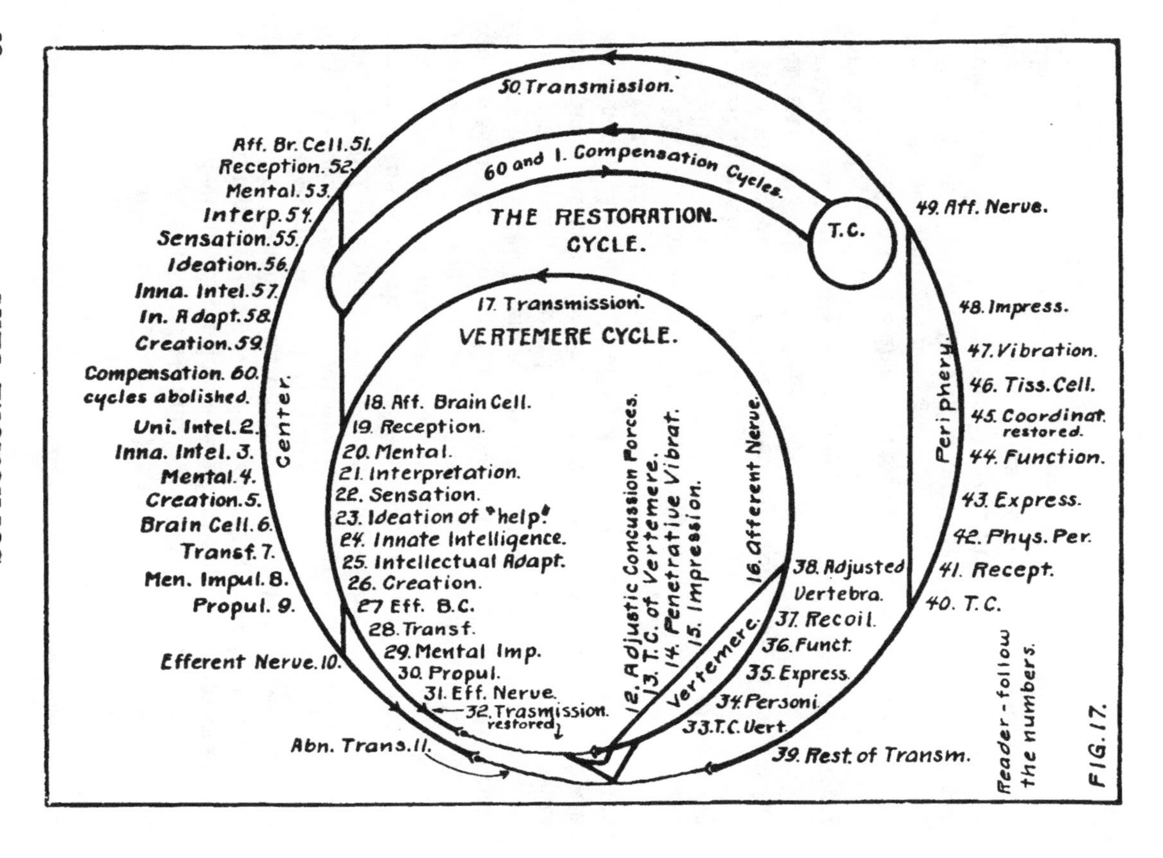
50. Transmission.
Aff. Br. Cell.51.
Reception.52.
Mental.53.
Interp.54.
Sensation.55.
Ideation.56.
Inna. Intel.57.
In. Adapt.58.
Creation.59.
Compensation. 60.
cycles abolished.
Uni. Intel.2.
Inna. Intel. 3.
Mental.4.
Creation.5.
Brain Cell.6.
Transf. 7.
Men. Impul. 8.
Propul. 9.
Efferent Nerve.10.
Abn. Trans.11.
Center.
60 and 1. Compensation Cycles.
THE RESTORATION.
CYCLE.
T.C.
17. Transmission.
VERTEMERE CYCLE.
18. Aff. Brain Cell.
19. Reception.
20. Mental.
21. Interpretation.
22. Sensation.
23. Ideation of "help."
24. Innate Intelligence.
25. Intellectual Adapt.
26. Creation.
27 Eff. B.C.
28. Transf.
29. Mental Imp.
30. Propul.
31. Eff. Nerve.
32. Trasmission.
restored
12. Adjustic Concussion Forces.
13. T.C. of Vertemere.
14. Penetrative Vibrat.
15. Impression.
16. Afferent Nerve.
Vertemere.
38. Adjusted
Vertebra.
37. Recoil.
36. Funct.
35. Express.
34. Personi.
33. T.C. Vert.
39. Rest. of Transm.
49. Aff. Nerve.
48. Impress.
47. Vibration.
46. Tiss. Cell.
45. Coordinat.
restored.
44. Function.
43. Express.
42. Phys. Per.
41. Recept.
40. T.C.
Periphery.
Reader - follow
the numbers.

FIG. 17.

and other accessory organs of intestinal digestion to do the work that the liver leaves undone, as far as it is possible for them to do so.

In explanation of this cycle, let us examine the Abnormal Complete Cycle (Art. 124 and Fig. 14). When Innate has made intellectual adaptation, she establishes the compensating cycles, referred to before. Also, knowing that there is interference with transmission on the main cycle in question, she does not attempt to send the same kind of mental impulses that she sent previously, but much more moderated ones. Assuming that the interference cuts down the conducting capacity of the nerve thirty-five per cent, Innate now sends only sixty-five per cent mental force (not an abnormal force) (remember that these percentages are only analogous). It requires some time for all the compensating and adaptative conditions to be established, and when that takes place, a state of *chronicity* exists. Before that, it is *acute*. When adjustments are given retracing begins and the compensation cycles are abolished. In Fig. 17 follow the step numbers from 1 (at center) to 60.

Art. 130. "Condition" and "Local."

Condition is the term used to indicate the state of organic matter, in health or dis-ease.

It is an important factor in major work; as, a major includes the "Local" and "Condition."

"Condition" pertains to the soundness of organic matter; indirect effect.

"Local" refers to the direct effect of a subluxation upon the tissues of the impinged nerves.

"Condition" is the effect of a subluxation or subluxations interfering with transmission to organ or organs, causing them to function abnormally, thus rendering the Serous Circulation abnormal, which in turn makes the effect of the "Local" worse.

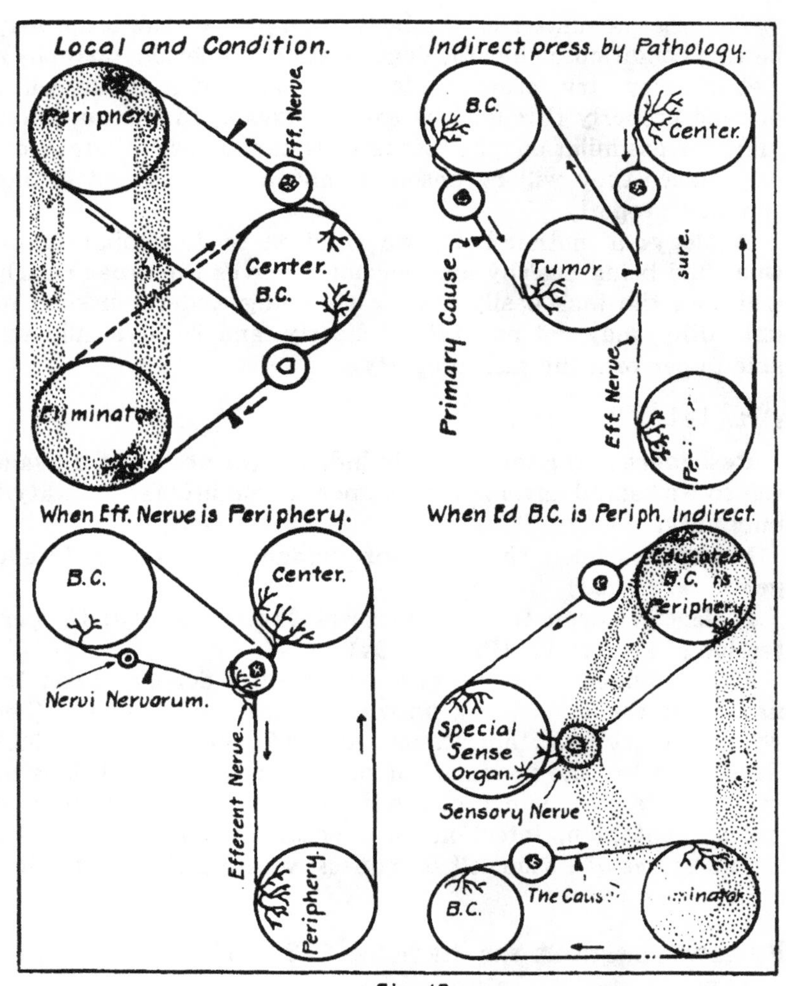
Local and Condition.
Periphery
Eff. Nerve
Center.
B.C.
Eliminator
Indirect press. by Pathology.
B.C.
Center.
Tumor.
Primary Cause
sure.
Eff. Nerve
When Eff. Nerve is Periphery.
B.C.
Center.
Nervi Nervorum.
Efferent Nerve.
Periphery.
When Ed. B.C. is Periph. Indirect.
Educated B.C. is Periphery
Special Sense Organ.
Sensory Nerve
B.C.

Fig. 18.

The organic matter of the body, or a part of the body, may be in a condition of health, degeneration, depletion (atrophy), wet insanity, dry insanity, etc. Obviously, if a tissue cell is not fed properly through the serous stream, the serum being unfit for assimilation, the tissue cells cannot assimilate properly, hence they will be unsound; and being unsound cannot function properly.

Analogy: a mother bids two children to do similar tasks. One child being healthy and normal, receives the order clearly and does the task easily; the other being undernourished or unhealthy, may not understand clearly, and is physically unable to perform the task properly.

Art. 131. Resistance.

Resistance is the term used to indicate the ability of a tissue cell to withstand adverse environmental conditions; "vitality," immunity.

It depends upon the constant guidance of Innate Intelligence. (Prin. 21)

It depends upon the soundness of the tissue cell; its perfection of structure. (Prin. 5, 24)

The soundness or perfection of structure depends upon Innate's success in adapting universal forces and matter. (See Evolution Art. 338; Inheritance, Art. 207; Survival, Art. 133.) Resistance to "the in-roads" of disease, adverse conditions or very trying environmental conditions, the rapid breeding of germs, contagion, infection, or mental and physical shocks, are questions of tissue cell soundness, wherein its adaptability is impaired.

Review Questions for Articles 122 to 131, inclusive.

1. What is the cause of dis-ease?
2. What is the physical representative of the cause of dis-ease?
3. How is dis-ease produced by the cause?
4. What is the Abnormal Complete Cycle?

5. What is the Complete Dis-ease Cycle?
6. What are Compensatory Cycles?
7. What is meant by "Local"?
8. What is meant by "Condition"?
9. What is Resistance?
10. Upon what two things does Resistance depend?
11. Upon what does the Soundness of tissue cells depend?

Art. 132. Insanity.

Insanity is the term used in Chiropractic to denote unsoundness of any tissue in the body.

If it concerns body tissues it is called "physical insanity"; if it concerns brain tissue, it is "mental insanity." (See wet and dry insanity in Serous Circulation, Art. 163, 164.)

From this and preceding articles, it is seen that the term insanity has a much broader scope than its medical meaning. In Chiropractic, it has reference to the unsoundness (imperfection in organic structure) of tissue, which of course weakens its resistance, impairs function, offers feeding ground for germs, etc. Of course, the Chiropractic meaning *includes* mental insanity, that is, unsound mind because of the abnormal functioning of unsound brain tissues. Chiropractic does not concern itself with the fine gradations of psychoanalysis, regarding this as merely the sorting, grading, and naming these classified effects. Chiropractic is a science of the cause—not effects. In mental insanity, the unsound brain cells are in the educated brain. Mental insanity may be direct or indirect effects of subluxations.

(See Figs. 13 and 18)

Art. 133. Survival Values.

Survival value is that positive value gained with every successful adaptation in organic structures.

That margin of organic success that is an element of evolution; the value given by parent to offspring.

As material resources in the body, it is the fundamental of major work.

The margin of value which survives subtraction; remainder.

Net gain in assets after the liabilities have been deducted.

It not only refers to condition or soundness of tissue cells, but to the racial gain in condition; "the resultant distillation of life."

Survival Value is the name of the **unit of adaptational success,** from a unit of mental force (mental impulse), in a unit of matter (tissue cell), when all losses have been deducted; therefore, **Survival Value is the unit element of evolution.**

NOTE:—This is not a discussion of religion or faiths, but a cold scientific study of matter and physics and of course the guiding power. Also, Chiropractic does not uphold the evolution theories of Darwin or Haekle; but our ideas of evolution are the result of deduction, not induction.

In the body, the cycle of construction and destruction always applies. When there is successful adaptation, there is no interruption in Innate's program; but when there are subluxations or unusual adaptation (Prin. 24) to adverse conditions, the law of destruction goes into effect, costing the organization a loss in construction. This is referred to in Art. 134. If, in the body, the advance is greater than the loss, there is a gain in construction which is called *Constructive Survival Value.* If there is no destructive action, the constructive advance is *net gain.*

Art. 134. Accumulative Constructive and Destructive Survival Value.

The accumulating of survival values of construction or repletion in a tissue cell.

The margin or remainder of constructive success, after losses due to destruction are deducted.

A "bank account" of construction after "losses" and "liabilities" are deducted; "net gain."

It refers to condition or sanity of tissue cells; has to do with both construction and repletion.

It is sometimes called *vitality,* **which is true, but it is not a storage of forces; it is a storage of material resources.**

It is the fundamental of major work.

When there is a failure of adaptation, there is no advance made by the tissue cell in living. In fact, if the lack of adaptation results in its becoming injured or unsound, that is a distinct set-back in its life, which must be regained, with the loss of time and effort. If, after balancing the constructive results with the results of destruction, there is no remainder, it is neither a good nor a bad state of affairs; but if, after balancing, there is a credit, the cell is well off indeed, or on the road to repletion, which it requires time and effort to stop. If, on the other hand, there is a debit, the tissue cell is in a bad way, or is being badly depleted, and it will require time and effort to turn affairs the other way. These conditions have an important bearing on the next act of the tissue cell; whether or not it falls behind in the "race of life."

ACCUMULATIVE DESTRUCTIVE SURVIVAL VALUE.

A negative value (algebraically) indicating the accumulating of the destructive or depletive effects of universal forces.

The remainder of destruction or "losses" after "gains" and "assets" have been deducted; "net loss."

It refers to condition or insanity of tissue cells; has to do with both destruction and depletion.

It is the result of unsuccessful adaptation; therefore an absence of evolution value. (See evolution Art. 338)

It is sometimes referred to (when it is severe) as "shock" (as after an operation or severe burn), but it is not a scarcity of forces; it is a drain upon material resources.

It does not refer to normal katabolism.

Of course, a lack of Constructive Survival Value results in a lack of ease. It is a lack of entity; lack of construction; lack of resource; lack of evolutionary value or advance—it is not surprising that there would be a lack of ease.

Art. 135. Momentum.

Momentum is the possession of motion; requiring effort and time to stop it.

Chiropractically, Momentum is the progress of dis-ease or health, requiring time and effort to stop it.

The Momentum of either health or dis-ease depends upon the survival values; which are material values requiring time to change. There is no process that does not require time. (Prin. 6)

Art. 136. Explanation of the Momentum Chart.

Let the length of the vertical lines indicate the survival values. Let the horizontal length of the diagram represent duration or time. The length of (a) represents health with no deductions of destruction; pure gain, no liabilities. The length of the line (b) represents death, with no deductions for health—total loss. The line (c) represents *fair* health. but not well. (d) represents a state of affairs where neither health nor dis-ease predominate. (e) represents very sick. Movement toward the right represents "getting worse," and toward the left, "getting better," indicated by the arrows (f) and (g). (h) is accumulative destructive survival value at that time, and is the remainder (net amount of destructive value) left after deducting (h') (the constructive value) from (h") (the destructive value). (i) is the accumulative constructive survival value at that time, and is the remainder (net amount of constructive value) left after deducting (i') (the destructive value) from (i") (the constructive value). Both of these, **(h)** and **(i)**, are the amounts of health or dis-ease. **(j, j, j, etc.)** are units of time, as days. At **(k)** the destruction is very small, completely overshadowed by construction, and perhaps represents the health of the average individual. At **(1)** the construction is very small, completely overshadowed by destruction, and represents a point very near death.

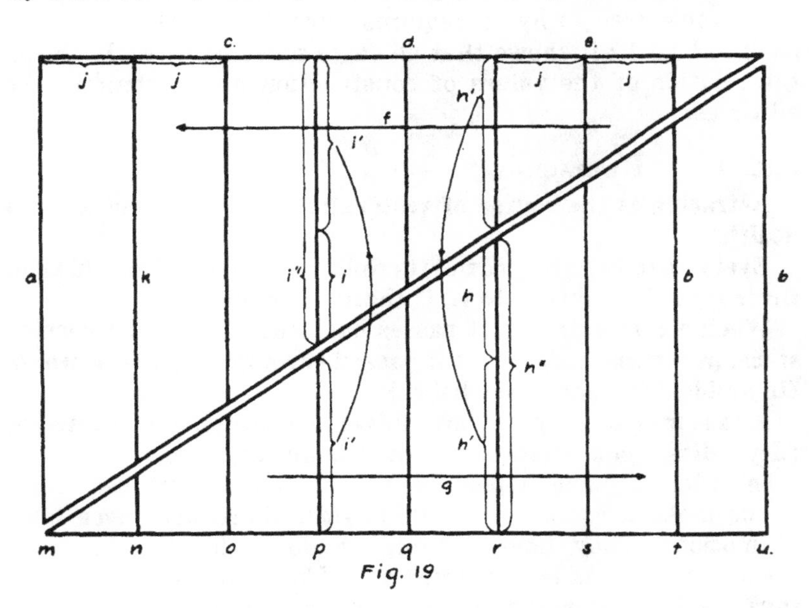

Fig. 19

Suppose for a hypothetical case, we assume that starting at **(m)** with a subluxation; at the end of the first day the accumulation is shown at **(n)**; the second day **(o)**; the third day **(p)**; the fourth day at **(q)**; the fifth day at **(r)**; the sixth day at **(s)**; the seventh day at **(t)**; if he goes to the end of the eighth day, **(u)**, there would be no use in adjusting the subluxation, even if it could be done. His state of health at any of these points of time is found by balancing the values.

If, at the end of the seventh day, an adjustment be given, he will begin to **retrace,** as shown by the arrow **(f)**, and successively passes back through the same stages reversed, having the same values (in an ideal case, see Retracing) through **t, s, r, q, p, o, n,** to **m.**

Thus, on the chart can be seen why it requires time to get sick people well; why it requires time to get them started back to health; it shows that all cases must retrace. It shows the relation of the values of construction and destruction at all times.

Art. 137. Retracing.

Retracing is the course of restoration from dis-ease back to health.

Every case retraces, for if there is a departure from health, there must be a return to it, if there is restoration.

When a case retraces, it passes back through the successive steps, in reverse order, that it passed through in getting worse (in an ideal instance—see below).

A case may or may not have adverse symptoms in retracing, (depending upon whether or not it is an ideal case.)

In order to make it plain what is meant by an ideal case, let us make a comparison. In physics there are three laws of motion. They have nothing to do with retracing, but *the way the second law is stated does.* The second law of motion says, "A body at rest remains at rest; a body in motion continues in motion in a straight line unless acted upon by other forces not parallel to its course, or opposed to it." Any one can see that the ideal example of this law would be the straight line action of a single force, not in the least bothered by any other forces. But, search the wide world over and you will not find a single instance of this.

When we say that a case retraces over the succesive steps, in reverse order that it passed through in getting worse, we are talking about an ideal case. Search the wide world over and you will not find such an ideal case of retracing; *but you will find* cases that approach the ideal so closely that *no new symptoms* are present, but there is a systematic return of the old; and many times these pass in such rapid succession as to be negligible, and we say that there are no adverse symptoms at all.

Referring to Fig. 19 again, we can see that in an actual case there will be factors enter into the problem of retracing, that are just as probable as the entrance of unexpected forces into the second law of motion. We have no assurance, that with ever-changing environmental conditions and new subluxations and passing pressures, that the same combination of circumstances will obtain that existed when we "sized up" conditions in the first instance; that there will be a mathematical reverse of the steps, with the same balancing of survival values at the same stated mathematical intervals.

Art. 138. Depletion.

Depletion is the abnormal shrinking of a cell that has once been normal size; or it is depreciation of soundness or construction.

Depleted cells can be repleted; they "can come back."

It is synonymous with *atrophy,* **if atrophy is used with the Chiropractic meaning.** (See Art. 139.)

The functions involved are: nutritive (trophic) and reparatory; and indirectly, others.

The student is referred to the Chiropractic theory of cell expansion, (Art. 70). When a cell is expanded and grows to its mature size and texture, it has a normal size, depending upon how large Innate wants it to be. In giants, there are no more cells, approximately, than there are in the average sized person, or dwarf, but they are expanded to a greater size. In a dwarf's body, the cells are not expanded so large as they are in the average person's body. When a cell is called upon to function, coordinately, it must expend some of its material contents in secretion and excretion. With ordinary adaptation, this would not impoverish the cell to any extent or affect its size and construction much. In rest, it soon recuperates. In extraordinary adaptation, however, as when called upon to expend great quantities of materials and action (which uses materials) the tissue cell is impoverished to the extent that it affects its soundness; hence it has suffered from the incoordination in the body. It takes time to recuperate and when that is done, it is almost as good a cell as before.

If the tissue cell has been affected to the extent that it is no longer useful in function, or metabolism, it is replaced by reparation. Perhaps glandular (visceral) cells "wear out" and are replaced more often than others, for with the exception of muscle cells, they are more active.

When cells are not used much, functionally, as when muscle cells are not used, they become somewhat depleted. On the other hand, much use causes them to build up more. If they are not used at all, Innate acts according to the law of evolution, deeming the muscle cells "excess baggage" when not used, tends to place them in the rudimentary state of depleting them, but keeping them in readiness to be repleted. Thus, there may be depletion from this cause.

Art. 139. Atrophy.

Atrophy, as used in Chiropractic, is synonymous with depletion and is due to lack of proper nutrition; or lack of coordinate functioning.

According to its Chiropractic meaning, it can "come back."

It does not refer to destruction of tissues; to degeneration.

Caution should be used when terms in medicine are also used in Chiropractic, for very seldom do they have the same meaning in both. In medicine, atrophy has its true meaning obscured by many different applications; but in Chiropractic it means the same always—a depreciated tissue that is not too far gone to be restored, which if the tissue were destroyed, it could not be.

Art. 140. Repletion.

Repletion is the restoration of a tissue cell to normal size and soundness, when it has been depleted.

It is not the same as expansion, which originally built the cell.

It is reparation, in the trophic or nutritional sense.

It is the "coming back" of a cell, which it cannot do if degenerated.

Repletion is recuperation from arduous adaptation or from sickness. After a long illness the body has many depleted cells and recuperation is usually a nutritional phenomenon. A muscle which has become smaller and weaker from lack of use, or when it has become atrophied because of direct interference with transmission, becomes filled out to full size and soundness in recuperation.

Art. 141. Degeneration.

The destruction of cells by abnormal disintegration; as, necrosis, suppuration, ulceration, etc.

Degenerated tissue cannot be restored by repletion; it cannot "come back."

If the expansional centers are destroyed by degeneration, there is no chance of restoration of the same kind of cells.

The place of the destroyed cells may be filled with scar tissue, but the same kind of tissue is not replaced.

Chiropractically, degeneration of tissue is not the same as atrophy, for atrophied cells can be repleted.

The repairing or "filling in" with scar tissue is by proliferation of connective tissues. It is called, in Chiropractic, reparation. If the degeneration has been so severe that the proliferation possibilities are destroyed, there is little likelihood that the ulcer will heal. A little inflammatory heat will cause the proliferation to be accelerated, but great destructive heat will hinder or prevent reparation because of the destruction of the expansional centers.

Review Questions for Articles 132 to 141, inclusive.

1. What is the meaning of the term Insanity, in Chiropractic?
2. What is the name of the material resources in the body?
3. Of what are material resources the basis, in Chiropractic?
4. What is the name of the unit element of evolution?
5. What does Survival Value refer to?
6. What is Accumulative Constructive Survival Value?
7. What is Accumulative Destructive Survival Value?
8. What is Momentum as used in Chiropractic?
9. What is Retracing?
10. Does a case always have adverse symptoms in retracing? Why?
11. What is Depletion of tissue?
12. What is Atrophy, as used in Chiropractic.
13. What is Repletion of tissue?
14. What is Degeneration of tissue?
15. Differentiate between Degeneration and Atrophy, as used in Chiropractic.

Art. 142. The Carrying Capacity of Nerves.

Ordinarily a nerve fiber does not conduct all the mental force of which it is capable.

There is always room for more adaptative current.

A pressure upon a nerve does not always interfere with transmission; it does when the disease is acute, and may not when it is chronic.

With the same degree of pressure, a chronic case passes into the acute stage when adaptation is increased through the nerve.

When the adaptative current suffers interference, part of it is transformed into heat. (If materialistic theory is used.) **Mental force is never dammed back.**

When there is interference with transmission, there is, at the place of impingement, an area of heat, known as the "hot box."

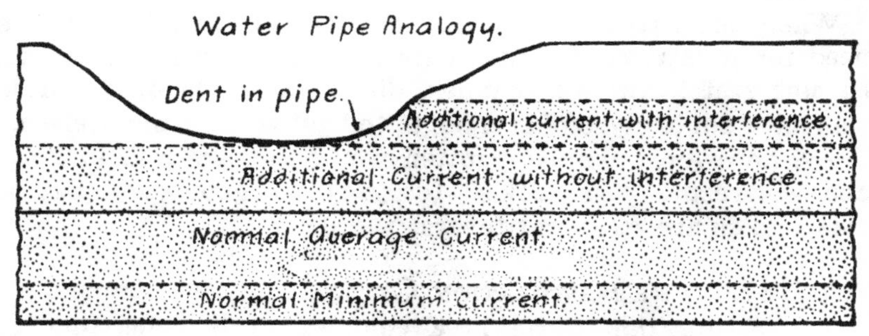

Fig. 20.

Using the analogy of the water pipe as shown in Fig. 20, it should be remembered, always, that it is only an analogy. Otherwise, one may be led into thinking that mental force can be dammed back in the nerve, as water can be in the pipe.

The figure shows the pipe dented down to the surface of the flowing water. It is obvious that the dent in the pipe does not interfere with the flow of water. Next, suppose that because of a greater demand for water at the discharge of the pipe, you adaptatively increase the flow of water through the pipe; then there will be interference with the transmission of the water.

In a chronic condition, where there is a constant pressure upon a nerve, ordinarily there is no interference after Innate has established her compensation cycles; but when the function in question calls for a greater amount of adaptation;

greater than the compensation cycles can take care of, Innate again tries to send more current through the impinged nerve and there is then, interference with transmission of this additional current. The hot box is acute; the abnormal transmission is acute; the lack of additional current is acute, and the again "scrambled" impulse is acute. The dis-ease is said to **recur.**

When the extra demand for adaptation subsides, or the need for it is removed, the acute condition subsides into the **chronic** state. In this manner, dis-eases are said, by those who have not analyzed far enough, to "get well by themselves." They, however, have not "gotten well," but are still lurking, and will recur. "Bad colds" (coryza) are good examples of this, and so are recurrent fevers.

Art. 143. The Restoration Cycle.

The Restoration Cycle is a complex cycle consisting of the abnormal, compensation, normal, and vertemere cycles.

It is the outline of the story of how abnormality is restored to normality, through the restoration to normality in the vertemere, and the removal of the compensation cycles. See Fig. 17. Follow the step numbers from 1 (Compensation) to 60, and the process can be readily understood.

Art. 144. The Practical Cycle.

The Practical Cycle is a Complex Cycle, consisting of the complete dis-ease cycle and all its parts, followed by the complete restoration cycle with all its parts.

It is a complete story from the beginning of disease to the accomplished restoration of health.

It shows that adjustments restore what has been taken away, and in no wise is anything added to the body; which is complete before the dis-ease, and is complete after restoration. When anything is complete, it cannot be more than complete.

Health is just simply completeness, everything restored, and restored from within.

Art. 145. The Serous Circulation as a Coordinator.

The ability of a tissue cell to coordinate depends upon its soundness as well as the functional impulses it receives. (Prin. 5.)

The tissue cell must not only have one hundred per cent mental impulses in order to function properly, but it must have one hundred per cent of soundness of structure in order to obey those impulses perfectly.

Since the serum is the means of the cells obtaining their nutrition, it is necessary that the Serous Circulation be perfect, in order that the cells coordinate perfectly.

A large part of the Sophomore work is devoted to the condition of matter which includes the Serous Circulation. The Serous Circulation is a very important part of major work.

Art. 146. The Serous Circulation. (317 Vol. IX) (260 Vol. II)

The Serous Circulation is the course of water through the body of an organism, conveying nutritional elements to the cells and carrying away from them, their used products.

Water circulates through all organisms. This pertains to any organism, from a cell body to greater organisms composed of cells. Plants draw water from the ground through their roots, pass it upwards through their trunks or stems to the branches; to the leaves, where it is evaporated into the air. In this manner, it carries nutrition to all parts of the plant, and leaving the plant, carries with it certain products that are no longer usable in the plant. An animal organism takes water into its body. It circulates to all parts of that body, carrying to the cells, food, oxygen, and other chemical elements. Leaving the body, the water carries heat, carbon dioxide, and other used chemicals. Uncombined water, then,

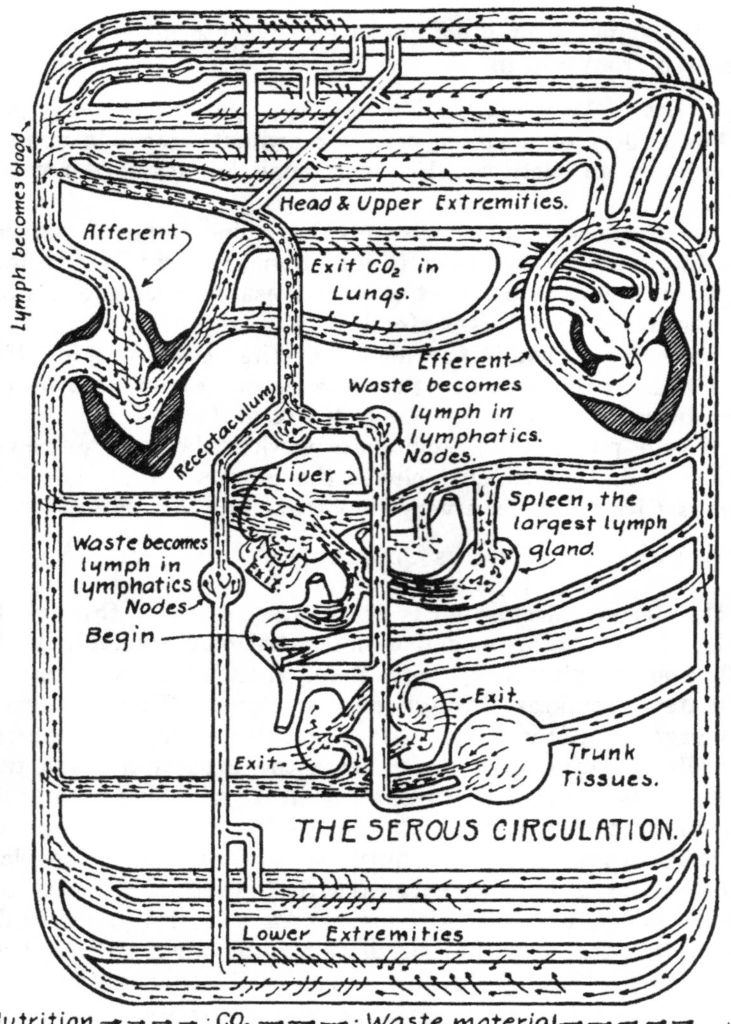

Nutrition →→→→; CO_2 ———; Waste material———
Reader-begin tracing with → to periphery; then follow—, and—o, and—.

Fig. 21.

is the vehicle for metabolism. This circulation of water from the environment through the body and back again to environment is the Serous Cycle.

It has been estimated that it requires about seventy-two hours for a complete cycle. That does not mean that all the water taken into the body follows the same channel, and that all of it requires seventy-two hours in the body. Some of it gets back to environment much sooner than that, while other amounts may be in the body for a much longer time. The water is taken into the body through the digestive tract, and leaves the body through the kidneys, skin, bowels, etc.

The body of a man averages about sixty-seven per cent water; the rest is solid matter, mostly proteids. This percentage is kept constant with great nicety, by balancing the intake and outlet of water by Innate Intelligence. If more water is taken into the body than is usable, there must be immediate elimination of it, to keep the percentage constant. If insufficient water is taken into the body to keep the percentage constant, there will be abnormal dryness, and the cells will suffer from lack of a vehicle to carry nutrition and waste materials. From this, it is seen that the "condition" of tissue cells depends very much upon the normality of organs concerned with the maintenance of the Serous Circulation.

Art. 147. Dr. Palmer's Analogy.

Dr. Palmer compares a man to a mud pie, which is composed of dust and water. In order to have the mud pie of the proper consistency, it must contain the right amount of water, mixed with the dust. Any more than this amount of water will make the mud pie too wet and any less will make it too dry. Also, this mud pie might be too wet or too dry in spots.

Man, also, is dust and water. The proper amount of water for man's body is sixty-seven per cent. Any more than that makes his body too wet in consistency, and less makes it too dry, also, a man's body may be too wet or too dry in spots. This we find in the study of cases and clinical work. Water uncombined, passes into organisms (and cells of course), passes through them, and passes out again. Dr. Palmer says they "sweat"; a cell sweats the same as the body sweats, and in doing so, heat and waste materials are carried from it.

Art. 148. "Condition."

One of the rules of major work states that the factors of a major are "location" and "condition." The term *Condition* in this case is used to indicate **the indirect effects of subluxations upon tissue cells via the Serous Circulation**; while *location* indicates the direct effects of a subluxation upon tissue cells at the periphery of the impinged nerve. The Condition or sanity of a tissue cell depends very much upon the quality of the serum; and its ability to coordinate can be lessened by subluxations which affect organs which have anything to do with the quality of the serum. (See Fig. 18 and Fig. 21.)

Almost every major has one or more subluxations included in it to be adjusted to take care of the Serous Circulation. An abnormal serum poisons any tissue cell, even when it is getting a high percentage of mental impulses, for this abnormal serum represents a very adverse influence which taxes to the utmost the adaptability of this small organism. If the tissue cell is already abnormal, because it does not receive one hundred per cent mental impulses, the abnormal serum will further aggravate it. It can be seen that an abnormal serum will show its worst effects at the weakest points in the body, sometimes very remote from the organ which is causing the abnormal serum. The abnormal serum tends to make all tissue cells unsound (and succeeds unless they are getting one hundred per cent mental impulses) and lessens their ability to obey Innate. (Prin. 4, 5.) It accounts for insanities, poisoning, non-im-

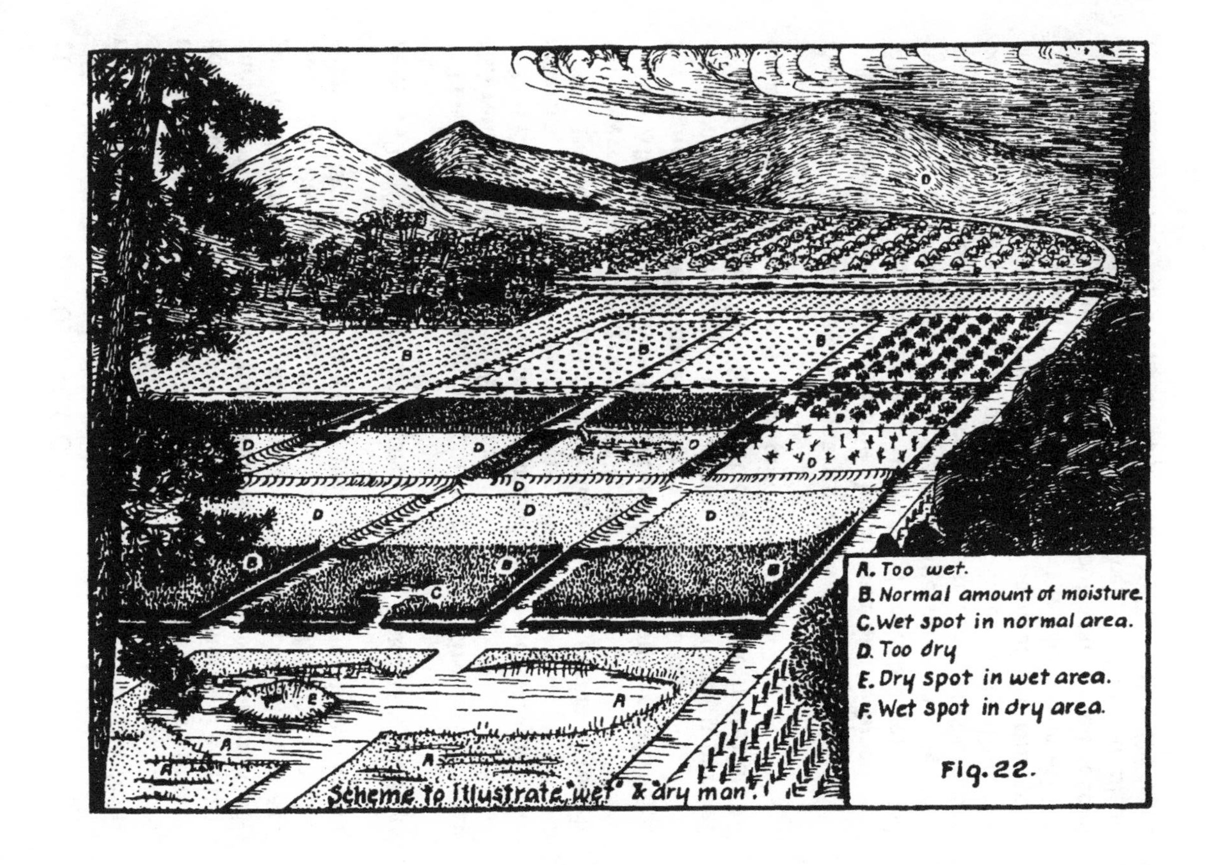
A. Too wet.
B. Normal amount of moisture.
C. Wet spot in normal area.
D. Too dry
E. Dry spot in wet area.
F. Wet spot in dry area.
Scheme to Illustrate "wet" & dry man".

Fig. 22.

munity, recurrent dis-eases, and what the physician calls "constitutional" diseases. Adjustments for condition are more natural and more scientific than the physician's tonic. Innate does not like tonics because the taking of tonic is the introduction of unadapted external forces. The most common adjustments are: K. P. for elimination of water, heat, or urea; Li.P. for the liver; Spl. P. for the spleen; U.K.P. for the suprarenals; or any organ whose primary function is secretion.

Art. 149. The Great Divisions of the Serous Circulation.

The three great divisions of the Serous Circulation are: Efferent, Peripheral, and Afferent.

The Efferent current is the plasma of the blood stream in the arteries, driven to the periphery by the heart.

The Peripheral division is the course of the serum through the intercellular and intracellular spaces.

The Afferent division is the return to environment through the organs which eliminate the urea from the body.

The afferent blood stream also may be considered a part of the afferent division, insofar as it conveys waste materials to organs, whose business it is to eliminate them.

Art. 150. The Efferent Serous Stream.

The Efferent Serous Stream is the plasma of the blood.

Chiropractically considered, true blood consists of blood cells, such as leucocytes and erythrocytes, etc. These cells must have a liquid vehicle to convey them to all parts of the body. It is a splendid example of Innate's economy that the serum which must be driven efferently, be used for this purpose. The liquid which is the vehicle for the blood, something to be pumped by the heart, is water; but water well loaded with nutritive materials for the tissue cells. The red blood cells also convey oxygen for the cells. Thus the Efferent

Serous Stream carries to the tissue cells carbon, oxygen, minerals, enzymes, and various blood cells and chemicals prepared by Innate.

Art. 151. The Peripheral Division of the Serous Circulation.

The Peripheral Division of the Serous Circulation is the flow of the serum through the inter-cellular and intra-cellular spaces.

The spaces around the cells (between them) are called the inter-cellular spaces; for brevity referred to as *inter spaces* The student is cautioned not to make the error of thinking of a group of cells always as a basket of apples. You will recall in your study of Histology that all cells do not have cell-walls. A cell may be a loose mass with its elements grouped closely about its center or nucleus; it may be a fibrous mass. Such cells may be vaguely separated from their neighbors by a matrix or a field of plasma. One can see, easily, that the serum is in such cells as well as around them. Even cells with cell-walls have serum within them, for it passes through the walls into the cells and out again. It takes nutritional elements into the cells, and conveys, as it goes out, the materials which are no longer usable in the cells. The spaces within the cells are called intra-cellular spaces—*intra spaces,* for brevity.

When the serum reaches the capillaries, it easily passes out through their walls into the inter and intra spaces. While in the blood stream it was called plasma, and in tissue spaces is called serum. We do not wish the student to think that all of the plasma of the blood passes out through the blood-vessel walls and becomes serum of the spaces, but that most of it returns by way of the veins to serve as the vehicle of the blood afferently. The amount that passes out of the blood stream is determined by Innate and is exactly the amount required by the cells—no more, no less, if normality exists.

In the blood stream the serum travels quickly, but in the tissues it moves slowly, seeping through the spaces. As it nears the beginnings of the lymph vessels and capillaries it moves faster, beginning to show in itself like the Gulf Stream in the ocean.

Review Questions for Articles 142 to 151, inclusive.

1. What is the name of an area of heat over the place of interference with transmission?
2. Does a subluxation interfere with transmission at all times?
3. How should we use analogies?
4. What is the Restoration Cycle?
5. What is the Practical Cycle?
6. What part does the Serous Circulation play in Coordination.
7. What is the Serous Circulation?
8. What are the proportions of water and solids in the body?
9. How does the Serous Circulation affect the Condition of tissues?
10. Name the three great divisions of the Serous Circulation.
11. What is the Efferent Serous Stream?
12. Describe the Peripheral Division of the Serous Stream.

Art. 152. Serum and Urea.

The Serum bathes the cells in liquid food, and is selected by them—the process of assimilation.

The cells do not admit every kind of serum or use all the nutritional elements in it. The cells as organisms have assimilation and select the substances needed in metabolism.

The fluid that approaches the cell is called Serum.

The cell throws into the serous stream the materials it has used. This is the exercise of its selective ability.

Each cell selectively takes something from the serous stream and puts something into it.

It is possible that if the resistance of a tissue cell is lowered, undesirable Serum (to the cell) will "penetratively" enter.

It is possible that some poisons in the Serum will "penetratively" enter in spite of the tissue cell's resistance, it being beyond the ability of the cell to defend itself in that case. (Prin. 24.)

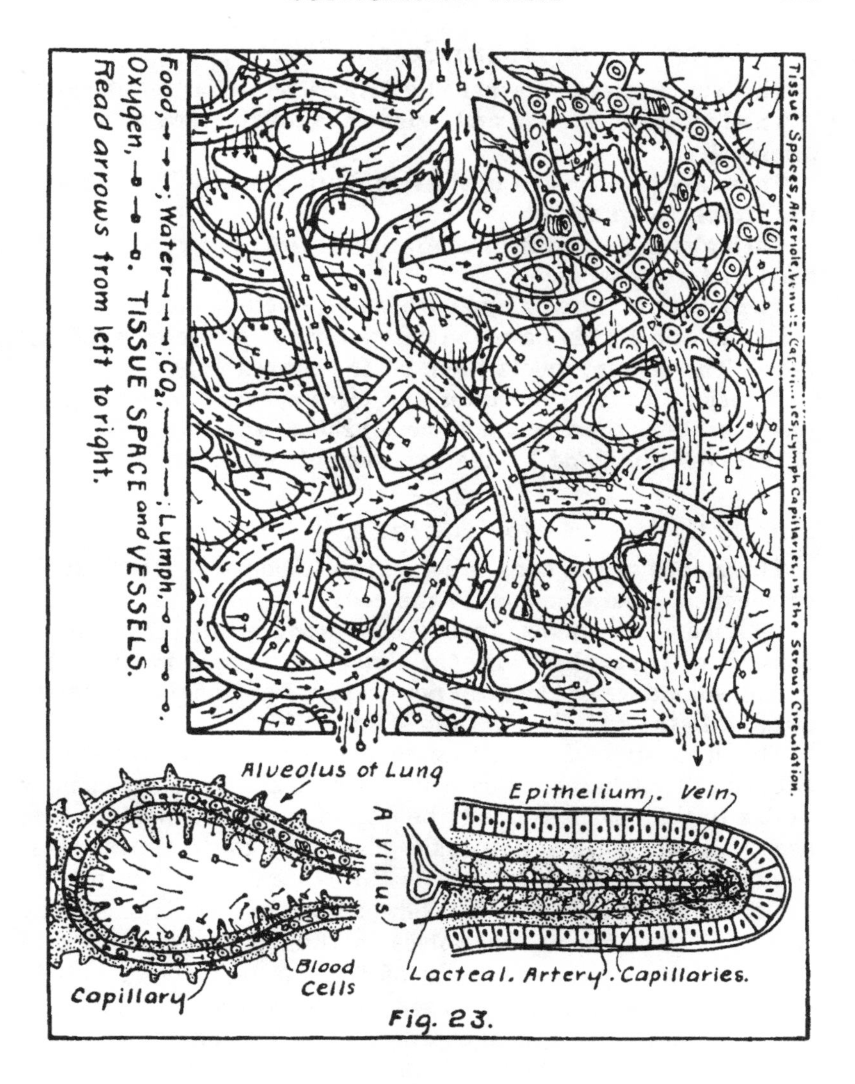
Food, ; Water ; CO_2, ; Lymph,
Oxygen, . TISSUE SPACE and VESSELS.
Read arrows from left to right.
Tissue Spaces, Arteriole,
Lymph Capillaries, in the Serous Circulation.
Alveolus of Lung
A Villus
Epithelium. Vein
Blood Cells
Capillary
Lacteal. Artery. Capillaries.

Fig. 23.

Art. 153. The Afferent Serous Stream.

The lymph streams gather like little rills into larger streams.

The lymphatic vessels and veins conduct the Serous Stream afferently.

There are many nodes in the lymphatic vessels. These nodes are lymphatic glands.

Each gland is a chemical laboratory to act upon certain waste matters for economy.

The larger of these glands are called *ductless glands*

Lymphatic glands have the characteristic shape of a kidney bean. The current meets them on the convex side.

It seeps through their inter and intra spaces and is changed in the process, thereby made more usable for tissue cells.

It leaves the gland by the concave side or hilum.

Art. 154. Innate's Laboratories.

The glands of the body are Innate's Laboratories for supply of chemicals and enzymes to the cells.

By means of glands, Innate can produce any chemical or substance (if supplied with the elements) needed in the body.

Any substance or chemical not prepared by Innate and introduced into the body is a poison. (Art. 166.)

The economy of Innate Intelligence is truly remarkable. A substance that has been used by a tissue cell and is no longer usable to that tissue cell may be usable to other kinds of cells; especially if clastic action takes place and the material reassembled. Thus, no substance is thrown away if it is needed somewhere in the body. A good example of this is shown by the ability of animals, as wolves in the far North, to thrive very well on a meager supply of food, it being very closely digested and economically used in the body. A starving animal's body will use substances that otherwise would be eliminated. In the body of an over-fed animal, there is a

tremendous waste of nutritional values, which not being required in bodily metabolism, are now rejected by Innate as in the poison class.

Art. 155. The Poison Possibilities of Serum.

Any substance that is no longer usable in bodily metabolism and retained in the Serous Circulation is a poison.

Any substance, even a food, that is in excess of what the body can use in its cells, is a poison.

Urea being retained by a cell or gland producing it is a poison to that cell or gland.

Any chemical not prepared by the cells or glands of the body is a poison.

Any glandular product in the wrong place in the body is a poison.

Any foreign substance in the body, liquid, solid, or gaseous, even if not chemically active, is a poison.

Too much water in the serum is a poison—serum too wet.

Not enough water in the serum—too dry— makes the serum abnormal and therefore a poison, for it cannot flow properly and soon becomes laden with urea.

Art. 156. The End of the Serous Cycle.

Full of used materials and heat, the serum arrives at the kidneys and skin.

These organs eliminate the heat and urea no longer usable, and excrete them from the body back to the environment.

Thus it leaves the whole body in a similar, though larger way, to that in which it leaves a tissue cell.

Art. 157. The Kidneys.

The Kidneys are the chief terminal glands of the serous cycle.

They have ducts leading from them, but not to them.

When the kidneys and the liver have finished working over urea, the last possible chemical combination of elements usable to the cells has been made. (The closest possible economy.)

If the kidneys excrete usable materials, it is because those materials are not then needed in metabolism, or have not been properly prepared for metabolism (as sugar in diabetes mellitus).

Urea is not urine. Urine is the secretion of the kidneys. It is prepared for the purpose of excretion from the body, and is made from urea; of materials that are a total waste.

The term *elimination* is used for this function; it indicates selection—an intelligently guided process. The term *excretion* is used to indicate the ejection of the eliminated material.

Art. 158. The Skin.

The Skin is an organ of the body containing many glands which are the terminal glands of the serous cycle.

These glands eliminate urea and are truly excretory because they eject the waste materials from the body.

They excrete water, waste, and heat.

Art. 159. "Wet Man."

***Wet Man* is the term used to indicate the condition when there is too much water in the serum.**

Wet man also is referred to as "wet insanity".

It may be local or general.

When there is too much water in the serum, it fills the inter and intra spaces too full and produces dropsy or edema. Dropsy is the term used to indicate a general wetness and edema, a local wet condition. In wet man the serum does not flow fast enough and becomes "stale", that is, laden with waste materials which in serious cases may begin to decompose and make worse poisons.

An analogy may be used to explain local and general wet man. An irrigated field may be equally and normally wet. The whole field may be too wet; or it may be too wet in spots. The same field may be too dry all over, or too dry in spots. Again, it may be very wet all over, except in spots which may be too dry, and vice versa. (See Fig. 22. Art. 147)

The symptoms of wet man are: edematous flesh, clammy skin which may be rather oily; oily hair, and general symptoms of poisoning. It is possible for wet man to exist with the skin normally dry; and possible for places in the body to be "wet man" locally, with the rest of the body normal.

The excretion of water must always balance the intake of water and the supply of water must be adequate for the bodily needs. Thus wet man may occur in the following ways:

1. Supply of water constant with lack of excretion of water.
2. Over supply of water with lack of excretion of water.
3. Over supply of water with excretion of water constant.

If normal, any of these factors will be adapted to coordinate or compensate for one or more that are not normal, in order to keep the percentage of water in the body constant, (at 67 per cent).

Art. 160. "Dry Man."

***Dry Man* is the term used to indicate the condition of the body when there is not enough water in the system.**

Dry Man also is referred to as "dry insanity".

It may be local or general.

When there is not enough water in the serum, the spaces are too dry and the serum flows too slowly and becomes laden with waste materials beyond the normal. Certain localities of the body may become too dry, producing friction and heat. The proper transportation of nutritive materials cannot exist for lack of a proper vehicle.

Dry man may occur in the following ways:

1. Supply of water constant with excess excretion of water.
2. Under supply of water with excess excretion of water.
3. Under supply of water with excretion of water constant.

If normal, any of these factors will be adapted to coordinate or compensate for one or more that are not normal in order to keep the percentage of water in the body constant (at 67 per cent).

Art. 161. Seredema.

Seredema is the name of the condition of tissues when supplied with too much serum or serum that is too rich.

It is sometimes called Efferent Poisoning, because too much serum or too rich a serum is forced upon the cells efferently.

It differs from edema in that it is not dropsy and the symptoms are widely different.

It may be local or general.

Seredema is likely to deposit too much fat in globules in the protoplasm of the cells. Most every cell with a protoplasm has some oily globules in it. Fat cells are those especially constructed to hold many such globules, but when other cells have more than a normal amount of oil, they are abnormal. These cells are not morbidly adipose, but it may develop into that state. The patient's cells are simply poisoned with too much food. The patient has good color; flesh and skin apparently have good texture. The patient looks well, but is not well. This shows us that one of Innate's rules is temperance in all things and that too much of anything in the body, even good things, is a poison.

Review Questions for Articles 152 to 161, inclusive.

1. **What is the difference between serum and urea?**
2. **What is the Afferent Serous Stream?**
3. **What are Innate's laboratories?**

4. What is a poison?
5. Name the poison possibilities of serum.
6. Describe the Ending of the Serous Cycle.
7. What part do the Kidneys play in the Serous Circulation?
8. Differentiate between Urea and Urine.
9. What part does the skin play in the Serous Circulation?
10. What is meant by "wet man"?
11. What is meant by "dry man"?
12. What are the ways in which Wet Man may occur?
13. What are the ways in which Dry Man may occur?
14. What is Seredema?
15. Differentiate between Elimination and Excretion.

Art. 162. Uredema.

Uredema is the name of the condition of tissues when the urea of cells is not removed from the cell bodies or from the immediate vicinity of the cells.

It is sometimes called Afferent Poisoning because waste matters are retained at the cell in its afferent current, which is not swift enough.

It differs from Edema in that, while it may be dropsical, it is studied from the standpoint of urea poisoning.

The patient does not look well, shows symptoms of poor elimination and is not well.

An analogy may be used to explain this. Plants have excreta as well as animals. They excrete water and gases into the atmosphere, which corresponds to respiration and perspiration of animals. Also, they pass excreta composed of solids into the soil by way of their roots. Many kinds of plants "foul" their own ground to such an extent that they are said to "kill out." A corn crop grown on the same field for a number of years, does not exhaust the soil so much as it "fouls" it, and after rotation of other crops, corn will grow very luxuriantly on the same field without addition of fertilizer. The excreta of corn is fertilizer for wheat and the excreta of wheat is fertilizer for corn. True, they both exhaust the soil to an extent, which must be replenished in nutritional elements.

Art. 163. Wet Insanity.

Wet insanity is unsoundness of any tissue, due to an abnormally wet serum; water poisoning.

Seredema, uredema, edema, dropsy, etc., are all forms of "Wet Insanity."

If it pertains to body tissues, it is wet physical insanity; as, dropsy.

If it pertains to the tissues of the educated brain, it is wet brain insanity; as, hydrocephalus.

Art. 164. Dry Insanity.

Dry Insanity is unsoundness of any tissue, due to an abnormally dry serum.

The condition of body cells in diabetes insipidus is an example.

If it pertains to body tissues, it is dry physical insanity.

If it pertains to the tissues of the educated brain, it is dry brain insanity.

Art. 165. A Chiropractic Discovery.

The Serous Circulation is a Chiropractic Discovery.

Chiropractic does not claim to have discovered the blood circulation, or the serum, as it has been known for a long time, in the inner and intra spaces; or the lymphatic stream and its vessels and glands. Chiropractic claims none of these, but it does claim the discovery of the cyclic connection of these three great systems, as has been explained in the foregoing articles.

Art. 166. Poison. (P. 287 V.)

Poison is any substance introduced into or manufactured within the living body which Innate cannot use in metabolism.

Art. 167. The Possibilities of Poison. (287, 291 V.)

Poison Possibilities are the different ways in which Poisons may occur.

The following four Possibilities are inclusive of any and every way that poisoning can occur; four blanket statements:

1. **Misplaced glandular products.**
2. **Excess glandular products.**
3. **Transported glandular products.**
4. **That which Innate cannot use in the general metabolism of the body.**

Glandular products are only usable in the places that Innate intended them to be used. If through incoordination these products are in any place where they should not be, they are just as surely a poison as any introduced poisons would be. (ex. jaundice.)

In any part of the body for any given time, a certain amount of glandular products are required, and as we have seen, they must be of the right kind. If there is an excess of a glandular product, even in the proper places for it, it is just as truly a poison as any foreign substance there. (Ex. biliousness.)

If a misplaced glandular product in a part of the body where it does not belong, is a poison, a glandular product that is not produced in that body is foreign to it and actually is a misplaced glandular product, for it is of use only in the body where it is made. Therefore, a glandular product taken from one body and introduced into another body, is a poison. (Ex. injected serums.)

Any substance in the body, whether glandular or not, which Innate cannot use in metabolism, is a poison. This includes both chemically active and inert substances. This fourth possibility will be explained fully in the following articles.

Art. 168. What "Educated" Knows About Poisons.

What "Educated" knows about poisons is the knowledge that tells us what substances are poisonous from accumulated experiences of scientists.

What "Educated" knows about poison constitutes the medical definition.

Medical definition: "Generic name for all substances which, when introduced into the animal organism, either by cutaneous absorption, respiration, or by the digestive canal, act in noxious manner on the vital properties, or textures of an organ." (Dunglison)

"Educated" groping this far, knows that such a substance has the "killing" or destroying property potential within it at all times; as carbolic acid in a bottle is known to be a poison substance which will act in the same manner. It gained this knowledge, not by chemistry, but by the experience of the race. Educated knows that it is not poison, actually, until introduced into the animal organism (see above definition), but has the educated knowledge of chemicals which tells it that substances *may* act harmfully if taken into the body, and of course this is useful knowledge. Moreover, by knowledge of chemicals, Educated might skillfully calculate what untried or new chemicals *may* be poison, if introduced into the body. However, this knowledge is limited and uncertain, as the definition shows, and Educated only knows about the *tried* substances.

Art. 169. What "Educated" Does Not Know About Poisons.

Educated does not know that a substance is a poison until Innate tells it; a tried substance; experience. After which, Educated calls that substance a poison.

Educated does not know, for certain, what substances may be poison until tried and Innate gives the decision.

Educated does not know if a newly discovered chemical (even if from knowledge of chemistry it calculates it should be) is a poison until it has asked Innate.

It does not know if a chemically inert substance is a poison until Innate decides.

Though these possibilities are told in a few words, instead of using volumes to tell them, they cover the entire situation, Chiropractically, showing that Educated does not know very much about poisons after all. Chiropractic does not scorn the educated knowledge of poisons; it makes use of it, of course. It is not content, however, to limit the science to the very finite knowledge of education, but prefers to refer the matter to Innate Intelligence.

Art. 170. How "Educated" Found Out About Poisons.

Educated knowledge of poisons is the sum total of experience of the human race for hundreds of years, as to what innates have said about substances. (Art. 321.)

Therefore, Educated only knows about such substances that have fallen into the experience of the human race. Of course this includes what human minds have observed about the innates of animals and plants. None of these poisons were determined for certain, by chemical analysis. History shows us how the somewhat morbid mind of Cleopatra was very interested in asking the innates of slaves (and sometimes friends and relatives) which were the most efficacious poisons. Therefore, Innate's judgment is the only criterion of a poison. She makes her opinion known by her expressions of contempt. (P. 288 V.)

Innate, however, does not record in the Educated Brain all that she knows, any more than you or I record all that we know on paper. If we worked every minute of our lives, we could not. When we realize that the educated mind is, after all, very finite, we can see that it is impossible for Innate, in a mere lifetime, to make educated records of her infinite knowledge. (Another instance of the limitations of matter, **prin. 24.**)

Therefore, there are many things that we do not know about poisons.

As we have remarked before, a chemist can make a very shrewd guess, by his knowledge of chemistry, that an untried substance may be a poison. But he finds that some substances may be harmless to one kind of organism and poison to others; harmless to individuals of a kind, and poison to others. We have plenty of instances. Seventy-five years ago, tomatoes were grown in flower beds for their red beauty, and children were warned not to eat them because they were poison. Today, we know that they are very good food, and refreshing; but still they are poison to some people. Some drugs are poison to some people, and not so noxious to others. (P. 287. V.)

Art. 171. What Innate Knows About Poisons. (P. 287, V)

Chirpractic definition: "Poison is any substance introduced into, or manufactured within the living body, upon which Innate Intelligence, after becoming cognizant of its presence through the interpretation of the vibrations set up in the tissue cells, and knowing that such a substance cannot be utilized, and if allowed to remain in the body will be absorbed by the tissue cells and do damage, begins a systematic process of elimination from the body." (Palmer.)

Any substance introduced into or manufactured within the living body, which Innate cannot use in metabolism, is a poison.

"Poison" is a word expressing the contempt that Innate has for a substance that she cannot use in metabolism. (p. 288, V)

The Innate Intelligence of a body knows all about what she does or does not want in that body. She knows what is a poison to that body. The Educated of a body does not know that much about it, for Educated is not an intelligence, but a physiological process of an organ, which is operated by Innate.

How could it know? It does not know anything about Innate's business in other matters! Does it know how to build a muscle? Or, how to operate a muscle? Innate is not to be compared with one of her functions.

It is easy to see that the Chiropractic definition of poison is more correct and much more comprehensive than the medical definition; containing all the truth to be found in the medical definition, and infinitely more.

REVIEW QUESTIONS FOR ARTICLES 162 to 171, inclusive.

1. What is Uredema?
2. What is "Wet Insanity"?
3. What is "Dry Insanity"?
4. Concerning the Serous Circulation, what is it that Chiropractic claims as its discovery?
5. Give the Chiropractic Definition of Poison.
6. Name the Four Possibilities of Poison.
7. Explain the Four Possibilities of Poison.
8. Give the medical definition of poison.
9. Explain how this definition is deficient.
10. In what manner was the medical definition formulated?
11. According to Chiropractic, how is poison determined as such?
12. Show in what way the Chiropractic definition of poison is superior to the medical definition.

Art. 172. SOME THINGS INNATES HAVE SAID ABOUT POISONS.

Medicine is a poison for it is substance that Innate does not prepare for use in the body. (293, 294, V.) If Innate accepts such a substance, showing no contempt, it is a food, even though it masquerades under the name of medicine. We mention this because it is a favorite argumentative point of the pro-medical or anti-Chiropractic people who seek to cloud the truth by starting the unwary chiropractor out on a false premise.

Medicine is a substance given to "stimulate" or "inhibit."

Substances which "stimulate" or "inhibit" are substances which "Educated" knows, because Innate recorded it, which, when given in larger doses will kill.

Substances which stimulate or inhibit are certainly chemicals with a "kick." They would be pretty poor medicines if they did not have. Do M.D.'s give inert, innocuous substances (except for psychological reasons) to their patients? They use minute quantities of powerful drugs. They search the forests for potent alkalines; manufacture powerful acids, grow plants for strong chemicals, and have hunters searching the jungles for the venom of tropical serpents.

Some things that Educated calls foods are sometimes poison. (Art. 170-172)

Some things that are good for one person, may be poison to another.

Some things may be food for a person, and poison to the same person at another time.

"Anything made or prepared artificially and then introduced into the body, against which Innate rebels, is a poison."

"Foods, air and water, when they have been 'doctored' are poisons." (294, V)

Art. 173. Food.

Food is any substance ingested into the body, which when digested and otherwise prepared furnishes wholesome nutrition to the tissue cells.

The necessary elements are demanded by Innate and made known consciously by normal hunger, thirst, and desire.

Given the demanded materials, Innate will make any combination she desires for metabolism.

Given the wrong materials, she will reject them or if they are unsatisfactory, but not poison, she will make the best of the circumstances.

Denied much needed elements, she will economize on what she has somewhere in the body; but if such a state of affairs exists chronically some tissues will become unsound.

Given too much food (usually because of educated fallacy), Innate will overwork the excretory organs in excreting and overstore tissue cells in order to dispose of it.

In any event, what Innate really needs cannot be regulated educationally, in either quantity or quality.

The Chiropractic standard of guidance in nutrition is to obey Innate's desires and restraints.

The person who incorrectly interprets these desires and restraints is technically a sick person, and is in danger from his "educated."

Art. 174. Diet.

Dieting, as commonly understood, is not Chiropractic.

Dieting is an educated attempt to regulate Innate or to regulate something against the wishes of Innate.

"A course of living or nourishment; also, what is eaten or drunk habitually; food; victuals; fare."

"A course of food selected with reference to a particular state of health; prescribed allowance of food, regime prescribed." (Webster.)

From these definitions we learn that dieting is "a course of living or nourishment," "a course of food selected with reference to a particular state of health; prescribed allowance of food; regime prescribed." We judge from these statements that there is something wrong with the state of health, else such attempts would not be made. If it is done to cure dis-ease, it will be unsuccessful, for **the cause of dis-ease is always in the spine.** (Prin. 30, 31.)

Prescription is a medical procedure, not Chiropractic. To attempt to cure a dis-ease by a prescribed allowance of food, is treating effects and not removing the cause. It may alleviate, and does, and to that Chiropractic has no objection; but in that case the cause still remains. **To pamper a weakness is to sidestep the cause. Why not meet the issue squarely and**

remove the cause? Then the patient can feel perfectly at ease in eating normal quantities of normal foods, according to the dictates of normal hunger and thirst.

When dieting is done with the idea of curing dis-ease, or as an arbitrary attempt to regulate the intellectual processes of metabolism, it is acting contrary to every fundamental principle of Chiropractic. A person who lives a simple life does not know how to do such things, much less think about them. Chiropractic is decidedly opposed to dieting, as studied in that light.

The reader and student is cautioned not to come to a conclusion about "the over-radical Chiropractic ideas," until he has read and studied further.

Art. 175. Common Sense, the Chiropractic Idea of Dieting.

If the body is given the elements that Innate requires, and in the quantities that she requires, and makes known that need by normal hunger or thirst, she can manufacture any combination needed. (p. 290 V)

Educated should not presume to determine the calories or determine which elements Innate should use.

People with abnormal hunger, or other abnormal desires, are technically sick people.

People with habitually abnormal appetites are victims of habit and are practicing a form of intemperance; not at all the expression of Innate Intelligence.

When dieting is done to offset or alleviate an adverse condition in living, brought on by "civilization" (an adverse state of affairs brought on by unwise precedents or human grooves of life), then dieting is not a battle between morbid educated mind and Innate; but between morbid "educated" and wise "educated." "Educated" versus "Educated"; "dog eat dog." In the latter case, Chiropractic approves, for *it is not truly diet,* but the coordination of a normal educated mind with Innate.

Therefore, **nutritional hygiene is not dieting but common sense.** It is simply the restoration of normal and natural environmental conditions. The restoration to normal, of conditions made abnormal by unwise educational living; restoration brought about by a wise, sane, and normal educated mind, coordinating with innate mind as it should, is nutritional hygiene. With this aspect of dieting, Chiropractic agrees. Consider diet in the light of common sense. **A sick person's abnormal educated mind will not allow him to use common sense, therefore somebody else's common sense must be used.**

Art. 176. The Fallacy of Trying to Regulate Innate Intelligence.

Innate Intelligence, the builder and warden of the body, with her infinite knowledge knows her own mind; knows what should be introduced into the body, both immaterial and material.

There is no educated mind, with only its finite gatherings of a lifetime, able to decide for an Innate Intelligence what is good for the body. This applies to forces and to matter. Innate makes known the needs for material by normal hunger and thirst; for the immaterial, by desire for movement or mental exercise, which desire might be called a kind of hunger.

The nourishment of the body should be governed by Innate Intelligence, with the cooperation of the educated mind.

The educated mind should serve as a cooperative function and not as a hindrance to innate mind, in the selection of food for the body.

No normal educated mind will try to oppose innate mind. When educated mind interferes with innate mind, it is abnormal. If it is abnormal, it is because of interference with transmission and the educated brain cells are slightly unsound;

consequently, instead of working in harmony with Innate Intelligence, it hinders in the efficiency of body operation as any other unsound organ would do.

Foods and water introduced into the body when not needed are poisons.

Foods and water denied the body, when the need is made known normally, is an insult to Innate and results in injury later, if not immediately.

Sterilized air and water, and artificially prepared foods are poisons for they are not natural; Innate's evolutionary structures are unacquainted with them as foods. Considered as medicines, they alleviate and sidestep, but they pamper the chemical abnormalities of the body so that this weakness grows worse, in exactly the same manner that a drug habit grows worse.

If one craves apples, one should eat apples, if they can be obtained. The function of educated mind is to obtain them; not to deny them. If one normally craves meat, educated should supply it; and not deny it, because a misguided dietitian has ruled it out.

The study of the human body shows that human beings are omnivorous. They should have both meat and vegetable foods. The teeth of carnivora are covered with enamel and they have fangs. The teeth of herbivorous animals are laminated and grow outward from the roots as they are worn off by use. The teeth of human beings as omnivorous animals, are covered with enamel and the human being also has fangs for the purpose of rending meat. Herbaceous foods require more grinding and chewing than meat foods and more processes of digestion. The human being does not chew the cud, nor is he provided with a series of stomachs (powerful laboratories with the action of powerful chemicals), as herbivorous animals are. But man has the digestive equipment to use both classes of foods.

The glands should secrete; if artificial foods make this unnecessary, the glands suffer from lack of use. The stomach is a muscular working organ. Take its job away from it by predigested foods, and the stomach gets lazy and weak. The bowels lose their peristaltic strength through the use of cathartics and pills; thus the "pill habit" is formed. Chiropractic is only urging the natural, but so unnatural has "civilization" made people, that the natural is greeted as something strange and radical.

If one takes the trouble to look into the question, it is easy to see that the natural foods of the human race are the foods upon which, for countless hundreds of years, the race developed. This great natural trend cannot be changed arbitrarily by dietitians in the space of a few years, without disaster to human beings. A few theorists have declared that there will be a time when a full meal will be concentrated to the size of a pill, and point out how convenient it will be to nourish the body and do it without the loss of time—a boon to business men, etc. It will be a sad day when the human race gets to the point where they have no time to eat naturally. The point we wish to emphasize is that Chiropractic is not a propaganda for a new method of dieting, but is a return to the old; a restoration of the natural. The digestive organs are made to do a certain amount of work—let them do it. As a muscle is strengthened by exercise, so are the digestive organs. The teeth are designed to rend and grind; they should be used for that purpose—it makes them stronger and better.

Chiropractic has nothing to say against dieting as a means of making fat people lean and thin people fat, except to say that it is not Chiropractic; and if people want to make sacrifices of that kind, it is more a science of martyrdom to fashion, than it is a science of healing. If a person wants to insult his Innate and injure his tissues for the sake of an educated ideal, mode, or fashion—it's his sacrifice! Chiropractic holds that it would be better, in every way, to eat the normal amounts and qualities of foods with the *normal* amounts of exercise. To be as thin as Innate wants you to be, reduce the amount of food *to normal* and step up the amount of exercise *to the normal* and natural amount. In this way, the body will be made as Innate wants it to be. Unfortunately for the vain, this does not always suit the "Gods of Mode." Some people are naturally fleshy and feel better in that condition, of course. For such people to forcibly make themselves thin by dieting, is injurious. Some people are naturally thin and feel better that way. To drive themselves to "a course of nourishment" to get fat, only poisons their systems.

Art. 177. Exercise.

Exercise is the natural and normal amount of movement of the body and its parts to obtain the normal amount of adaptation that is due to every part of it.

Natural demand in order to obtain the normal supply, of adaptation. (Prin. 33)

If exercise conforms to the above definition, Chiropractic is "strong for it." Any part of the body, whether muscles or any other part, requires a certain amount of movement daily, in order that it gets its share of survival value.

Natural exercise obtains a natural and beneficial tiredness. Unnatural or over exercise produces a fatigue or exhaustion which is not beneficial. Exercises calculated to develop or reduce parts of the body are beneficial if not driven to excess. If this is over done, it produces abnormally developed organs and that is not beneficial. Athletes' bodies are very abnormally developed, and sometimes it reaches the state of pathology. Outdoor exercise is much better than indoor, for one gets fresh air while doing it, and sunlight, which is very necessary to the human organism. The even and natural bodily development by exercise, natural exercise, is what

Chiropractic favors. Again, we point out that this should be restoration of natural environment by "educated," of that which "educated" has taken away.

Art. 178. HYGIENE. (Vol. III)

Hygiene, Chiropractically, is the restoration of natural and healthful environmental conditions which have been made abnormal by the necessities of civilized life.

In many instances, where it is impossible to restore natural conditions, compensation must be made.

Civilization is the sacrifices that individuals must make, in the matter of personal likes and dislikes and even of necessities, in order to have community living; to avoid infringing upon the rights of others; to give service in coordination.

The student is not to think, by this, that we mean that to have a perfectly natural environment for the body, we must restore jungle conditions and that we must live like Tarzan of the Apes. We mean that we aim to give the body properly balanced foods, suitable for omnivorous animals, fresh air, suitable light, and sanitary surroundings. All of these things one can have without living like Tarzan; in fact, can be much more hygienic and sanitary than that fictitious character could possibly be. We do not mean that the cooking of food is an unnatural preparation; but we do mean that the foods over-prepared lose natural food values. We do not mean that clean water is unnatural, but that water with injurious chemicals in it "to sterilize" it is unnatural; also distilled water is not a fit beverage. We need to realize that civilized life imposes conditions that are not healthful unless compensated for. Long hours of unnatural living because of industries; improper food, lack of sunshine and fresh air for economic reasons; necessary inhibitions for decency, are all factors that deprive us of natural living. There must be restoration, or at least compensation so far as possible, to make up for this.

The writer is not belittling civilization — it is necessary of course, if people are to live in tribes, communities, etc. It is necessary though, to realize that what naturalness civilization takes away, civilization will have to restore, if the human race is to be well. We are obliged to make a normal use of our educated minds to get out of, or to compensate for the abnormal difficulties that our educated minds got us into. Civilization is necessary, and as civilized beings we must make sacrifices of many personal comforts and likes, and even needs, to avoid infringing upon the rights of others. That is the real meaning of civilization. A strawberry, by itself, may be plump and luscious looking; but put into a basket with others, it becomes squeezed out of shape. Too bad! But necessary. However, as human beings, being equipped with the most competent organs of environmental adaptation of any living creatures, we are fully able, if we will, to compensate for what we lose in naturalness, by educationally restoring naturalness. The restoration of natural conditions, as far as possible, in the midst of civilized circumstances, is the meaning of the word *hygiene* in Chiropractic.

Art. 179. The Poisons of Environment.

Abnormal or extremely adverse environmental conditions for the human body are important in the study of the cause of dis-ease.

They affect the health by making normal adaptation more difficult if not impossible.

They are not considered the cause of dis-ease, or even secondary causes, but they further limit the limitations of matter. (Prin. 24.)

Poor environmental conditions can affect the health by making adaptation very difficult; especially if one is not acclimated to those conditions. If subluxations exist, and in most people they do, especially those affecting the eliminating organs, the effect is still worse. Some environmental conditions would poison a healthy person; as very unsanitary surroundings. Some environments are downright impossible. If there are subluxations causing poor elimination, the adverse conditions act more readily upon the tissue cells, there being some accumulative destructive survival values already. Even if there are not such subluxations, the bad environment may call for more adaptation than a body can afford. (Prin. 24.)

In our studies of environmental poisoning, the Serous Circulation is the main factor in the consideration of indirect effects.

Environmental poisoning is made possible because of necessity, or carelessness, or ignorance. Normal educated mind usually receives warning, and Innate knows there is danger. However, warnings are frequently disregarded for the foregoing reasons. Perhaps necessity, or economic reasons are the most numerous; office work, factory employment, property in or near a swamp, poverty in a tenement. All these are difficult to overcome; they exist nevertheless and in such, troubles lurk.

The utterly impossible conditions mentioned are: water, extreme heat, and poisonous gases in which the human body cannot live, no matter how perfect the transmission of mental impulses.

The possibilities of environmental poisoning are: impure water, air, food, bad climate, poor sanitation, poor hygiene, personal and environmental, effluvia and germs.

Art. 180. Water as an Environmental Factor.

Water may poison a body of lowered resistance when it is impure; impregnated with injurious minerals, stagnant, charged with poisonous gases, etc.

Pure water for human consumption contains none of these, but may have a harmless and normal amount of minerals and germs.

Impure water may contain putrid matter, poisonous gases, or other matters, harmful materials which, when introduced into the body, poison the Serous Circulation. External application of such water may poison the skin. If stagnant, it pollutes the air. Water charged with excess mineral or minerals injurious to the body is apt to irritate the bowels.

Innate warns educated mind by smell, taste, and sight, and depends upon educational adaptation for safety.

Art. 181. FOOD AS AN ENVIRONMENTAL FACTOR.

Abnormal food may poison a body of lowered resistance when it is impure or contains impurities; as, poisonous chemicals in it, poisonous gases, has changed chemically, decomposed, etc.

Pure food for human consumption must be free from any of these impurities.

If food contains chemicals, or gases that cannot be used in metabolism, these foreign substances, not the food, are poison. Of course, such food is unfit for use. If what was once a good food undergoes a chemical change, it is no longer the substance that it was when educationally named a food. Fermentation is a good example of this. If what was once a good food decomposes or partly decomposes, it is unfit for use as a food. For the human economy uses organic matter for food mostly. It is first raised in the scale by organisms which of course lose their lives in order that the human organism may live. This is true of both vegetable and animal life. A little thought will show us how true this is. If we could live by using the inorganic foods, we could exist like a tree or a cabbage. Although we move in an ocean of protein, we must buy it at so much per pound at the butcher shop or at the grocer's. The organic food must be in a clean state, because the human body is not prepared to use decomposed matter in metabolism. If compelled to eat it from necessity, poisoning is likely to take place. Races of people who, from necessity, like the Digger Indians or the Terra del Fuegans, are obliged to use decomposed food, show the effects of such food in their inferior physique and low mentality. It requires entirely too much adaptation for the human mechanism, to raise the grade of these foods, therefore poisoning of the Serous Circulation occurs.

Review Questions for Articles 172 to 181, inclusive.

1. Why are medicines poison?
2. Are harmless substances used as medicines?
3. When is a food a poison?
4. What is food?
5. How is food determined as such, Chiropractically?
6. Does dieting remove the cause of dis-ease?
7. Granting that dieting alleviates, what harm does it do in the long run?
8. How does Innate Intelligence make known the needs for food?
9. What is the cause of abnormal hunger and thirst?
10. Does Chiropractic object to regulating the diet of sick people? Why?
11. What proof have we that man is an omnivorous animal?
12. Is Chiropractic a propaganda for a new method of dieting or is it for restoration of the natural?
13. On what grounds does Chiropractic object to predigested and other "artificial" foods?
14. What is the Chiropractic view of dieting to get thin or fat?
15. What is the Chiropractic policy of exercise?
16. Why is it a fallacy to prescribe certain foods to produce fat and others to produce leanness?
17. What is the Chiropractic definition of Hygiene?
18. According to the principles of Hygiene, what is Civilization?
19. What evolutionary evidence have we that we should not interfere with Innate's processes of naturalness?
20. What are the possibilities of environmental poisoning?
21. What part do environmental poisons play in dis-ease?
22. State which Fundamental Principle applies to the foregoing question.
23. Name some utterly impossible environmental conditions.
24. Why do people persist in living in unhygienic surroundings?

25. Explain water supply, or surroundings, as an environmental factor.
26. Explain food as an environmental factor.
27. What is the character of practically all foods used by human beings?
28. Why is the human organism not prepared to use decomposed foods in metabolism?

Art. 182. Air as an Environmental Factor.

Air may poison a body of lowered resistance when it is impure; containing too much carbon dioxide; not enough oxygen; too much oxygen; substances injurious to the lungs; or effluvia of dead things.

Air containing too much carbon dioxide or not enough oxygen, poisons by asphyxiation. It may contain injurious germs or poisonous gases. It may contain solid materials that injure the lungs; as, the air in factories, mines, and smoky cities. The effluvia of dead things is unfit to enter the lungs of the human. Such an environment is unfit for the human organism; it requires too much adaptation. Innate warns educated mind by smell, sight, etc.

Art. 183. Climate as a Factor of Environment.

Adverse climate can poison a body with lowered resistance by imposing extraordinary adaptation.

A rapid change of temperature closes the pores of the skin too suddenly and before compensation can be made via the Serous Circulation (which as you remember, requires seventy-two hours to make a complete cycle) some tissue cells have been made unsound by the retained poisons. When the weather is extremely hot, overheating the body calls for extreme adaptation, and besides, the heat cannot be dissipated fast enough. Tissue cells are, after all, very delicate structures and it does not require much above the normal temperature to injure them. In order to dissipate great heat from the body into an overheated environment, the adaptability of the human body is often overtaxed. The attempt by

Innate to do this causes excess traveling of water through the body, which is not good for the tissue cells. Adverse climate may make the atmosphere too humid, lessening the amount of oxygen in a cubic foot of atmosphere, and making it difficult for the body to perspire, since perspiration depends upon evaporation. This also retains too much heat in the body. All in all, it requires too much adaptation or too sudden adaptation to be healthful.

Art. 184. Hygiene and Sanitation as Environmental Factors.

Poor Hygiene and bad Sanitation can poison the body with lowered resistance, by imposing too much adaptation, if not by actual direct poisoning.

They can poison the air or pollute the water and taint the food. In such environments, poison germs breed. Human excreta, if kept on the body or kept too near it, has the same effect upon the body that the excreta of a cell has upon the cell, if not removed from it. Keeping perspiration and other waste materials from leaving the surface of the body, poisons the Serous Circulation. If the body does not get enough light, it is injurious, for light gives something to the body that is almost as necessary as air. Innate warns educated mind by discomfort, sight, smell, etc.

Art. 185. Effluvia as an Environmental Factor.

Effluvia is poisonous gas from putrid and decaying organic matter.

We pointed out that Innate cannot use decomposing matter in metabolism when introduced by impure foods. It is just as true in regard to air. The poisonous gases entering the lungs can poison the Serous Circulation. Innate certainly warns, not only by sight and smell, but by an innate fear of the dead.

Art. 186. Germs as a Factor of Environment.

Germs can poison a body of lowered resistance when they are too numerous, or by their excreta when they are numerous, or when they are the poisonous kind.

There are such things as germs. Chiropractic does not deny their existence as is so frequently reported. It would not deny them any more than it would deny any other laboratory finding (Arts. 10 to 13, incl.). As in regard to other laboratorical findings, the Chiropractic view is different from that of the medical world. Chiropractic recognizes that some germs are beneficial and necessary. Some are necessary to human life; necessary as food; parts of the human body are germs. The body develops from a germ, itself. Water is better for drinking when it has some kinds of germs in it; but all germs are not beneficial to the body. Some are poisonous. Some are harmless scavengers, but their excreta may be poison. Some of the scavengers are harmless enough when not numerous, but poison the body by the presence of great numbers. There are both vegetables and animal germs. **Chiropractic holds that germs are scavengers;** that they gain no foothold in the body in sufficient numbers to poison it as long as there is no abnormal tissue or abnormal secretions for them to thrive upon. As scavengers, they are beneficial to the body and cause no harm as long as there are not too many. **They do not cause the abnormal tissue upon which they thrive.** The dis-eased condition comes first, offering a breeding ground for them.

Art. 187. Parasites.

Parasites are organisms that feed upon their host or materials that the host has prepared for its own use.

Unlike the scavenger germs in the foregoing article, they do not thrive upon dead tissue or abnormal secretions, but require live flesh or good food materials intended for the metabolism of the host. As there are both sheep and wolves among the animals, so there are both sheep and wolves among the micro-organisms. They enter and thrive, in and upon apparently healthy bodies, but their presence indicates a lowered resistance, for these undesirables are driven out by Innate in a healthy body, by means of secretions. These secretions act as poison to that particular parasite. An example of this is shown by the killing of the tapeworm by Innate when adjustments are given. This is also shown by the adaptation of the body against the attack of mosquitoes.

Art. 188. Epidemics.

Epidemics are adverse environmental conditions which in spreading attack those with similar lack of resistance.

These adverse conditions may be bad water, bad weather, bad food, bad air, or poisons of various kinds, including germs. An "epidemic" attacks those who cannot make sufficient adaptation. This lack of adaptation is due to subluxation. (305 V.) If the adverse conditions are exceedingly over and above the adaptative resistance of healthy people, the tribe had better move.

Art. 189. Contagion and Infection.

A contagious disease is one transmitted from one person to another by direct or indirect contact.

An infectious disease is one transmitted from one person to another without direct contact necessarily; but one caused by the multiplication of pathogenic germs.

These are not Chiropractic definitions.

Chiropractic states that germs are transmitted from one body to another, and that poisons of a dis-ease in a person may be transmitted and poison another person with lowered tissue resistance; but Chiropractic claims that the germs and

the poisons do not cause the dis-ease. The cause of the dis-ease is always in the spine.

Interference with transmission causing tissue cells to become unsound gives a breeding ground for germs. They may or may not be present. If they are, they will breed in great numbers if there is enough abnormal tissue, and perhaps further poison, by the presence of so many of them. Dr. Palmer's analogy of the dead horse and buzzards will apply here. The buzzards are present around the dead horse, but they did not kill the horse. Germs are present around dead tissue, but they did not kill the tissue. They are scavengers in the same sense as the buzzards.

Art. 190. Blood Poison. (305 V.)

Blood Poison is not a tenet of Chiropractic.

Chiropractic does not believe in blood poisoning as the physician does, that is, that the blood can be diseased as a connective tissue; but believes that the blood, as part of the Serous Circulation, can be laden with poisons. This applies whether the poisons are introduced into or are manufactured within the body.

Art. 191. Immunity.

Immunity is the adaptative resistance of tissue cells because of the constructive survival value they possess.

Immunity is the high percentage of adaptability of tissue cells, because of their perfection in "condition" which requires time and effort to tear down.

This perfect condition is dependent upon the perfect transmission of mental impulses. (Prin. 5, 28).

When tissue cells are thus very sound, they are able because of their adaptability and material resources, to withstand the invasion of poison better than those not so fortunate. A body so equipped does not "catch diseases." The

Chiropractic way of saying this is, that a body immune is not susceptible to poisons of the epidemic kind.

Review Questions for Articles 182 to 191, inclusive.

1. Explain Air as an environmental factor.
2. Explain Climate as an environmental factor.
3. Explain Sanitation as an environmental factor.
4. What is effluvia and explain it as an environmental factor.
5. Explain Germs as an environmental factor.
6. Does Chiropractic deny the existence of germs?
7. What is the Chiropractic philosophy of germs?
8. What are Parasites?
9. Give the Chiropractic explanation of parasites.
10. Give the Chiropractic definition of epidemics.
11. Give the Chiropractic philosophy of epidemics.
12. Give the Chiropractic philosophy of Contagion and Infection.
13. Give the Chiropractic idea of "blood poisoning."
14. Give the Chiropractic explanation of Immunity.

Art. 192. Periodical and Recurrent Dis-eases.

Periodical and Recurrent Dis-eases are those which alternate with periods of apparent recovery and in some cases the periods are regular.

There are several kinds, but most of them belong in the poison family. The toxins or poisons accumulate over and above the amount of elimination which of course, in these cases, is abnormal. When this accumulation reaches a point where it is dangerous, Innate brings about a crisis of some kind; as fits in epilepsy, high fevers as in dengue or ague. The analogy of the geyser can be used here. A geyser tube slowly fills with water until its hydrostatic pressure is over-balanced by the superheated steam from volcanic fires, then it bursts forth with violence and is relieved.

There are other types, as hay fever, which is seasonal and comes on at certain seasons because there is a chronic subluxation which does not offer inconvenience and does not interfere with transmission until the season comes when more adaptation is required.

Coryza or head cold is another example. One has a chronic subluxation impinging the nerves leading to the tissues of the nasal pharynx. Through the summer weather, while it is warm, there is no interference; but when in the fall or winter the colder weather calls for more adaptation in those tissues, there is interference with transmission, hence incoordination.

Art. 193. The Philosophy of Fevers.

This explanation pertains to febrile conditions.

Through lack of proper elimination of toxins and waste materials, poisons accumulate in the Serous Circulation.

The ordinary channels of elimination are not available to Innate.

Accumulation of poisons always chills the body. (p. 300 V.)

Innate plans to eliminate the poisons through the lungs in the form of carbon dioxide.

She starts to oxidize them.

Calorific function, unfortunately, is abnormal.

Therefore, the process of oxidation (burning) gets beyond control.

Too much heat is developed, which is made worse by the ordinary channels of elimination not being available; viz., kidneys, and skin.

The temperature goes above 98.6 degrees and the condition is called fever or febrile dis-ease.

Because of lack of proper elimination through the ordinary channels for that purpose, namely, the kidneys, skin, and bowels (E—, K.P.), toxins and waste materials accumulate in the Serous Circulation and poison the tissue cells of the body. Such poisons produce coldness and as their amount grows serious they produce what is known as *chill.* Then Innate plans (I.A.) to eliminate these poisons via the lungs in the form of carbon dioxide, for the poisons are composed mostly of carbon, hydrogen, and oxygen, which can be made into gases. However, before the lungs can handle these toxins, they must be changed to the gaseous state. Therefore, Innate starts to oxidize the carbons—a chemical process that produces very much heat, for it actually burns. All goes well, and not too much heat is produced by this adaptation and there is no evidence of febrile trouble *if* the calorific departments are normal. Unfortunately, in febrile dis-eases, they are not. (C+, C.P.). The process of oxidation, so nicely started by Innate, gets beyond control; the C+ is evidence of that. Not only is the process of oxidation (burning) out of control, and the temperature of the body raised above normal from that source, but the temperature goes still higher because of the usual excretory channels (E—, K.P.) being out of order, ordinary heat dissipation cannot take place, not to mention the dissipation of the extra heat which should be done. Thus the lungs are the organs that Innate is depending upon and their action is much accelerated adaptatively as well as that of the heart. The lungs carry off the oxidized materials as well as great quantities of heat. In time, if the amount of poison is not too great and the subluxations not too severe, the poisons will be oxidized and carried away and the febrile conditions subside. It is commonly said that the fever "wore itself out." Its cause still remains and it is apt to recur. If, however, adjustments are given, the proper use of the eliminating organs restored, the poisons quickly will be eliminated, so there is no use of further burning toxins. There also is no further unusual demand upon the calorific department and therefore there ceases to be interference with transmission, especially if C.P. be adjusted with the K.P. (Art. 199). Such adjustments are followed by profuse sweat and the almost immediate "breaking" of the fever. Whereas, without the adjustments allowing that the condition does not become fatal, it may last for days before it subsides, with consequent damage to the delicate tissue cells which are not able to stand much heat.

Art. 194. B. J.'s Fever Cycle.

This complete cycle is condensed to three steps which have each three different aspects or names and are here given side by side.

1. Invasion.	**1. Chill.**	**1. E—, Concussion of forces.**	**K.P.**
2. Incubation.	**2. Fever.**	**2. C+, Subluxation.**	**C.P.**
3. Recuperation.	**3. Sweat.**	**3. O Adjustments.**	**C.P., K.P.**

Art. 195. The Poisons of Strong Emotions.

These have references to the poisoning of the Serous Circulation by strong emotions; as, worry, fright, anger, hate, nervousness, shock, etc.

There are several theories; we present three.

1. Theory: Strong emotions produce a shock with the effect of penetrative forces that act upon the tissues in the vertemere region.

This of course, may produce dis-eases directly by "local," or indirectly through the Serous Circulation.

2. Theory: Strong emotions have an effect upon secretions of the body which enter the Serous Circulation and are poisonous to the tissues.

Those who favor this theory point out instances of nursing babies being poisoned by the mother's milk after the mother having undergone anger, fright, or worry.

3. Theory: Strong emotions cause excessive carbon dioxide and other waste matters in the brain, which enter the Serous Circulation.

Brain tissue requires an enormous blood supply at any time. Note the comparative size of the blood vessels supplying it. Sudden or violent use of the brain produces a hard strain upon it, which if continued will injure it. Naturally its already large blood supply will have to be increased. Study, worry, or long protracted heavy work of the brain not only requires a great blood supply, but produces a heavy amount of waste matter which entering the Serous Circulation acts in a very noxious manner.

Art. 196. The Poisons of Fatigue.

Any exercise produces waste materials, which if not eliminated but retained in the Serous Circulation, act as poison.

Either brain exhaustion or physical exhaustion poison the whole body in a way that it requires time to restore.

Everyone knows how hard it is to think clearly when physically exhausted; or to work physically when very much mentally exhausted. We are also acquainted with the cramping effects of toxins in the muscles after we have had a very exhausting tramp as, a difficult march or a long hunt.

Art. 197. Stimulation.

There are two kinds of Stimulation: the direct and indirect; or the true and the false.

The direct or true Stimulation is the action of stimuli upon dead tissue, driving it to an unadapted activity resembling function.

The indirect or false stimulation is really not stimulation at all. It is the adaptative response of live tissue to invading stimuli. (300 V.)

The direct or true stimulation is shown when stimuli are used in prepared muscle, as dead frog legs. It causes dead tissue to act in a manner resembling function, but this movement is wholly unadapted; one could produce no definite governed action with it. The indirect or false stimulation calls for unusual adaptative action of tissue cells, which because of the fact, such action resulting from applied stimuli, is apt to mislead one into thinking that the stimuli caused the action. This unusual or even violent adaptative action is in defense of the tissues against the stimuli which are penetrative forces (Art. 117). Such action over-works a tissue cell, leaving it exhausted depleted, and poisoned. The cell must recuperate at the expense of survival value.

Innate Intelligence neither stimulates nor inhibits; and for the reason that the student is apt to make the error of believing so, Dr. Palmer objects to the use of these words in Chiropractic. Innate does not create stimuli. Mental impulses are not stimuli, for stimuli have none of the characteristics of adapted forces. Neither does stimulation take place in the body; only in dead tissue. What really takes place when a stimuli are applied to the living body, is usual adaptative action. One might reason that if a stimulus will act upon a dead muscle cell it will act upon the same muscle cell in the living body. The answer to that is, if a stimulus acts upon a cell in a living body, causing it to act in an unadapted manner, it is because interference with transmission leaves the cell "partly dead." This is a part of the explanation of excess function.

Art. 198. Inhibition.

Inhibition is the name for the suppression of the action of a tissue cell, by penetrative forces (as of a drug) at the same time loading it with more work to do.

As there is no real stimulation in live cells, so there is no real inhibition in live cells. A drug which inhibits is a poison and as such causes the tissue cells to make violent efforts to eject it, followed by extreme exhaustion. There is no difference in the action of any poison (stimulating or inhibiting) upon a tissue cell except that a poison which inhibits is more deadly and damages the cell more. (See p. 299, 300 Vol. V.)

Art. 199. Application of the Cycles to Successful Adaptation to Poison.

In this example there are two cycles involved simultaneously showing the cycles of the "local" and the "condition."

Example used: the stomach and ingested poison.

1. Poison.
2. Tissue cell of stomach.
3. Penetrative chemical vibration.
4. Impressions of vibrations.
5. Afferent nerve.
6. Transmission of impressions.
7. Afferent brain cell.
8. Reception of impressions.
9. Mental.
10. Mental interpretation.
11. Sensation of poison.
12. Ideation of poison.
13. Innate Intelligence.
14. Intellectual adaptation.
15. Uni. Intel. supplying the forces.
16. Creations of foruns.
17. Efferent brain cell.
18. Transformation of foruns.
19. Mental impulses.
20. Propulsion.
21. Efferent nerve to stomach.
22. Transmission.
23. Muscle cell of stomach.
24. Reception.
25. Physical personification.
26. Expression of Innate.
27. Functional movement.
28. Poison ejected.
29. Coordination.
    Cells working in harmony.

1. Poison.
2. Tissue cell of stomach.
3. Penetrative chemical vibration.
4. Injured tissue cell.
5. Equivalent impressions.
6. Afferent nerve.
7. Afferent transmission, of equi. impress.
8. Afferent brain cell.
9. Reception of equivalent impressions.
10. Mental.
11. Mental interpretation.
12. Sensation of injury and pain.
13. Ideation of damage.
14. Innate Intelligence.
15. Intellectual adaptation.
16. Uni. Intel. supplying the forces.
17. Creation of foruns.
18. Efferent brain cell.
19. Transformation of foruns.
20. Reparatory mental impulses.
21. Propulsion.
22. Efferent nerve to stomach.
23. Transmission.
24. Tissue cell of injured stomach.
25. Reception.
26. Physical personification.
27. Expression of Innate.
28. Reparatory functional movement.
29. Coordination.
    Cells being repaired—recuperating.

Tissue Cell is the representative of tissue cells; the cells constituting the organ. The student is not to make the error of thinking that we are stating that just one cell became injured, or that one cell ejected the poison from the stomach. **The cell of a cycle is always a *representative cell,* with the proper name, Tissue Cell.**

Art. 200. Application of Cycles to Unsuccessful Adaptation to Poison.

This is a complex cycle, showing the complete disease cycle followed by the restoration cycle (complete).

Tissue cell is the representative cell in this system of units.

Example used: the stomach and ingested poison.

1. Poison.
2. Tissue cell of stomach.
3. Chemical penetrative vibrations.
4. Impressions of chem. vibrations.
5. Afferent nerve.
6. Transmission of impressions.
7. Afferent brain cell.
8. Reception of impressions.
9. Mental.
10. Mental interpretation.
11. Sensation of poison.
12. Ideation of poison.
13. Innate Intelligence.
14. Intellectual adaptation.
15. Universal Intelligence.
16. Creation of foruns.
17. Efferent brain cell.
18. Transformation of foruns.
19. Mental impulses.
20. Propulsion.
21. Efferent nerve to stomach.
22. Transmission of impulses.
23. Tissue cell (damaged by poison)
24. Reception of impulses (difficult)
25. Physical personification (not good).
26. Expressions of Innate (not perfect).
27. Motor function (crippled).
28. Unsuccessful reaction.
29. Violent shock.
30. Vibrations to the vertemere.
31. Concussion.
32. Tissue cell of vertemere region.
33. Penetrative vibration.
34. Impressions of vibrations.
35. Afferent nerve of vertemere.
36. Transmission of impressions.
37. Afferent brain cell.
38. Reception of impressions.
39. Mental.
40. Interpretation.
41. Sensation of concussion.
42. Ideation of vertemere.
43. Innate Intelligence.
44. Intellectual Adaptation.
45. Creation of foruns.
46. Efferent brain cell.
47. Transformation.
48. Mental Impulses.
49. Propulsion.
50. Efferent nerve to vertemere.
51. Transmission of impulses.
52. Tissue cell of vertemere.
53. Physical personification.
54. Unbalanced expression.
55. Unbalanced function.
56. Unbalanced resistance.
57. Subluxation.
58. Interference with transmission in both cycles.
59. Tissue cell of stomach.
60. Reception.

61. Abnormal personification.
62. Abnormal expression.
63. Abnormal function.
64. Incoordination; perhaps the drug habit, brought about by lack of chemical balance. A permanent adaptation to that is the drug habit.
65. The compensation cycles established and perhaps a continual manufacture of antidote.
66. Compensation made in the main cycle of our story.
67. The Restoration Cycle can be applied in the usual way, showing how recovery may obtain by giving adjustments and with the assistance of the will, break the drug habit. (196 V)

Art. 201. How Poison Kills.

Poisons impair the condition of tissue cells so that it limits Innate's expression. (Prin. 5, 24) This action may be so great that death will occur.

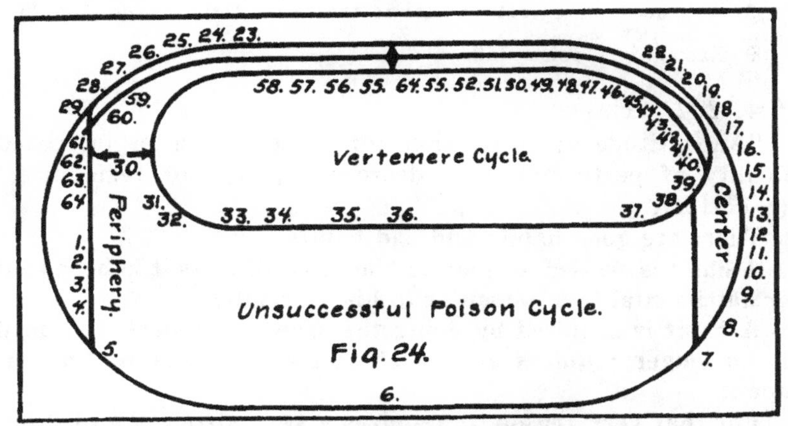

Fig. 24.

If Poisons injure innate brain, death is immediate. (317, V)

Poisons produce a shock as any other penetrative force, causing subluxations which may be severe enough to cause death.

Poisons do not "bite" Innate.

Violent poisons, such as cyanide of potassium, produce extreme "stimulation" which produces violent contractions. This affects the vertemere regions, causing subluxations and injury to vital organs. Some believe that it injures innate brain by acting upon all nervous tissues. Some believe that the violent "stimulation" injures or destroys the metabolistic nervous system.

Review Questions for Articles 192 to 201, inclusive.

1. Give the Chiropractic explanation of Periodical and Recurrent diseases.
2. Give the Chiropractic explanation of Febrile Conditions.
3. Explain the poisons of Strong Emotions.
4. Explain the poisons of Fatigue.
5. Does Innate Intelligence stimulate?
6. Explain "stimulation" according to Chiropractic.
7. Explain "inhibition," Chiropractically.
8. Why does Chiropractic object to the terms "stimulation" and "inhibition"?
9. Explain how poison kills.

Art. 202. Habit.

"An aptitude or inclination for some action in increased facility of performance or decreased power of resistance." (Webster).

There are good habits and bad habits.

A habit is classed as good or bad, according as it is beneficial or detrimental to a person or to his associates.

A habit is acquired by doing the same act repeatedly, until it no longer requires an act of "conscious" will to bring it about.

For that very reason, it requires a very strong act of "conscious" will to change a habit.

If there are subluxations affecting the normal exercise of educated will, it will be much harder to change a habit or to break a bad habit. In Article 200 is shown a condition that is impossible to change without adjustments, especially if the educated mind is weak in will. It does not necessarily follow that if a person has a strong habit which he has not the will to change, he is weak willed in all things, for it is the cardinal characteristic of a habit, that it requires more will to change it, than any other act. According to some psychologists, a habit is the very tiny evolutionary beginning of an instinct, and it is easy to understand that an instinct is not easily changed.

Art. 203. The Philosophy of the Drug Habit.

Drug Habits are such as smoking, tobacco chewing, snuff habit, coffee, tea, alcohol, stimulants, and opiates.

The example used here is the acquiring of the tobacco habit.

The poison is first taken and Innate shows her contempt and displeasure by ejecting the contents of the stomach and vigorous elimination through the excretory organs. Some tyro smokers notice that the action of the bowels is accellerated. The first repulse is shown in Article 199. If the dose with some drugs is strong enough, the result is shown in Article 200. A subluxation will result in the latter case. Immediately the mechanical demonstration of Innate's displeasure has taken place, she begins to form an antidote for the poisons that have remained in the system.

Then the drug dose is repeated. Innate again may rebel. In the beginning of smoking, she does not always do so mechanically. Having started making antidotes, she continues the process. As the doses are repeated, Innate just as repeatedly creates the antidote so that the serum will be chemically balanced even with the presence of the nicotine. In time, the manufacture of antidote is a continuous process, in expectation of the regular or constant repetition of the drug.

A failure to take the drug, therefore, leaves an unbalanced antidote, which then becomes a poison and the habit victim becomes distressed because of it. Innate makes an imperative demand for the drug; it seems strange that Innate would demand a poison, *but now* it is something that she requires in metabolism to neutralize the poison already there. From this demand of Innate's, made known by strong desire for the drug, arises a craving that is very difficult to deny. It requires a vigorous effort of the will, even with strong willed persons, to deny it. If, however, this is done and the body gets no more of the drug, Innate will proceed to destroy the antidote and cease making it. But, during that time, the case suffers the torments of craving.

One of the factors that makes it so easy to give in to the craving and so hard to deny it, is the force of habit. Thus there is a double battle for the will: the will to deny the craving and the will to change a habit.

Subluxations play their part in all this, in the matter of incoordinated educated mind, poor elimination, and inadequate adaptation in the matter of balancing drug and antidote for every day's struggle.

Art. 204. Medical Habits.

A Medical Habit is the habitual use of a treatment to the detriment of the body.

This includes the habitual use of pills, patent medicines, opiates, cathartics, enemas, and artificial foods.

The use of pills and cathartics accustoms the intestines to profuse secretion in order to dilute the poisons and flush the bowels of them. These drugs are poisons; Innate does not want them there and gets rid of them in this manner. "Salts do not move the bowels, but the bowels move the salts." (Palmer) Repeated doses of this get the bowels into a habit; a habit of heavy secretion of fluids and lessened peristaltic action. The muscles of the intestines of chronic pill users are almost entirely inert. The too frequent or continuous use of the enema also has the same effect upon the muscles of the rectum.

Some users of patent medicines have made of themselves drunkards and drug addicts. True, they did not have that reputation, but they had to have, regularly, their particular patent medicine, with its high alcoholic content or its opiates, or other poisonous drugs.

The users of over-prepared foods (artificial foods) can become addicts to them, for they get certain digestive organs into the habit of shirking, which causes them to become abnormal, weakened, or depleted through non-use, and then, when they are called upon to do their natural work, they suffer a great deal.

Art. 205. Intellectual Adaptation. (155, V)

Intellectual Adaptation is the mental process of Innate Intelligence to plan ways and means of using or circumventing universal forces.

This mental process is made manifest or expressed through change in organic matter.

It is the universal law of change which governs adaptation.

Organic matter is the only kind that requires adaptation to protect its structural values.

The "essence" of this intellectual process is preserved in the race of the organism, in an accumulative manner, called survival value and is the fundamental principle of evolution.

We study Intellectual Adaptation by its expression, manifestation, namely adaptation.

Art. 206. Adaptation.

Adaptation is the movement of an organism or any of its parts; or the structural change in that organism, to use or to circumvent environmental forces.

Adaptation is a continuous process — continually varying.

It is never constant and unvarying as are other universal laws.

Adaptation is a universal principle—the only one of its kind. It is the principle of change, and the changes are always according to law, which is Intellectual Adaptation.

For an exhaustive treatise on Intellectual Adaptation and Adaptation, the student is referred to (155, V). It cites many good examples. The acclimatization of plants and animals; the growth of hair on bodies for protection; the forming of callouses on hardworked hands; the strengthening of tree roots on the windward side—these are all examples of adaptation to forces which if they had not been thus opposed or circumvented, would have proven destructive. These organisms strengthened their structure where it was most needed (that is, their Innates did it), so that they were able to withstand future stresses of that kind. Note that the organism successfully meets the stresses for a given moment, but the strengthening of the structures is not done instantaneously for that particular moment; *it is done to provide for the next time.* This gives a positive value that is transmitted to posterity.

Art. 207. Inheritance of Dis-ease.

Inheritance of dis-ease is not a Chiropractic tenet.

Chiropractic holds that dis-ease cannot be inherited because it is not a value but a lack of value.

Dis-ease is lack of adaptation. There is no constructive survival value, no evolutionary values to inherit, in that case.

Diathesis is not a dis-ease; it is but the inheritance of type; of forms of family characteristics, the same as one could "inherit" the shape of nose belonging to his father or grandfather.

If one has a diathesis for tuberculosis, that does not mean that he has tuberculosis or that he is obliged to have it. The term is used to indicate that such a person has a body with a low resistance to that kind of dis-ease. True, this one's parents may have had tuberculosis. The offspring of those parents with a family resemblance will have the same kind of tissues with a likeness in strength and resistance. He will have the same type of spine, subject to the same subluxations. If subjected to the same environmental conditions that his parents had, perhaps living in unhygienic or unsanitary quarters, he will have the same adaptative battles to fight that they did. He is likely to be overcome in the same way they were. If, however, he seeks to improve on the hygiene and sanitation of his family, he is no more likely to have tuberculosis than anyone else.

There is another question that is commonly presented. How about leprosy, syphilis, etc.? Are not the germs inherited, and do not the children of syphilitic parents have this disease? Yes, but not always. A mother supplies the foetus with nutrition by serum (not blood) through the placenta. That is one of the functions of the placenta. It provides a serous nutrition upon which the foetus thrives and grows. Obviously, the environment of a developing foetus must be normal and natural, supplying clean food, by the same principle that the adult human must have a suitable environment. We have seen that a human adult body cannot use impure or putrid or poisonous food; neither can the foetus. If the mother's serum conveys the germs of a dis-ease, as syphilis, to the foetus, of course it is possible for the foetus to have them in its body. From this point on, it depends upon the resistance of the tissues of the foetus. The germs very seldom get a start then. If there are subluxations in the child, they do. If not, the germs lie dormant. The child may grow to adulthood, and often does, before the disease shows. It would not then, if at some time the tissue resistance were not lowered. Just think, how many people reach the age of twenty or twenty-five without having sickness of some kind which lowers resistance. How many people are without K.P. subluxations or subluxations of some kind? Even then, the tissue resistance may be too great for the germs to gain a foothold and the person may live out his life untroubled. True, it may be said that the child inherited the germs. For that matter, he may inherit many kinds of germs, but germs are not dis-ease. He may have inherited the diathesis, but that is not dis-ease. Without the subluxations that lower his tissue resistance in that particular respect, he will never have the dis-ease which is said to be inherited.

Review Questions for Articles 202 to 207.

1. Explain Habit.
2. Give the philosophy of the Drug Habit.
3. Explain Medical Habits.
4. Explain Intellectual Adaptation, as is given in Art. 204.
5. Explain Adaptation as related to Survival Value and Evolution.
6. What is the value produced by Adaptation which is transmitted to posterity?
7. What kind of adaptations are inherited by posterity?
8. What is the explanation of Acclimatization?
9. Is dis-ease a value or lack of value?
10. Can a dis-ease be inherited? Why?
11. Explain the inheritance of Diathesis.
12. Is Diathesis a dis-ease?
13. Answer the question in regard to "inheritance" of syphilis, leprosy, etc.

Junior Section

Art. 208. Introduction.

The Junior Textbook consists of the explanation of normality and abnormality and the practical application of principles in analysis. These embrace the study of the meric system, function, abnormal function, dis-ease, pathology, compensatory adaptation, equations, major methods, analysis and etiology.

As a basis for this, the Freshman Textbook explained the normal working of Innate Intelligence in the body and the natural laws, and presented a number of fundamental principles. This was built upon, as a further preparation for Junior work by the Sophomore Textbook, which took up the study of cycles and the condition of matter. It embraced "condition," one of the main factors of major methods.

Art. 209 The Brain. (The Center) (Vol. IX) (Art. 350)

The brain is an organ of nervous tissue located in the cranial cavity.

It is used by Innate as the headquarters of control.

It is the central point for coordination.

It is the "clearing house" for the operation of the Law of Demand and Supply.

All the mental force transmitted to tissue cells is sent from the brain. There are no substations or tributary brains, as ganglia. The brain is the one mathematically absolute place from which Innate governs the body and coordinates all its actions. A body with subsidiary brains, supposing that such a one existed, could not have perfect coordination, for while the subdivisions might have harmony within themselves, they would be cut partially off from the one unitary management, which is the only way for one hundred per cent management as regards the whole body. All nations recognize this fact, for in times of stress, as in war, the management is put into the hands of one person in order to obtain perfect coordination. In the United States, the President becomes Commander-in-Chief, in time of war. Subsidiary brains, or more than one point of control, make for more individuality of parts. More individuality means less cooperation, less mutuality. It is a law that shows itself in the character of people and in nations. In order to have perfect coordination which is perfect cooperation of parts to make a perfect organization, one manager must have all the reins in hand and control from one point, every detail of function. Of course the manager must be perfect if this great natural principle is to apply to a nation, a community, or a body. Such control is not thought to be best for nations, except in time of war; not because the principle is bad, but because the human managers may be. In the body, though, there is not this difficulty, for Innate is a perfect manager and is always virtuous. She controls from one point—the brain. There is no question whether there is a good, bad or indifferent manager of the body. Innate is always one hundred per cent quality—perfect. (Prin. 9, 27)

Art. 210. INNATE BRAIN. (Universal Diagram, Fig. 4. Art. 38)

That part of the brain used by Innate as an organ, in which to assemble universal forces into foruns.

It is supplied with mental impulses directly from Innate Intelligence, whose headquarters it is.

For that reason it is a vital spot and cannot be dis-eased (317, V)

Its existence is actual but its location is theoretical.

There is no transmission of mental impulses from Innate Intelligence to Innate brain. There is no necessity for it,

Innate being right there. Therefore, it always has one hundred per cent mental impulses. This being true, it has perfect function, perfect metabolism, and never has incoordination. It does not assimilate poisons from the serous stream, which other tissues with less than perfect supply of mental impulses do, when they depend upon imperfect transmission. It can of course be damaged by trauma as any other tissue. A virulent poison can penetrate it, in spite of its resistance. If it is damaged by trauma, is poisoned, is subject to anemia—lack of blood and nutriment, death speedily ensues, for it will not endure dis-ease or injury. Although Innate's management is nothing short of miraculous, she is after all, limited in what she can do, on account of the limitations of matter. (Prin. 5, 24)

Review Questions for Articles 208 to 210, inclusive.

1. What is the nature of the studies in Junior work?
2. What is the brain, anatomically?
3. What is the brain, philosophically?
4. What is the necessity of having one central management in such an organism as the human body?
5. According to the principles stated in Art. 208 why is the human organism superior to the grass in your lawn or to a jellyfish?
6. What is Innate Brain, philosophically?
7. Can Innate brain be located exactly, anatomically?
8. Why is Innate Brain a vital spot?
9. How does Innate Brain get its mental impulses?
10. In what manner do the cells of Innate Brain take their nutrition and why?

Art. 211. Educated Brain. (See Universal Diagram, Fig. 4. Art. 38)

That part of the brain used by Innate as an organ for reason, memory, education, and the so-called voluntary functions.

The seat of Educated Mind.

It is supplied with mental impulses over nerves as other tissues are.

It is liable to incoordination as any other tissue; it is not a vital spot.

Its existence is actual but its location is theoretical.

It is the chief organ of adaptation to environmental conditions.

The educated brain is an organ used by Innate for a certain purpose just as the liver and stomach are organs used for certain purposes. We must not let the fact that it is an organ confuse us, though it is made of nervous tissue and happens to be located within the cranial cavity. We must never conceive of it as a Power which can create thoughts or as a Thing that can govern the body. It is merely a piece of flesh, and therefore matter. Matter does not create force—it only expresses it. It is only the physicists who believe that by the clashing of its atoms, physically and chemically, thoughts are born of it. Like many other organs of the body, the liver for example, it has multiple purposes. It is used by Innate, by virtue of experience and training stored within it, as an organ to so "tincture" impulses that they are *consciously* guided—called voluntary functions. It is used by Innate to receive percepts concerning the environment of the body, obtained by her able scouts, the Five Senses. The constant comparison of these percepts with former percepts and with each other, enables Innate to avoid actual or threatened dangers and to guard the body for its comfort and welfare. The Educated Brain used by Innate to store away percepts, by a physiological change in its structure, and the accumulation of stored percepts is what makes education. At birth it is a "clean slate" for Innate to record experiences upon. (See philosophy of Education in the Senior Text)

Art. 212. The Spinal Cord.

The Spinal Cord is a bundle of nerve axons which is used by Innate as a main cable to conduct mental forces from and to the brain.

Within the spinal cord are axons which supply every tissue cell in the body.

The spinal cord is the main conduit from the brain to the peripheral nerves. Its branches, the spinal nerves, emit through the intervertebral foramina and ramify to all parts of the body. While some tissue cells have nerve supply that does not pass through the spinal cord, yet **the coordinative action of all cells is dependent upon impulses which must arrive via the spinal cord.** This is accounted for by the fact that all tissues are subject to incoordination, if the spinal nerves or the cord are impinged—a clinical finding.

Art. 213. Spinal Nerves.

Spinal nerves are the branches from the spinal cord which leave the neural canal by way of the intervertebral foramina in pairs.

Each segment of the spinal column has a pair of nerves superior to it.

There are thirty-one pairs of spinal nerves.

There are both efferent and afferent nerve axons in each spinal nerve.

Each pair is said, arbitrarily, to belong to the vertebra below it.

A nerve is a bundle or group of nerve axons or axis-cylinders. An axon is a very minute filament or branch of a nerve-tissue cell which transmits the impulse to the Tissue Cell. When a nerve is "impinged," it means that one or more of the axons is impinged and there is interference with transmission in the nerve, not the whole nerve necessarily, but in one or more axons. A nerve may be considered as something like a conduit filled with electric wires — much like the lead cables we see strung overhead in the cities, or the iron pipes that lead from a central point or the meter, conduct electric wires all over the building. A more complete description of nerves is given in Senior work. (See Fig. 34)

Art. 214. The Periphery.

Periphery is the term used to indicate the tissues at the ends of efferent nerves (Axons); or at the beginning of afferent nerves (dendrites).

The tissues which are supplied with mental impulses.

Nerve tissue itself may be periphery.

The brain is the central nervous system; the spinal cord, spinal nerves, cranial nerves, and the visceral nerves are the systems of distribution; and the tissues supplied are the periphery. This might be called the Physical Triunity. It is the physical representation of "Brain Cell" and "Tissue Cell" and the "Link" between them as spoken of in Freshman work.

The spinal nerves divide into superficial and deep branches. (Note—This refers to division of conduits; of whole nerves, not axons.) The superficial branches divide and supply the superficial tissues. The branches supply the deeper tissues and there are branches of the latter which communicate with the visceral system, which supply the viscera of the trunk and head. Thus we see that all parts of the body are supplied with mental impulses by certain nerves and their branches from the spinal column; each pair of spinal nerves has a definite division to supply.

Art. 215. The Inferior Meric System.

The Inferior Meric System is a system of dividing all the periphery of the body into zones according to distribution from the spinal column.

It is used for clinical purposes to trace from effect to cause or from cause to effects. Theoretically, we trace from cause to effect; and clinically, we trace from effect to cause.

The division is exact but varies with each individual.

Its divisions are Zones and Meres.

There are just as many zones as there are pairs of spinal nerves, that is, thirty-one.

There are thirty-one pairs of spinal nerves; seven cervical, twelve dorsal, five lumbar, five sacral and two coccygeal. However, since the five segments of the sacrum are immovable (in relation to each other) the five pairs are usually classed as one group. The zones are numbered from above downward from one to thirty-one, or from one to twenty-six according to the way the sacral and coccygeal nerves are classed. Thus, the zone supplied by the pair of nerves belonging to seventh dorsal vertebra is called the Fourteenth Zone. Its number is obtained by adding the seven cervicals to the seven dorsals counted.

Think of the body as being divided into horizontal sections or bands or zones; or in slices as a cucumber is sliced. Then think of each of these slices of the body as having a double nerve (pair of nerves) supplying its every particle. So far, this is only analogical and not realistic. To make it realistic, visualize the segments as overlapping or rather as being well blended; a segment running into or merging with its neighbors but still retaining its identity and still with its own nerve supply. If slicing is a "system of division" so the identification of parts by nerve supply is no less a system of division. The customers of Jones, the grocer, do not have to live in a different part of the city from the customers of Smith the grocer; they can intermingle freely and still retain identity of supply.

This division of the body is not theoretical; it is actual. By this system we are able to know quite certainly which nerves are impinged by knowing the anatomical nerve supply of organs. Hence which foramina, approximately, to examine for impingements, therefrom find which subluxations to adjust. If the nerve itself is incoordinated and shows strong symptoms of it, the task is very much easier. In such cases nerve tracing and taut fibers show us which neuromere is affected.

Review Questions for Articles 211 to 215, inclusive.

1. What is Educated Brain, philosophically.
2. Why is it not a vital spot?
3. How does Educated Brain get its mental impulses?
4. Why are organisms with good educated brains superior to other organisms with educated brains not so well developed?
5. Can Educated Brain rule the body?
6. What is the spinal cord, anatomically?
7. What relation does the spinal cord have to the functional coordinating of the body?
8. What are spinal nerves, anatomically?
9. How are the spinal nerves classified and named in Chiropractic.
10. When impingement occurs are all the axons affected, necessarily?
11. Anatomically, is a nerve one axon or a bundle of axons?
12. What is Periphery?
13. What nerve tissue, only, is not periphery?
14. Is the nerve tissue mentioned in Quest. 13, periphery (as to supply from the blood stream or Serous Circulation)?
15. What is the Inferior Meric System?
16. Is the Inferior Meric System an anatomical division?
17. What is the method of division in the Inferior Meric System?

Art. 216. Zones.

A Zone is a vertebra, the pair of nerves superior to it and all the tissues supplied by those nerves.

A Zone is a section of the body determined by a pair of spinal nerves.

The zones overlap or merge, for the branches of different spinal nerves intermingle.

An organ may be in different zones.

A tissue cell can be in only one zone, for it is a specific unit with a specific nerve supply.

Zoning is a classification of tissues according to anatomical nerve supply and not according to kind. While location does coincide with this division in a general way, location of tissue cells in the body have nothing to do with zone division. Every zone has within it, every kind of tissue. There are tissue cells belonging to other zones among them or near them. Each of the tissue cells is definitely in one zone or another and never is in two or more zones. This is because, anatomically, it has its definite nerve supply from a certain spinal nerve.

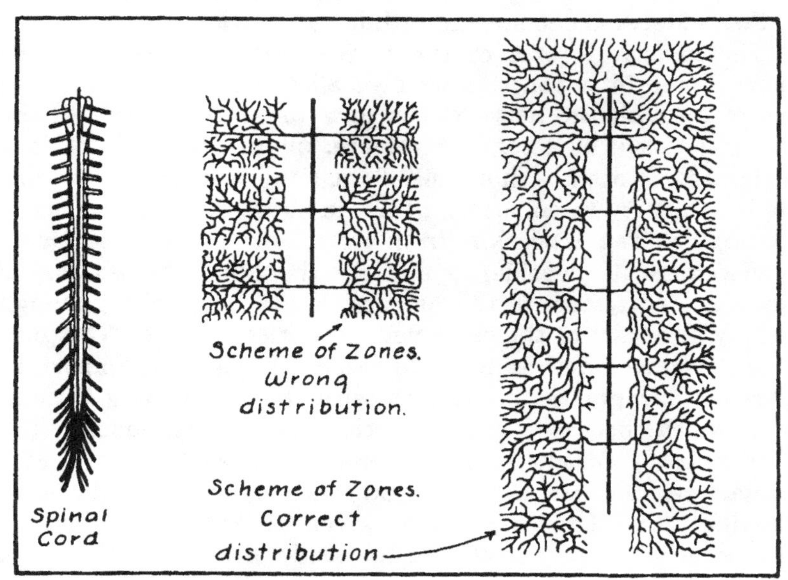

Fig. 25.

In general, these zones are horizontal or oblique belts of division, though they overlap, they have their more concentrated portions wherein there are comparatively few cells belonging to other zones. Thus the zone is a more apparent division at that place. The zoning of the body according to nerve supply has a clinic value in making analysis, enabling the chiropractor to trace from effects to causes with fair certainty.

Art. 217. Mere. (342, Vol. II) (220, Vol. XV)

A Mere is all of any one kind of tissue in a zone.

A Mere is a subdivision of a zone determined by kind of tissue.

A zone has as many special functions as there are meres in it.

Some Meres are named according to function.

The names of some of the meres are: osseomere, all the bone tissue in a zone; myomere, all the muscle in a zone; neuromere, all the nerve tissue in a zone; viscemere, all the visceral tissue in a zone; deramere, all the integument in a zone. If one needs a more specific naming of meres than this, he is at liberty to do so; as, in the integument if he wishes to distinguish the true skin from its underlying tissues, or in a viscemere, to consider separately the other tissues in the viscera. **Vertemere** is the name given to a vertebra, though it may be a part of the osseomere in the same zone. This one, then, is named according to function. It plays an important part in Chiropractic, because it, with its surrounding tissues, is so much concerned in subluxations and adjustments. (See Senior Text) Olfamere, gustamere, audimere, optimere, etc., pertain respectively, to the special sense organs of smell, taste, hearing, etc. They are names given according to function. All meres are closely related to the study of Primary Function.

Art. 218. Anatomical Study of the Zones.

The study of the individual zones is anatomical and the student is referred to Orthopedy, Vol. XV. by Craven, for this work and to Vol. II by Palmer. However, in order to show what such study is, we give an example:

THE FIRST ZONE CONTAINS:

The First Neuromere, which supplies all the tissues of the First Zone.

The Osseomere, which consists of the eight cranial bones, the atlas, and the ossicles of the ear.

The Viscemere, of this zone is the brain.

The Dermamere, is the integument of the scalp, the upper ear, and the upper forehead.

The Myomere, is all the muscles which are covered by the dermamere.

The Vertemere is the atlas, although this is not always the vertebra which, when subluxated, affects the above meres most.

Art. 219. Description of the Generic Table.

The Generic Table is a tabulated listing of tissues according to their anatomical nerve supply from the spinal column, together with the names and symbols of the "places" in the spinal column.

They are the "places" on the patient's back where subluxations may be found which affect given tissues. This table was compiled according to the results of adjustments or clinical findings, and the Meric System. It is accurate anatomically, but later developments proved that while it is a good Meric Table it is too limited for a Generic Table. Note:—A detailed study of the Meric System is to be found in Vol. II, page 342 and Vol. XV, page 220.

The letter Names of the table are as follows:

At. P.	= Atlas place.	A. P.	= Arm place.
Ax. P.	= Axis place.	H. P.	= Heart place.
M. C. P.	= Middle cervical place.	Lu. P.	= Lung place.
L. C. P.	= Lower cervical place.	Li. P.	= Liver place.
V. P.	= Vertebra Prominens.	C. P.	= Center place.
U. P.P.	= Upper lumbar place.	S. P.	= Stomach place.
M. P. P.	= Middle lumbar place.	Pan. P.	= Pancreas place.
L. P. P.	= Lower lumbar place.	Spl. P.	= Spleen place.
Sac. P.	= Sacrum place.	U. K. P.	= Upper Kidney place.
Cc. P.	= Coccyx place.	K. P.	= Kidney place.

The classifications in the following Generic Table are according to anatomical nerve supply, verified by clinical findings and nerve tracing. They, however, are based upon nerve supply *after the nerves have emitted from the neural canal,* therefore does not show the possibilities of cord tension, or any of the multiple pressures.

Art. 220. THE GENERIC TABLE.

Generic Title	Vert.	Zone	Anat. ratio of weakness	Clinic ratio of weakness	Tissues involved. *All zones blend with their neighbors, therefore an organ is not squarely in any one "place."*
At. P.	1c	1st	6th	2nd	Brain, optic tract to commis., 8 cranial bones, scalp, atlas, upper ear, ossicles, upper forehead.
Ax. P.	2c	2nd			Blends with 1st zone; brain, portion of face, back of neck.
M.C.P.	3c 4c 5c	3rd 4th 5th	1st	4th	Trifacial nerve, nasal passages, retina, teeth, cheeks, optic nerve (ant. to chiasm) cornea, 14 bones of face, mouth, gums, tis. of face, nasal pharynx, post. nares, eustac. tube, jaw, outer ear, hyoid bone, eye, nose, face, post. & lat. neck musc.
L. C. P.	5c 6c	5th 6th			Larynx and adjacent tis., lower part of neck & shoulders, thyroid gland, post. of mouth, palate, tonsils, voc. cords, reg. of sterno-mastoid, ant. of arm, sup.. bronchii, post. neck musc., upper part of arm, deltoid musc. trachia, radius.
V. P.	6c 7c 1d 2d	The spinous process of one of these vertebrae is more prominent than the others. When the head is in its normal upright position the *vertebra prominens* is the most prominent ' bump." It is used as a landmark for counting in prone palpation after having been carefully established by analysis. It should never be adjusted unless it is subluxated.			
A. P	6c 7c 1d 2d	6th 7th 8th 9th			Shoulder, arm musc., humerous, bronchii, scapula, clavicle, manubrium, 1st rib. ulna, carpal metacarpal.
H. P.	1d 2d 3d	8th 9th 10th			Heart, pericardium, aorta, lower arm, hand, bronchii, radius, ulnar, carpal, metacarpal, 2nd rib.
Lu P	2d 3d 4d	9th 10th 11th			Lungs, pleura, lower heart, ribs, lower sternum, breast, nipples, chest.
Li P	3d 4d 5d	10th 11th 12th			Liver, gall bladder, bile ducts, 4th ribs, lower part of lungs.

Art. 220. THE GENERIC TABLE—Continued.

Generic Title	Vert.	Zone	Anat. ratio of weak-ness	Clinic ratio of weak-ness	Tissues Involved. *All zones blend with their neighbors, therefore an organ is not squarely in any one "place."*
C. P	4d 5d 6d	11th 12th 13th	4th	3rd	General heat mere, brain, spi. cord, nerves, fifth ribs.
S. P	5d 6d 7d 8d	12th 13th 14th 15th			Stomach, esophagus, pharynx, omentum, uvala, tonsils, palate, tongue (dorsum ant.) mouth glands, stomach glands, 7th ribs, eyeballs, iris, pupils, cornea, salivary glands, muc. membrane of mouth and stomach, and many other tissues.
Pan. P.	7d 8d	14th 15th			Pancreas, upper spleen, duodenum, omentum, 8th ribs.
Spl. P.	8d 9d 10d	15th 16th 17th			Spleen, duodenum, omentum, pancreas, 9th ribs
U. K.P.	9d 10d	16th			Supra renals, kidneys, eyes, 10th ribs.
K. P	10d 11d 12d 1l	17th 18th 19th 20th	2nd	1st	Kidneys, supra renals, ureters, serous circulation, end of spinal cord, 11th & 12th ribs, eyes.
U. P P.	1l 2l	20th 21st			Upper small intes., peritoneum, loins, ureters, leg musc., verm. appendix, ovaries, caecum.
M.P.P.	2l 3l 4l	21st 22nd 23rd	5th	5th	Sex. organs, bladder, lower small intes., appendix, caecum, colons, abdominal musc., ant. thigh, knee, broad lig.
L. P. P.	4l 5l Sac.	23rd 24th 25th			Large intest., post. thigh, legs, feet, leg bones pelvis, colons, bladder, uterus, sex organs, urinary tract, prostate gland.
Sac. P	Sac.	25th			Rectum, bladder, urinary tract, uterus, buttocks pelvic organs, lower abdominal organs, legs and feet.
Cc. P.	Cocc.	26th	3rd	6th	Rectum, anus, urinary tract, pelvic organs., prostate gland, buttocks, cord tensions.

Art. 221. THE MODERN GENERIC TABLE.

This table is the result of amplification by the study of modern anatomy, (Gray, 1924). This table is extended still more by multiple pressures, in which a major for any part of the body is liable to be found anywhere in the spine, particularly in the cervical region.

Cervical Place: 1, 2, 3, 4, 5, 6, 7 Cervicals and 1st dorsal.

By Superficial System, to tissues of the head, neck, shoulders, ribs, arm, etc.

By Visceral System, to tissues of cranial viscera, cranial nerves, Special Sense organs of head, viscera of neck, thorax, abdomen and pelvic cavity.

By Cord and Multiple pressures to any part of the body.

Thoracic Place: 2, 3, 4, 5, dorsals.

By Superficial System, to arms, hands, shoulders, neck, chest, breast, walls of thorax, etc.

By Visceral System, the heart, lungs, bronchi, trachea, larynx, etc., via Cranial Nerves, esophagus, stomach, kidneys, spinal cord, cranial viscera, mouth, eyes, ears, head and neck glands.

By Post. Ganglionic, vasomotor and skin of cranium, head and neck, arms, hands, etc.

By Cord and Multiple pressures, any part of the body.

Abdominal Place: 6, 7, 8, 9, 10, 11, 12, Dor. and 1st Lumbar.

By Superficial System the walls of abdomen lower ribs, abdominal and back muscles (lower.)

By Visceral System, viscera of abdomen, as, stomach, pancreas, blood-cells, liver, spleen, suprarenals, small and large intestines, etc.

By Post. Ganglionic, the vasomotor and skin of trunk.

By Cord and multiple pressures, any part of the body.

Mesenteric Place: 2, 3, 4, Lumbar.

By Superficial System, walls of abdomen, lower ribs, abdominal and back muscles, etc.

By Visceral System, Large intestine, rectum, kidneys, bladder, sex organs and external genitalia.

By Post, Ganglionic, vasomotor of trunk, and lower limbs.

By Cord and multiple pressures, any part of the body.

Sacral Place: 5 lumbar, 1, 2, Sac. segments.

By Superficial System, lower limbs and superficial tissues and walls of pelvis, and hips.

Pelvic Place: 3, 4, 5, sacral segments.

By the Great Pelvic Nerve, large intestine, rectum, kidneys, bladder, sex organs, and external genitalia.

Coccyx Place, by local nerves, superficial tissues of the region.

By Cord Tension, and Multiple Pressures any part of the body.

This table may be difficult for Juniors if they have not studied neurology but will be no trouble for Seniors. However it is preferable to put it in this place because the subject of generic tables is not repeated in Senior work.

Art. 222. The Superior Meric System.

The Superior Meric System is a theoretical division of the Educated Brain into zones which correspond to the Inferior Meric Zones, showing the clinical relationship between them.

The zones number from the supraorbital ridge from before backward to the foramen magnum.

When there is incoordination in an inferior zone, there is always an associated discomfort in the corresponding superior zone.

This discomfort may amount to a headache.

The associated discomfort is a conscious sensation, in the same way that pain is. Therefore the division is of the educated brain. Since the location of the educated brain is theoretical (Art. 211) likewise the division will be theoretical. The administration centers of Innate brain do not suffer discomfort, (Art. 43) though Innate will be cognizant of the trouble which is in the inferior zone. However, she makes this known consciously in educated mind, so that we know pain or headache. In pain we are conscious of discomfort in the inferior zone; in headaches we are conscious of pain in the superior meric zone.

Whether "the associated discomfort amounts to a headache" or not, depends a great deal upon the temperament of the individual. To some it would be a mere dull feeling, logginess or "chuffiness." To others the same condition would be the source of much complaint.

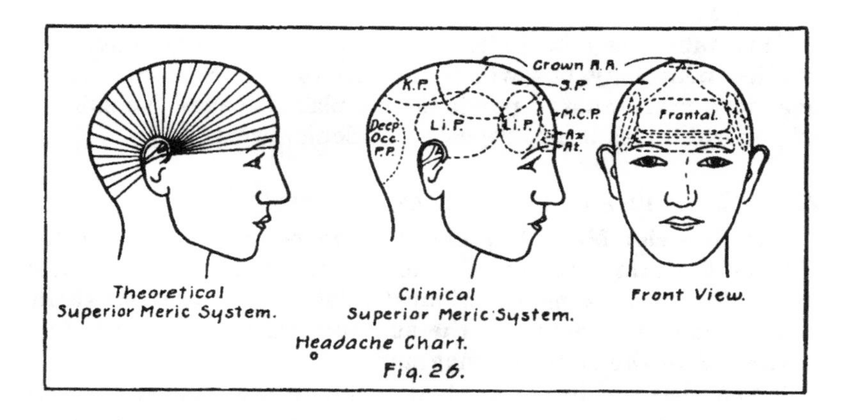

Headache Chart.
Fig. 26.

The only tissues concerned in the Superior Meric System is brain tissue; even that is in the inferior system, so far as metabolism is concerned—its material aspect. In no case is any other tissues of the head concerned in true headache, though they may be in false headaches, (See Art. 223).

In the theoretical division the head is visualized as sliced into zones or segments from the periphery of the skull to the ears. (See Fig. 26.) These segments are numbered with the numbers corresponding to those of the inferior zones. Clinical findings show that these areas are closely approximate.

Art. 223. The Clinical Division of the Superior Meric System. (Headaches.)

The Clinical Division of the Superior Meric System is the location of actual (not theoretical) areas according to clinical findings.

True headaches are in the brain.

False headaches are in other tissues of the head.

Direct headaches are parts of educated brain suffering incoordination, because it, itself, is the incoordinated periphery.

Indirect headaches are the ones associated with incoordinated inferior zones; namely, true and false.

All parts of the head, including the educated brain as tissues, are in the inferior meric system; that is, in the periphery.

The Superior Meric System is but a functional consideration. (Art. 114)

Headaches.	Direct.	Not associated with, but is the inferior zone which is suffering incoordination.
	Indirect.	True: in tissue of educated brain.
		False: in other tissues than the brain.

When a part of the brain is suffering incoordination as periphery, another part will be in discomfort because of it, as an axis subluxation may cause a frontal headache and an occipital headache at the same time.

Art. 224. Efferent Nerves.

The route from brain cell to tissue cell.

The path of nerve axons from brain cell to tissue cell.

Efferent nerves, anatomically, are bundles of histological axons of neurons which lead out from the brain. They leave the cranial vault by various foramina. Most of the cranial nerves leave by small openings in the cranium, but the spinal cord makes its exit by way of the foramen magnum. The efferent nerves have their cells arranged so that their axons extend from the cell body toward the periphery. The nerves are bundles of axons enclosed within the nerve sheath. Philosophically, when we say Efferent Nerves we do not mean, necessarily, the whole nerve, as in anatomical language, but the route of mental force from brain to tissue. In many cases this may concern a single axon or a chain of axons. The nerve, anatomically, branches and re-branches so as to supply the tissues of its territory. (See Senior Text.)

Art. 225. Afferent Nerves.

The route from tissue cell to brain cell.

The path of nerve axons from tissue cell to brain cell. (If it is a sensory nerve under consideration.)

Sensory nerves are the afferent nerves from the special sense organs.

In the Normal Complete Cycle the Afferent Nerve is theoretical.

In the Normal Complete Cycle the afferent mental current, (Impressions) suffers no interference with transmission.

Afferent Nerves, anatomically, are bundles of histological axons of neurons which lead from the tissues to the brain. They enter the cranial vault by various foramina. Most of the cranial Afferent nerves enter by small openings in the cranium, such as, the sphenoidal fissure, foramen rotundum, optic foramen, etc. The spinal cord, which contains afferent axons, enters by the foramen magnum. The Afferent nerves have their cells arranged so that their axons extend from the cell body away from the Periphery to the Center. These Afferent nerves, like the Efferent, are composed of axons ensheathed, the nerve being like a conduit. When we speak of Afferent Nerve, philosophically, however, we do not mean this anatomical conduit nor especially the histological chain of neurons with their connecting branches, but the route from Periphery to Center. (See Senior Text)

Review Questions for Articles 216 to 225.

1. State the definition of Zone.
2. Are the Zones clearly separated or do they merge?
3. What is the method of zoning?
4. For what purpose are zones used in Chiropractic?
5. Give the definition of Mere?
6. Name some of the tissue Meres.
7. Name some of the functional Meres.
8. What functional Mere is very important in the study of Chiropractic Art or Technic?
9. What is the Generic Table?
10. For what purpose is the Generic Table used?
11. How does the Modern Generic Table differ from the old one?
12. For what purpose is the Superior Meric System used?
13. Be able to draw the headache chart.
14. What is the Superior Meric System?
15. What are Efferent Nerves, anatomically?
16. What are Efferent Nerves, philosophically?
17. What are Afferent Nerves, anatomically?
18. What are Afferent Nerves, philosophically?

Art. 226. Sensory Nerves.

Sensory Nerves are afferent nerves leading from the Special Sense Organs to the brain.

The function is Sensory and this is a conscious (educated) function.

Their dendrites have special construction as receptors of environmental vibrations.

Most of the special senses have cranial nerves as their Sensory Nerves. (See Figs. 12 and 13.)

A study of these diagrams will show that a special sense organ must always be periphery in the Normal Complete Cycle. The special Sense Cycle is a special cycle concerning a subject entirely different from that of the Normal Complete Cycle. The impressions from the special sense organs are concerning an entirely different set of circumstances than the impressions from the same organ via the afferent side of the Normal Complete Cycle (See Fig. 27). That the afferent sides of both cycles use the Sensory Nerve is not likely, for Special Sense can suffer interference and General Sense cannot. The current of the General Sense impressions seems to be the more intimate property of Innate, as the Innate Brain is.

The impressions from sensory organs reach Innate Brain in any case, whether we are asleep or awake. The educated brain is only the recording place of percepts. If this were not true, we could not be awakened by noise or any other circumstance that affects the special senses. Educated mind sleeps; Innate mind never does. (See Senior Text)

Art. 227. Special Sense. (See Chiropractic Physiology)

Special Sense is the functioning of the special sense organs; namely, optic organ, olfactory organ, gustatory organ, auditory organ and the organ of feeling.

Special Sense is Sensory Function, one of the Nine Primary Functions.

There are Five Special Senses, namely, sight, smell, taste, hearing and feeling.

There are several kinds of Feeling, namely, touch, pressure, heat, cold and muscular.

Art. 228. Some Other Special Senses.

The Sense of Equilibrium is that which enables a person to sense bodily position and balance.

The Sense of Orientation is the sense of direction and location.

There are thought to be other special senses, which are very latent or rudimentary. (See Chiropractic Physiology.)

Art. 229. General Sense. (Art. 242, 244.)

General Sense is information which Innate receives over the afferent half of the Normal Complete Cycle.

Normally, they are the indications of normal needs of the tis-

sue cells; such as, hunger, thirst, comfort, satisfaction, pleasure, etc.

They are made known educationally through the Interbrain Cycle. (See Fig. 13.)

Pain, itching, and the like are educated consciousness of abnormalities in the periphery, via the Interbrain Cycle and the Normal Complete Cycle.

Pain, itching, etc., are not special senses, Chiropractically.

Art. 230. Organization.

An organization is an assemblage of ideas, principles, or material, in which each part has an office to fulfill in the maintenance of the whole unit.

The human body is a very close organization with definite centralization at the brain.

Every tissue cell and organ has an office to fulfill as a part of the organization.

Therefore every part must render to the whole unit a necessary service. (Prin. 19, 21.)

Let us consult Webster for the definition of *organize*: "To analyze or constitute in interdependent parts, each having a special function, act, office, or relation with respect to the whole; to svstematize; to get into working order." (Webster.)

We know from this definition that an organism is the logical result of *organize*, or creation. An organism consists of interdependent parts. An independent part could not be a true part of the organism, but would be something not needed or wanted there—foreign material. All the parts have common needs, common supply of these needs, common interests, common mission in the Universe, and common justification for existing at all. Therefore, each part has a duty to perform in the organism, (a function) which is for the common good of all the parts. Examination of the definition again, shows us that our reasoning is correct, "Each having a special function, act, office, or relation with respect to the whole—" These duties are not haphazard, or just what the part happened to be or do; it is something the organization (or organism) needs or it would not have been incorporated. Its presence in the organization, normally, is its justification for existence, for it is to produce something or do something for the benefit of the whole. Again the definition bears us out; "to systematize; to get into working order." Then, there is a great principle that accounts for the existence of this creation which has been created (organized) and that principle is system. Now we know by reasoning and examination of many definitions, that system can be nothing less than a process of intelligence, (just as selection in the Signs of Life is a process of intelligence). Therefore there is intelligence throughout the organism, and each part has an amount proportional to its state of organization. Then what is Innate Intelligence? Scientifically, it is the Law of Organization. (This is by no means a view of the physicists but is squarely in Chiropractic.)

Review Questions for Articles 226 to 230, inclusive.

1. What are Sensory Nerves?
2. Does the Special Sense Cycle work while we sleep?
3. What is Special Sense?
4. What Primary Function is Special Sense?
5. Name the different kinds of Feeling.
6. Name some Special Senses not named in the usual list.
7. What is General Sense?
8. Name some normal General Senses.
9. Name some abnormal General Senses.
10. Why are we educationally conscious of abnormal General Sense sometimes?
11. Differentiate between General Sense and Special Sense.
12. What is an organization?
13. In an organization, what is the relation of a part to the whole?
14. Is anything truly a part of an organization unless it is serving it?

Art. 231. Coordination. (Prin. 32)

Coordination is the perfect harmonious action of all parts of the body in fulfilling their purposes, so that all parts will be benefitted by the united efforts.

It is the perfect operation of the Law of Demand and Supply. (Prin. 33)

It is the perfect cooperation of organs for mutual caretaking and benefit.

It is called health because every tissue cell is sound when the organization takes care of it.

It is necessary by this time, that the student should at least begin to understand why Chiropractic uses the term *incoordination* instead of *disease* for sickness. If he thinks of sickness as incoordination, then everything said about Chiropractic will appear more clear, logical and reasonable. To understand the Principle, Coordination, is to possess the key to most difficult questions of Chiropractic study; for instance, "excess function" which we shall soon meet. (See Art. 85, Freshman Text)

Art. 232. Function and Functioning.

Function is the office or purpose of anything in the Universe.

Functioning is the fulfillment of that purpose.

"Office, duty, calling, operation or the like. The normal and special action of any organ or part of a living animal or plant; as, the function of the heart or limbs; the function of the leaves." (Webster)

As a member of an organism any part of that organism has an office, duty or purpose to fulfill. That is its justification for existence, and normally, for its presence in the organism. It is not properly a part of the organism unless it is, when called upon, fulfilling its purpose. Every tissue cell, as the unit organ, has one or more functions. It may not be an active unit (as a muscle cell) but a passive unit (as a bone cell) yet be an important part of the function, else it would not be there. When this cell is fulfilling its purpose whether active or passive, it is functioning. The products of its function, whether material (as a secretion) or immaterial (as motion or support) is the service desired in the body by the Law of Demand and Supply.

Art. 233. Innate's Function. (Prin. 23)

Innate's function or purpose is to assemble or adapt universal matter and forces for use in the body.

To create adaptative forces for use in the body.

As everything in the universe has a purpose, so has Innate. There is only one justification for the existence of an Innate Intelligence, and that is an aggregation of units of matter, which are to be put into organized form and kept in that condition. To adapt continually is the only way to do this. Whereever there is organization, there is need for adaptation; whereever there is adaptation, there is necessity for an Innate Intelligence.

Art. 234. The Function of a Body.

The function of a body is to serve as a unit of organic matter to complete the scheme of universal existence. (See Universal Cycle, Art. 398)

As everything in the universe has a purpose so has the unit of matter called the body. It is not for the finite educated mind to say just what the purpose of man is, except in a general way, as above. In an economical or political way, a human is a unit of a nation or of some other organization. As the units grow more specific, so does the function being studied, become more specific.

Art. 235. The Function of an Organ.

The function of an organ is to serve a purpose or to perform an active service for the good and welfare of the whole organism; that is why it is called *organ*.

The function of any anatomical part of the body is to serve the whole body cooperatively.

An organ is an instrument used by Innate to do a certain class of work for the whole body, coordinately.

Review Questions for Articles 231 to 235.

1. What is coordination in anything?
2. What is coordination in the body?
3. State Principle No. 33.
4. What is function?
5. What is functioning?
6. When a part of an organization is acting, but the action is not service to the organization, is that action function?
7. When a thing is present in an organization but is not serving it, has it function?
8. What is the name of foreign materials in the body, which do not in any way serve it?
9. What is the name of foreign forces in the body, which do not in any way serve it?
10. Why is function the same as cooperative service?
11. What is Innate's function in the body?
12. What is Innate's justification for existence?
13. What is the function of a body?
14. What is the function of man as a unit?
15. What is the function of an organ as a unit?
16. When an organ is considered as a functioning unit, what is the larger unit which it serves?

Art. 236. The Function of a Tissue Cell.

The function of a tissue cell, which is the smallest organ in the body, is to give service to all the rest of the parts, for the welfare of the whole body.

The cell is the smallest definite part of the body and therefore is the smallest organ. It is, within itself, a definite unit like the whole body itself. The parts of a cell are the cell's organs, as the parts of the cell functioning for its benefit, are not functions of the whole body, directly, but are functions for the tissue cell's body. The manifestations of these we call signs of life. The service that each cell renders to the whole body is called Primary Function, and of course the manifestation of these, in general are signs of life, though we seldom use that application.

The cell is a very highly specialized instrument to be used by Innate for a particular kind of work. Its structure and location is always according to the kind of work it is required to do. Each tissue cell may be used for more than one kind of work, but the purpose it serves normally is always service of function. Not all tissue cells are mechanically active in fulfilling their offices; as, bone cells, cells of ligaments, etc.

All cells are in a state of vibratory motion, expressing the energy which is in them. These energies are universal forces which are in all matter. (Prin. 1) It is without specifying, universal function and therefore universal life. This universal life has none of the characteristics of organic life; but while in the body, if the body is normal it is adapted, and therefore becomes organic life. (Prin. 1, 14) When these universal forces are adapted and governed by Innate, being used to produce service for the body, they become functioning forces; when they act without the control of Innate they are not functioning, but are the forces which produce, what is called for convenience, "excess or minus function." (Prin. 23) (Arts. 262 and 263.)

The unclassified services that tissue cells render the body are called General Functions; when the services are classified, they are called Primary Functions.

Art. 237. THE FUNCTION OF EPITHELIAL TISSUE.

The function of epithelial cells depends upon their location and what is required of them by Innate.

The variations in their structure are according to the kind

of work required of them. In glands it is secretory; in integument, protective; in ducts and tubes it serves as lining; and the ciliated kind has motor function. In the parenchyma of active organs, as viscera, it has active function; as parts of protective or supporting organs, its function may be passive. Active or passive it renders a service to the other cells.

Universal function gives to it energies for dynamic purposes, and for strength where strength is required. (Prin. 16) Each cell has a nucleus which represents the centralization of its own intellectuality; and it has adaptability to respond to the urges of the Law of Demand and Supply, which are called mental impulses. (See Fig. 9)

Art. 238. The Function of Connective Tissue.

The functions of connective tissue depend upon its location and kind and what is required of it by Innate Intelligence.

The variations in its structure are according to what is required of it. Its most common function is support, that is Connective Function. Its function is mainly passive. As parts of active organs, indirectly, it has active functions. Active or passive, its function is to give service to all other tissues of the organization.

When not particularly classified into Primary Functions, its service is called General Function and is always Connective. Universal Function gives its molecules energies and cohesion for strength. Each cell has a nucleus which represents the centralization of its own intellectuality; and it has adaptability to respond to the urges of the Law of Demand and Supply, which are called Mental Impulses.

Art. 239. The Function of Muscle Tissue.

The function of muscle tissue is motor.

Its purpose is to deliver mechanical service to the body or its parts.

Its function is always active. It may, as parts of larger organs, be said to have other primary functions. When not especially classified into primary functions, its service is called General Function. Universal Function gives to it dynamic energies for adaptative use in producing motor function, as steam is regulated by the engineer to give an engine motor function.

Each cell has a nucleus which represents the centralization of its own intellectuality; and it has adaptability to respond to the urges of demand and supply which are sent to it from Innate's clearing house. (See Fig. 9)

Art. 240. The Function of Nerve Tissue.

The function of nerve tissue is to transmit mental force.

As the parenchyma of special sense organs, its function is sensory. As the brain, it is mental. Its function is active like that of glandular tissue, but not mechanical as that of muscle tissue.

When not especially classified into Primary Functions, namely, Transmission, its service is called General Function. Universal function gives to it dynamic energies to activate it under the management of Innate and supplies Innate with an inexhaustible source of energy from which to create foruns. Each cell has a nucleus which represents the centralization of its own intellectuality, and it has adaptability to respond to the urge of the Law of Demand and Supply, given to it by the "Boss," very analogous to the way of the boss and clerk or messenger in a clearing house. (See Fig. 8)

Review Questions for Articles 236 to 240, inclusive.

1. What is the function, generally, of a tissue cell?
2. Is a tissue cell an organ?
3. What is the name of the service that a tissue cell renders to all the other tissue cells?
4. What are unclassified, generalized services of organs in the body called?

5. When the services of the organs of the body are specifically classified, what are they called?
6. Name some of the functions of epithelium.
7. Name the main functions of connective tissue.
8. When does it have other functions which can be specified?
9. What is the main function of muscle tissue?
10. When does it have other functions which can be specified?
11. What is the main function of nerve tissue?
12. When does it have other functions which can be specified?
13. When the dendrites of nerve tissue cells form the parenchyma of special sense organs, what is its function called then?
14. When it is the parenchyma of the mental organ, what is its function called?
15. Do the cells of the Center require mental impulses?
16. When the functions of the above named primary tissues are not classified specially as Primary Functions what are they called?
17. Where do the primary tissues get their vibratory energy?
18. Do these energies act according to universal law or innate law, while in the normal body?
19. Where does Innate get her supply of universal energies wherewith to balance or adapt the energies mentioned in Quest. 17?
20. Is the cell an organism?
21. What is the purpose of the nucleus of each cell?

Art. 241. Universal Function in the Body.

Universal Function in the body is the vibration of atoms and molecules which gives them continual motion; which cannot be prevented by Innate. It, however, is adapted by Innate for use in function.

Innate adapts them to her uses by balancing, opposing, augmenting, etc., by the application of other universal forces. (Prin. 23)

Adapted, they act as Innate wishes them to and the tissue cells act coordinately. Unadapted, because Innate's control is absent, the cells act as they please, according to the urge of universal forces alone. Action, therefore, is not function unless it serves the body. (Prin. 11)

Universal Function is the expression of Universal Life. (Prin. 14) It is the expression of that energy which Innate

uses to activate active organs and strength for passive organs. In the body of a cell the chemical and physical forces are at work, which must be controlled if their action be coordinative.

Art. 242. General Function in the Body.

General Functions are the unclassified, or non-specialized functions in the body; the general name for coordinative services of all the organs (tissue cells) of the body.

Unless the signs of life are very latent, the protoplasm of all cells is in constant motion. This is the expression of the life within them; evidence that they are really alive and distinguishable from inorganic matter. This, their "response" (see Signs of Life, Freshman Text) is to the forces which greet them from the external. These forces which come to them are either universal forces, or universal and Innate forces combined. If the body is normal it will be both with nice balance. This universal form of motion is called by physicists, "motor function." Dr. Palmer also calls it by the same name at times, but the student must not be confused by the application of the medical term to General Function. Dr. Palmer also says: "A mental impulse is a thought in motion; motion is function; and function is life." This is absolutely true and well said but one must analyze epigrams. "Coordination is health," also, but if these very general statements were all that we put into a book, it could not be a textbook for study.

The report to Innate is over the afferent half of the Normal Complete Cycle (not the Special Sense Cycle) and is General Sense. Note that General Sense goes with General Function.

Art. 243. Primary Function in the Body.

Primary Function is the cooperative service which the parts of the body render to each other.

Since the tissue cell is the smallest organ, it is the basic unit in the study of function. General Function is Primary Function considered generally without specifying the kind of expression. Primary Functions are arbitrarily divided into nine specific kinds for convenience in making analyses. Two others might be added, namely, Transmission, and Connection. But as they have never been used with symbols, the writer will not attempt to add them to the nine. The student should keep them in mind however, in making analyses and can give them the symbol for General Function—(O).

Art. 244. PRIMARY FUNCTIONS AND THEIR NORMAL SYMBOLS.

0. General Function,	O.
1. Motor Function,	M.
2. Calorific Function,	C.
3. Sensory Function,	S.
4. Secretory Function,	T.
5. Excretory Function,	E.
6. Nutritive Function,	N.
7. Reparatory Function,	R.
8. Expansive Function,	X.
9. Reproductive Function	Y.

These are the names of the nine specific kinds of coordinative service that tissue cells give each other. Some of these are mostly (considering each separately) the service of one kind of tissue, as Motor; but most of them are the concerted actions of many tissues.

Think of the Primary Functions as products (and in some cases the service is in material form) necessary for exchange in the Law of Demand and Supply. The conveyor of the material service is the Serous Circulation.

The reports to Innate over the afferent half of the Normal Complete Cycle, is not divided into nine classes to correspond to the Nine Functions but are considered as one class, just as though all the nine afferent reports were gathered into one bundle for them all. This afferent side of the Nine Functions is called by Dr. Palmer, "The Wife." (See Fig. 27) This is, (See Art. 241) after all, General Sense which has been described before. It suffers no interference with transmission and therefore the sensation obtained by Innate is always cor-

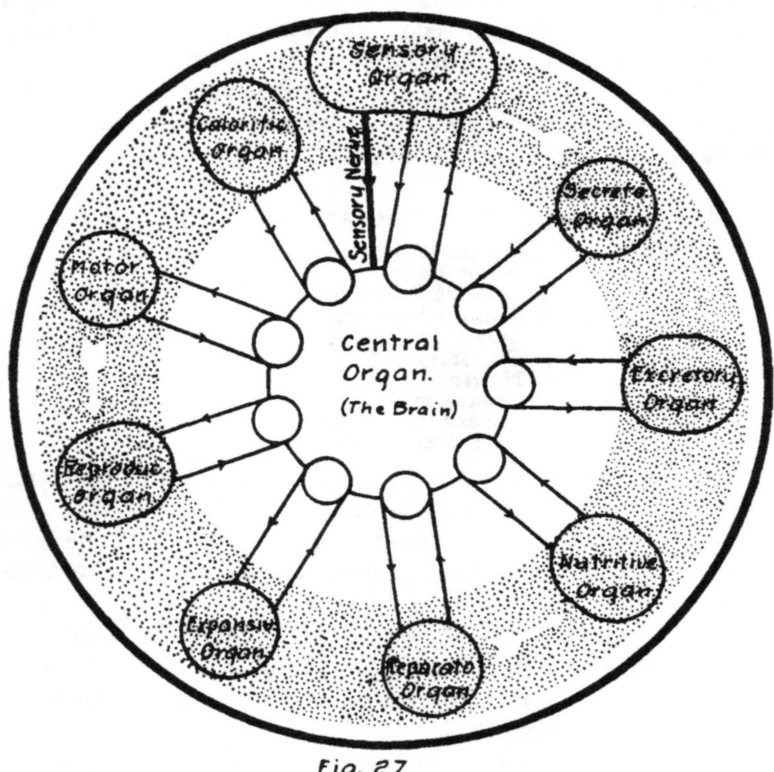

Fig. 27.

rect. The student is cautioned not to confuse General Sense with Sensory Function, one of the Nine Primary Functions, for Sensory Function, as one of the Nine is itself reported on by The Wife.

Art. 245. The Law of Demand and Supply. (Prin. 33.)

When the tissue cell needs something, either material or immaterial, this need is equivalent to a variation of forces locally. The energy waves of this variation is picked up by the sensitive tentacles of the afferent nerve. It is then known as Impressions of Vibrations, which it really is. The behavior of the afferent nerve cell (adaptability of nerve tissue cell responding to forces) informs Innate of the condition at the tissue cell, (sensation). Innate, cognizant of the needs of the tissue cell, issues demands to the cells which she knows can deliver the supply. If the cell needs materials, they are later delivered through the Serous Circulation. If the cell needs forces, Innate assembles them and sends them direct. The supply of forces reaches the tissue cell immediately and is used to balance the obstreperous universal forces, which made the demand necessary. It takes longer to ship the material supplies which the cell needs. If the (supply houses) cells cannot furnish the materials there will of course, "be a famine somewhere." This is incoordination. (Prin. 23)

Review Questions for Articles 241 to 245, inclusive.

1. What is Universal Function?
2. What is its characteristic outside the body?
3. What does Innate do with it in the body?
4. What happens if they are not adapted in the body?
5. What is General Function in the body?
6. What is the difference between General Function and Universal Function?
7. What is General Sense?
8. Differentiate between General Sense and Special Sense.
9. What is Primary Function in the body?
10. What is the difference between General Function and Primary Function?
11. How many kinds of function (specific) is General Function divided into?
12. What other two specific functions might well be added to the Nine Primary Functions?

13. Are the Primary Functions of the body actually limited to nine?
14. Name the Nine Primary Functions, in the order given.
15. Give their normal symbols.
16. What great law in the body is a fundamental principle?
17. What is the report to Innate over the afferent half of the Normal Complete Cycle, called?
18. Is this the same as Sensory Function?
19. What is the law of Demand and Supply?
20. Explain the working of the Law of Demand and Supply in the body.
21. In what way does a tissue cell make a demand?
22. In what way is its demand answered?
23. What kind of demands require a longer time to be supplied?

Art. 246. Normal Function.

Normal Function is the perfect cooperative service which an organ gives to the body.

It is accomplished by perfect adaptative variations according to the Law of Demand and Supply.

It is dependent upon perfect transmission and perfect condition.

An organ may act and does act under "stimuli" but stimuli are not mental impulses and the action they cause is not function, for function is cooperation. While perfection is hard to obtain, yet perfect normality is no less than that standard, and it is that ideal which we desire everything to approach. No function can be normal if it never varies, for circumstances and demands vary. Hence, normal function is never constant but shows that adaptation is the Law of Variation (See Fig. 10). Function, in order to be normal, must always meet the ever changing demands of bodily requirements. The demands of bodily requirements cannot be met by any organ if it fails to receive the "urge" and failing this Innate Control, the never ceasing vibration of its parts, (for it *will* vibrate) (Prin. 1, 14) will drive it to action not pleasing to Innate. Besides this, the organ must have perfect structure (Condition) in order to obey a mental impulse. By lack of perfect structure Innate may be hindered. (Prin. 5, 24)

Art. 247. Motor Function. (Primary Function)

Motor Function is the production of mechanical motion as a coordinative service to the body as a whole or for any of its parts.

All living cells have motion. This is not Primary Function necessarily but their individualistic motion. Motor Function is the action of definite cells especially constructed for the production of mechanical motion. The most common tissue used by Innate for Motor Function is muscle tissue. Other tissues which have Motor Function are: ciliated epithelium, erectile tissue, etc. The body and parts of the body require mechanical movement from one place to another. This is accomplished by organs made of muscle tissue. Each muscle cell like other cells, has a protoplasm that is constantly moving. By coordinated control whole phalanxes of such cells are compelled to shift their protoplasm at the same time and a sum total of movement is obtained in the same direction. No other example of coordinated movement is better than this one. All the cells of a muscle pull together at the same time and relax at the same time; or oppose each other at the right moment. The cell being an elongated string-like cell, has the power to shift its protoplasm to make it longer; and again shift it to make its length shorter. Having natural elasticity, and alertness of protoplasm (tonicity) it is capable of using the heat and chemical agencies of universal energies. It has its individualistic movements as its signs of life. But any part of a very highly organized unit, like the body cannot be entirely individualistic for it must "fulfill its office" and entirely independent movements would be out of order. It is easy to see why there must be management or functional control from the Center to make all parts work together.

Art. 248. Calorific Function. (Primary Function)

Calorific Function is the production of heat for maintenance of normal bodily temperature.

The production of heat, for use in the body, is a coordinative service to the body.

All active cells produce heat as a by-product of their actions but that is not, necessarily, Primary Function, and a great deal of the time it is necessary to dispose of by-product heat by thermolysis. The tissues most concerned in the production of heat, as direct Calorific Function, are glandular; especially the liver, which not only acts as the "furnace room" of the body, but stores its fuel to be doled out to the rest of the body for local oxidation. However, any other tissues used by Innate to produce heat for bodily use, whether momentarily or constantly, locally or generally, may be said to assist in Calorific Function.

Art. 249. Thermogenesis.

Thermogenesis is the generation of heat, whether considered as Primary Function or not.

It may be the production of heat by Calorific organs or the production of heat as a by-product.

If made by calorific organs coordinately, it is Calorific Function. If by-product heat is saved and made use of by Innate coordinately, it then is also classed as Calorific Function. A good example of the latter is shown by the following: a person who is out in very cold weather, upon becoming chilled because the loss of body heat is great and the calorific organs are not able to keep the supply up, has an Innate desire to exercise. He stamps his feet, runs, or otherwise uses his muscles, thereby deputizing the muscles as calorific organs, to warm up the body by oxidizing carbons.

Art. 250. SENSORY FUNCTION. (Primary Function)

Sensory Function is the service which certain cells and organs give to the body, by reporting environmental conditions and in some cases information concerning the actions of other cells of the body. (See Fig. 27)

This function is a protective service for the whole body; it is the Innate method of obtaining information of possible dangers or benefits existing in "the external."

It also, as muscular sense, is the fundamental of skill, art, dexterity and the like; and in other instances we are able to know educationally about involuntary functions going on in the body.

Sensory Function is the action of definite tissue cells, namely, nerve tissue. (See Art. 242, 244.)

Since Sensory Function is a conscious function, the educated brain may be said to have Sensory Function. All cells have general Sense; the ability to report to Innate concerning themselves, and things which concern them. The special sense organs, which are tissue cells themselves, must also report to Innate concerning themselves. The report to Innate concerning the condition of cells engaged in Sensory Function, is General Sense (See Fig. 27.) If a cell's ability (nerve tissue of course) to send impressions to Innate becomes so specialized that it takes it out of the general class, that cell may be said to have Sensory Function and to be a Special Sense Organ. (See Special Sense Cycle Art. 109, and Fig. 12)

REVIEW QUESTIONS FOR ARTICLES 246 to 250, inclusive.

1. What is normal function?
2. What two important things is it dependent upon?
3. Is the action of an organ produced by stimuli, function? Why?
4. Why is normal function ever changing in rate and quantity?
5. If it remains normal does the quality ever change?
6. While we speak of "perfect function," "perfect health" and the like, are we likely to find them absolutely perfect in the body?
7. What is Motor Function?

8. What are the chief organs of Motor Function?
9. In what manner are the individual muscle cells of a muscle caused to lengthen and shorten in unison?
10. What would happen if the individual muscle cells moved their protoplasm according to their own pleasure?
11. When muscles do not act in unison, what is the reason?
12. Could muscle cells which are undernourished, depleted, or injured, act coordinately?
13. What is Calorific Function?
14. How is by-product heat disposed of?
15. What is Thermogenesis?
16. When is the making of by-product heat, Calorific Function?
17. What is the chief organ of Calorific Function?
18. What is Sensory Function?
19. What is its purpose?
20. What Sensory Function is necessary to skill, dexterity and the like?
21. Is Sensory Function an Innate or an Educated function?
22. What Cycle is used to explain Sensory Function?
23. What tissue is concerned in Sensory Function?
24. When a sensory cell reports its metabolistic condition to Innate, what kind of sense is it?

Art. 251. Secretory Function. (Primary Function)

Secretory Function is the coordinative action of certain cells with appropriate structure to produce chemical combinations for various uses in the body.

All cells secrete substances as the Serous Circulation passes through them, but this is not necessarily Primary Function, it merely being the action of the cells in excreting their own waste materials, as a sign of life. Secretory Function, as a Primary Function, concerns the making of those materials which are to be used in and for the body. Of course this is an arbitrary classification, but that is the way we classified Primary Function in the beginning. (Art. 243) If Innate uses the excretory matter of some cells as nutriment for others in the body, then that material is called secretion. This material is a poison to the cell which excretes it, if retained in it or near it, but may be very good material for assimilation some other place in the body. Thus, the secretion of the thyroid gland is a necessary secretion for metabolism of the body but the thyroid secretion is excretory material to the gland which made it. The secretion itself is the product of Secretory Function, a material product, but the act of producing it coordinately is a service to the body and therefore is a Primary Function.

The kinds of tissue most concerned in this function are glandular epithelium, lymphoid and the like. The secreting glands for Primary Function are: the liver, spleen, pancreas, thyroid gland, lymphatic glands, etc. Other tissues and structures, as part of secreting glands, may be said to assist in Secretory Function.

Art. 252. Elimination.

Elimination is the selective process of Innate Intelligence, expressed through tissue cells, which separates the usable materials from waste matters or toxins, or vice versa.

Elimination is performed in every cell. (See Signs of Life, Arts. 64, 65, 66) When the body is considered as the unit organism, elimination is performed by Innate through certain organs for that purpose; as, spleen, liver and kidneys. We make a differentiation between Elimination and Excretion in the body. Elimination in the picking out of the desirable or the undesirable, which is the process of selection. Selection requires judgment on every item; and judgment is the prerogative of intelligence.

Art. 253. Excretory Function. (Primary Function)

Excretory Function is the coordinative action of certain cells, with appropriate structure, in ejecting from the body certain waste matters, poisons and heat.

All cells excrete eliminated materials from their own bodies, but the excretion from the whole body is the coordinative service rendered by excretory organs. The thing eliminated may be either material, as urine; or something not matter as, heat. The tissues which assist excretory organs constantly or are deputized at times, may be said to assist in excretory function. (Example, the muscle of the stomach in vomiting.)

Art. 254. Thermolysis.

Thermolysis is the action of excretory organs in the dissipation of unnecessary heat.

The surplus heat is usually the by-product of functioning or an adaptative condition. When it is abnormal, it causes the body to be too cold or too hot. Thermolysis is just as important as thermogenesis in keeping the temperature of the body normally constant, i.e. ninety-eight and six-tenths degrees. Heat dissipation is accomplished by conduction, radiation, and convection. The skin is most active in this form of excretion, though much of the surplus heat is carried away with excreta from the lungs, kidneys and bowels. The creation, circulation and excretion of heat is just as important in bodily metabolism as any other cycle of the body. (See Art. 105)

Art. 255. Nutritive Function. (Primary Function)

Nutritive Function is the action of certain cells in preparing nutriment for assimilation in the body.

All cells have assimilation but that is not Nutritive Function as a primary act; it pertains to the private affairs of the cell, while Primary Function is service for the body as a unit, by the cell as a functioning unit. All cells secrete as individual cells (see Serous Circulation) as a process of excretion but that is not Nutritive Function, considered as a Primary Function in the body. There are many physiological processes concerned in Nutritive Function. Digestion, a process of mechanical and chemical breaking down of food materials into simple compounds, which are thus rendered soluble, easily transportable by the blood and serum, and easily available by the cells in assimilation. Secretion also plays an important part in Nutritive Function; hence it is seen that Secretory Function and Nutritive Function are dependent upon each other. The cells most concerned in Nutritive Function are glandular but when the structure of the digestive organs is considered, it can be seen that many other tissues are engaged in this important service to the body.

Review Questions for Articles 251 to 255.

1. What is Secretory Function?
2. Do all cells have Secretory Function?
3. What are secretory organs?
4. When cells or larger organs have Secretory Function what unit of matter do they serve?
5. What is the difference between secretion and excretion?
6. To what cells are secretions poison?
7. What is Elimination?
8. What is the difference between Elimination and Excretion?
9. What is Excretory Function?
10. What is Thermolysis?
11. What organs are chiefly concerned in Thermolysis?
12. What is the normal heat constant of the body?
13. In what three physical ways is heat taken from the body?
14. What organ is chiefly concerned in heat excretion?
15. What is the Heat Cycle and what is its purpose?
16. What is Nutritive Function?
17. What is the difference between Nutritive Function and assimilation?
18. What physiological process is most important in Nutritive Function?
19. What is digestion?

Art. 256. Reparatory Function. (Primary Function)

Reparatory Function is the action of certain cells with appropriate structure in providing cells to repair tissues which have been injured, those pathological, or to supply normal anabolism and catabolism.

It is also the process of repletion. (Art. 140)

All cells have the ability to repair themselves, but that is not directly Primary Function in the body. It applies more nearly to the fundamentals of repletion and in that sense the private actions of tissue cells are indirectly concerned with Primary Function.

Reparatory Function is very dependent upon Expansive Function, for in order to obtain new cells for Reparation, cells must be expanded in the developmental or expansional centers. Reparatory Function is a very arbitrary grouping of several functions and physiological processes.

Reparatory Function is the name of a coordinative service that relates to specific disposal of certain expansional and nutritive products.

Art. 257. Expansive Function. (Primary Function)

Expansive Function is the action of cells with appropriate structure for reproducing new cells of their own kind to be used in growth or reparation.

It is the coordinative service of certain cells, appointed by Innate for that purpose, in expanding new cells for growth and reparation.

All cells expand to maturity but only in the sense that this serves the whole body, can these private actions of tissue cells be construed as Primary Function. The tissue cells which are concerned in true Expansive Function are the developmental centers all over the body which represent the "scattering" of the blastoderm, (see Arts. 70 to 78, incl.) the origin of all embryonic centers. In the study of physiology, these expansional centers can easily be found and the connection between Physiology and Philosophy made clear. The expansional centers are of all kinds of tissue, since all kinds of tissue are necessary in growth and reparation. But all tissue cells are not allowed by Innate to reproduce themselves, for that would not be coordinative. In such a case there would be no control of the amount, shape and extent of the body. On the other hand we know that there is a very decided plan for the body in both growth and maintenance, and in order to manage the signs of life of the individual cells, Innate must be ever vigilant to have new cells when she wants them and at no other time; and where she wants them and at no other place; and the number that she wants—no more or less.

The analogy of the bee hive may be used here to advantage. Let the hive of bees represent the cells of an organization and the queen bee the expansive center or developmental center. The queen bee is the only reproducing unit of the hive, (with the exception of the male bee of course). The queen bee is allowed by the laws of nature to reproduce, while hundreds of worker bees (the females) and the drones (the males) are not. If all of them reproduced there would be no close organization which enables the bees to have strong and efficient colonies. If any one will take the trouble to study these interesting insects a little, he will see that they have very close organization; very centralized. (Art. 70)

Art. 258. Reproductive Function. (Primary Function)

Reproductive Function is the action of certain cells in secreting germs for the propagation of the race.

The tissues most concerned in Reproductive Function are glandular. Expansive Function refers to reproduction of cells as units; Reproductive Function refers to the reproduction of the whole body; to the secreting of its germ. From this germ, which contains cell possibilities of the future body, the housing of the new life is developed. The blastoderm, the union of the spermatazoon and ovum, contains the cell possibilities for all the tissues of the body during its life time; and the blastoderm, originally a cell of double chromoplasm, develops cells with double chromoplasms, and in this manner two races are propagated, namely, the male and female. The germs that arise in the blastoderm by cell division, become germinating centers all over the body, to expand new cells for growth and reparation. A certain division of these becomes the parenchyma of the reproductive organs, for the purpose of secreting new germs, which will carry within them the possibilities of all four primary tissues.

Art. 259. Incoordination.

Incoordination is the lack of harmony in the actions of the parts of the body, due to lack of Innate control.

It is the condition of unbalanced service; or rather the unbalanced actions of tissue cells, which then fails to be service. The actions of tissue cells are not coordinative service unless they act in obedience to the Law of Demand and Supply. (Prin. 33) Incoordination is called disease because tissue cells will become unsound when they are neglected of caretaking by the organization.

Art. 260. Lack of Adaptation.

Lack of adaptation is the failure of the management of universal forces in the tissue cell, by Innate Intelligence.

The cause of this is interference with the transmission of mental impulses; interference with Innate control, which mental impulses represent. The purpose of mental impulses is Innate balance or control of universal forces, which are always in the tissue cell. (Prin. 1, 14, 16.) Lack of control allows universal forces to act more according to the unadapted laws of physics and chemistry; very much as they do outside of the body. The actions of unadapted universal forces are not cooperative and therefore are not function. It should be remembered that it is not necessary to have total lack of adaptation to produce some incoordination. Any deviation from the perfect, in adaptation, means a proportional deviation from the perfect in function.

Review Questions for Articles 256 to 260, inclusive.

1. What is Reparatory Function?
2. What other Primary Function is it a branch of?

3. What two main physiological processes compose it?
4. What is Expansive Function?
5. What is the disposal of the products of Expansive Function?
6. Explain the centers of expansion.
7. Why is it necessary that cell expansion be under close control of Innate?
8. What is Reproductive Function?
9. What is the difference between Reproductive Function as Primary Function and Reproduction, the Sign of Life?
10. What becomes of the blastoderm?
11. What is the characteristic of the expansion of cells to reproduce the race?
12. What is Incoordination?
13. Why is Incoordination called dis-ease?
14. What is lack of adaptation?
15. When Innate adapts, what does she adapt?
16. How much lack of adaptation is necessary to produce incoordination?

Art. 261. Abnormal Primary Function.

Abnormal Function is the arbitrary term used to indicate the production of more or less action of a given kind, than Innate desires for coordination, in any part of the body.

Since Primary Functions are coordinative, the existence of abnormal functions is ascertained by comparison with other functions, and the comparison is made regardless of whether the others are normal or abnormal, for any function is abnormal if it does not vary at an adaptative rate. The action of any organ is not normal if it fails to accommodate itself to the actions of the others, whether the others are doing right or not. (See Fig. 10)

Abnormal function, which really is not function at all (wholly or in part) is of course due to a lack of adaptation, which is in turn due to interference with transmission, which is caused by a subluxation in the spinal column. (Prin. 31) When the interference is directly on the Efferent Nerve, it causes the organ in question to function abnormally; it is suffering direct effects and is named **Local.** When the interference is on the Efferent Nerve supplying an organ, whose business it is to keep the Serous Circulation in order, the tissue in question is said to be suffering indirect effects and this condition is named **Condition.** A tissue is not apt to suffer from an abnormal serous circulation when it is normal, being quite able to defend itself. (See Resistance, Arts. 130 and 131) Therefore we find that a Major Condition is the result of both Local and Condition. (See Fig. 18)

As General Sense is the report to Innate from every tissue cell concerning its function and metabolism, so General Sense, also, gives a report to Innate Intelligence concerning any abnormality of tissues. It shows to Innate, in Sensation and Ideation, the exact proportions of normality and abnormality. This is called Equivalent Sensation and gives Equivalent Ideation. It was derived from Equivalent Impressions from Equivalent Vibrations of an abnormal tissue cell. (See Abnormal Cycles in Sophomore Text)

Art. 262. Minus Function. (Lack of Function)

Minus Function is the arbitrary term used to indicate the production of less action of a given kind than Innate desires for coordination in any part of the body. (See Art. 261.)

There is in this case, probably, some action of the kind in question but it is not sufficient for Innate's needs. This lack need not be very much, in order to produce incoordination. On the other hand, it may be totally lacking and then it is indeed, Lack of Function, or Minus Function as it is called. This does not mean, necessarily, that the tissue is dead, for other functions may not be deficient there. Death is the total absence of all functions, and not the total absence of one function. The term Minus Function or Lack of Function happens to be literal for there is actual lack of service, hence lack of function.

Art. 263. Excess Function.

Excess Function is the arbitrary term used to indicate the production of more action of a given kind than Innate

desires for coordination in any part of the body. (See Art. 261)

The name Excess Function is employed for something which is not function because it is abnormal action which resembles a Primary Function, just the same as a cell in a tumor can and does resemble a useful cell in the body. Excess Function resembles function, therefore is called function; but since it is not coordinative service in the body it is not really function. The excess action need be very little to produce incoordination —ever so little is a deviation from the perfect. A tissue cell is always in motion and it also has motion from the universal forces within it. (Prin. 1, 14, 16) Innate cannot prevent this motion but she can control it, if she has no interference. (Prin. 23, 24, 26, 29) In Excess Function, the action of universal forces in the cell is making it produce what otherwise would be service, if there were not so much of it. It is action, but any action which is in excess of Innate's requirements, cannot be function. Sometimes normal adaptative conditions resemble excess function; as, ankylosis.

Sometimes normal adaptation resembles excess function; as, fast breathing when in violent exercise.

Excess Function is never the result of excess mental impulses; there is no such thing as excess mental impulses.

Art. 264. PARALYSIS.

Paralysis is the condition of any part of the body which is suffering incoordination.

Paralysis is any dis-ease of any degree.

Paralysis is any degree between life and death and is neither.

Paralysis may be the slight abnormality of one function, either in excess or lack; or it may be a great degree of the foregoing. But the student is advised to use the simpler way and think of Paralysis as:

Any degree of deviation from the normal of General Function is Paralysis, for Paralysis is a term of generality which naturally goes in the same class as General Function, General Sense and the like.

Art. 265. Life and Death.

Life is one hundred per cent function; perfect coordination; absolute adaptation.

Death is zero per cent function; absence of coordination; total lack of adaptation, which brings the matter of the body under the sway of universal forces, the same as any other "dust."

A comparison:

100% function is Life.
100% minus any degree is Paralysis.
0% is Death.

Review Questions for Articles 261 to 265, inclusive.

1. What is abnormal Primary Function?
2. Is there actually such a thing as abnormal function or is that an arbitrary classification?
3. What produces abnormal function?
4. What produces lack of adaptation?
5. What produces interference with transmission?
6. What is the meaning of the term Local?
7. What is the meaning of the term Condition?
8. What is Lack of Function?
9. Why is the term Lack of Function not so arbitrary as it may seem in the definition given in Art. 262?
10. What is Excess Function?
11. Why is the term absolutely arbitrary, unlike Lack of Function?
12. How is it possible for a lack of mental impulses to allow excess function?
13. When may normal adaptation resemble Excess Function?
14. When may adaptative conditions resemble Excess Function?
15. What was the reason for using the term function at all in the name Excess Function?
16. What is Paralysis?
17. Why is it best in explaining Paralysis, to speak in terms of General Function?
18. What is Life?
19. What is Death?
20. In death, what is the state of matter?

Art. 266. DEGREES OF PARALYSIS.

Any degree of deviation from the normal is paralysis.

The amount of Innate's expression is normally, an ever varying amount; a fixed quantity would be abnormal but since Innate's function is perfect (Prin. 27) it must be the function of matter which is imperfect, when imperfection is present. (Prin. 5, 24, 29)

A fixed quantity of function of matter would also be abnormal, (see Fig. 10) and the normal would be an ever varying quantity.

The normal function of matter in the body is likewise an ever varying quantity, and a fixed or constant rate would average either more or less than Innate requires for coordination, therefore would be abnormal. This average amount of excess or minus could be one degree or many and the cause is always the same for one degree or many, namely, the interference with transmission. Therefore the adjustment of subluxations is in about the same place in the spine (according to the Old Generic Table) for all kindred dis-eases (see Families) whether they be of one degree or many.

In the case of Minus Function, let us assume that health is zero degree of abnormality; then the degree of abnormality can be numbered as far as Death, which is one hundred degrees. Then any amount less of abnormality would, in degrees, be from one to ninety-nine, inclusive. In case of Excess Function, let us assume that Health is zero degree abnormality and we can number the degrees as far as Destruction, which would be Death, and that number would of course be one hundred. Then any Excess Function less than Destruction or Death would, in degrees, be from one to ninety-nine, inclusive. Any dis-ease could have this range of severity; its Minus Functions and its Excess Functions involved, be anywhere between zero degree and one hundred degrees and the adjustment for it in any case would be the same. The physician, on the other hand, takes into consideration all these degrees of severity, dividing them still further into fractions of degrees till he has over twenty-five thousand things to name, each of them with certain treatment. We think Chiropractic much simpler.

Art. 267. Paralysis. Chiropractic and Medical Definitions Compared.

Medical Definition: "Abolition or great diminution of the voluntary or involuntary motor functions and sometimes of sensation in one or more parts of the body. Immediate cause is generally pressure, either by blood effused or by serum or vascular turgescence. It generally admits of palliation and is extremely apt to recur."

Quotation from Dr. Palmer (Page 327, Vol. V)

"We have been taught by medical and osteopathic work that paralysis is distinctly that phase of abnormal phenomena wherein muscles (voluntary and involuntary) are unable to move. I make a different interpretation carrying the idea that **every function is the expression of an Innate Intelligence which personifies the intelligence behind it, and the lack of that energetic intellectuality is what makes paralysis."**

Art. 268. Compensatory Function and Compensatory Conditions.

Compensatory Function is the extra work thrown upon a Normal organ (and perhaps an abnormal organ) to compensate for that which an abnormal organ fails to do.

Its symbol is I. A. meaning Intellectual Adaptation.

This produces "adaptative symptoms" of a case; and seventy-five per cent of the symptoms are of that nature.

It sometimes resembles Excess Function but absolutely is not.

Prolonged Compensation results in Compensatory conditions

which resemble pathology, and which in time may become real pathology. (See Art. 144)

When an organ fails, because of interference with transmission, to do its work, Innate causes other organs, when that is possible, to do extra work in addition to their own, to make up for the loss. This gives rise to symptoms that are often symptoms of dis-ease, or at any rate that is what they are called, but it would be a mistake, if they are adaptative, to tamper with the organ producing them, for that organ is only doing its duty. If the organ called upon to do the extra work is abnormal, or if the functional nerves leading to it are not in perfect order, a complication arises and a new interference appears. (See Transmission, in Senior Text) When the dis-ease becomes chronic, Innate may find it necessary to make a change in tissues; as, exostosis, ankylosis, and enlarged lung, etc. This appears as pathology, but the tissue in them is normal, and remains so, unless the organ called upon is abnormal itself. In this case the change in tissue is apt to be not just what Innate wants, and therefore really pathological.

Art. 269. Symbols Used in Chiropractic Equations.

Symbols are signs used in Chiropractic to represent each of the normal Primary Functions, each when in excess, each when minus, and for General Functions.

Symbols without plus and minus signs represent normality; they do not represent Species of families.

List of symbols commonly used:

For the Nine Primary Functions when normal; M. C. S. T. E. N. R. X. Y.

When the same are in excess: M+, C+, S+, T+, E+, N+, R+, X+, Y+.

When the same are minus: M—, C—, S—, T—, E—, N—, R—, X—, Y—.

For General Function, normal and abnormal: O, O+, O—.

For area involved: A, A+, A—.
For depth involved: D, D+, D—.
For Power, P. For Force, F.
For Intellectual Adaptation, I. A., always normal.

Art. 270. Abnormal Motor Function.

Abnormal Motor Function is the production of more or less mechanical motion, in any part of the body, than Innate requires for coordination.

It is due to lack of mental impulses, which allows unadapted action of universal forces, in motor tissue cells. (Art. 239, 241, 247.)

Symbols of direct effects are M+ and M—, and are forms of paralysis.

Other direct and indirect effects are explanation in Families.

Review Questions for Articles 266 to 270, inclusive.

1. What difference would there be in your adjustment for one degree of severity and fifty degrees of severity, of a dis-ease?
2. What is the main difference between the Chiropractic idea of paralysis and the medical idea?
3. What is Compensatory Function?
4. What symptoms does it produce?
5. What does it resemble?
6. What is prolonged compensation apt to result in?
7. What happens when the organ called upon to compensate, is itself abnormal?
8. Name the symbols for normal functions.
9. Name the symbols for excess functions.
10. Name the symbols for minus functions.
11. Name the symbols, normal and abnormal, for General Function.
12. Give the symbol for Compensation, and what the letters stand for?
13. What is abnormal Motor Function?
14. To what is it due?

Art. 271. Abnormal Calorific Function.

Abnormal Calorific Function is the production of heat in excess of, or less than Innate's requirements for coordination.

It is due to lack of mental impulses which allows unadapted action of universal forces in heat producing organs.

Symbols of direct effects are C+ and C—, and are forms of paralysis.

Other direct and indirect effects are explained in Families.

It may be a general condition; as, a febrile dis-ease, or general coldness.

It may be a local condition; as, inflammation or a local coldness.

Art. 272. ABNORMAL THERMOGENESIS.

Abnormal Thermogenesis pertains to abnormal Calorific Function; also to any other source of heat in the body in which the production of it is uncontrolled.

An example of the latter is seen in febrile dis-eases; (Art. 193) in which the burning of toxins, which should have progressed smoothly, as in "spring fever," is beyond control of Innate Intelligence. More heat is produced than can be taken care of by thermolysis, especially since the organs of excretion are not normal in febrile diseases.

Art. 273. ABNORMAL SENSORY FUNCTION.

Abnormal Sensory Function is the abnormal action of sensory organs, (cells) in which they give false information to Innate or fail to give enough.

It is due to lack of mental impulses from Innate, and that lack allows unadapted action of universal forces which make the special sense organs send impressions that are either false or meaningless. This is "excess sensory function;" or, the special sense organs are lacking in action of any kind, good or bad, and that is "minus sensory function." Remember that the terms Excess and Minus Function are names of something and the names are not always literal. (Art. 262, 263)

The direct effects are indicated by S+ and S—, and are forms of paralysis. For explanation of other direct and indirect conditions see Families.

Art. 274. Abnormal Secretory Function.

Abnormal Secretory Function is the action of secretory cells (organs) which produces more or less secretion than Innate desires for coordination in the body.

It is due to lack of mental impulses and that allows unadapted action of universal forces which makes the glands secrete at a rate that is not according to the Law of Demand and Supply.

It is ascertained by noting the quantity of secretions and if they are disposed of by the other parts of the body properly. The direct effects are indicated by T+ and T— and are forms of paralysis. Other direct and indirect effects are explained in Families.

Art. 275. Abnormal Excretory Function.

Abnormal Excretory Function is the abnormal action of excretory organs which causes them to eject substances from the body which Innate wishes retained; or fail to eject from the body that which Innate wishes to discard.

It is due to lack of mental impulses which allow the unadapted universal forces to act in an unadapted manner. The direct effects are indicated by E+ and E— and are forms of paralysis. Other effects are explained in Families.

Review Questions for Articles 271 to 275, inclusive.

1. What is abnormal Calorific Function?
2. To what is it due?
3. Differentiate between general and local abnormal calorific conditions.
4. What is abnormal thermogenesis?
5. What is abnormal Secretory Function?
6. What is abnormal Sensory Function?
7. What is abnormal Excretory Function?

Art. 276. Abnormal Thermolysis.

Abnormal Thermolysis is the abnormal action of eliminating and excretory organs, which dissipate heat faster or slower than Innate desires for coordination.

It pertains to Excretory and not to Calorific Function. If too much heat is dissipated it leaves too little heat in the body, which must be compensated for; or it leaves the body too cold. If the heat is not dissipated fast enough, the by-product heat accumulates too fast and makes the body too hot. In order to coordinate, Excretory function must thermolyze faster or slower, adaptatively, to balance thermogenesis, sufficiently to keep the bodily temperature at ninety-eight and six-tenths degrees.

The direct effects are indicated by E+ and E— but often C+ and C— are used, which is convenient but erroneous. Other functions may be concerned indirectly.

Art. 277. Abnormal Nutritive Function.

Abnormal Nutritive Function is the action of nutritive organs, in which they physiologically prepare nutrition in more or less quantity than Innate requires for the needs of the body.

It is due to lack of mental impulses and is a form of paralysis. It of course, depends upon the cooperation of other functions, for nutritive organs cannot supply prepared nutriment unless they are supplied with "raw materials." Therefore these cells may fail to coordinate because of remote causes, whose effects reach the nutritive cells through the Serous Circulation. Direct effects are indicated by N+ and N—. Other functions may be concerned indirectly.

Art. 278. Abnormal Reparatory Function.

Abnormal Reparatory Function is the action of certain expansional centers in producing cells in more or less quantity than Innate requires for normal reparation.

In another sense, also, it is the abnormal extension beyond repletion, of certain body cells because of lowered resistance, due to interference with transmission.

Direct effects are indicated by N+ and N— and is a form of paralysis. Many other functions may be concerned in a case indirectly, as explained in Species and Families.

Art. 279. ABNORMAL EXPANSIVE FUNCTION.

Abnormal Expansive Function is the action of the cells in developmental centers in producing more cells than Innate requires for growth or reparation.

It is due to lack of mental impulses and there is lack of control of expansional centers. Direct effects are indicated by X+ and X—, and are a form of paralysis. Other functions may be concerned indirectly.

Art. 280. ABNORMAL REPRODUCTIVE FUNCTION.

Abnormal Reproductive Function is the action of the reproducing organs, at a rate which is not coordinative with Innate's requirements.

It is due to lack of mental impulses which prevents adaptation of universal forces. Direct effects are indicated by Y+ and Y— which are forms of paralysis. Other functions may be concerned in a case, indirectly.

REVIEW QUESTIONS FOR ARTICLES 276 to 280, inclusive.

1. What is abnormal thermolysis?
2. Is abnormal thermolysis the fault of abnormal calorific organs or abnormal excretory organs?
3. What is abnormal Nutritive Function?
4. What is the cause of all these abnormal Primary Functions?
5. In what manner does the cause of abnormality produce abnormality?
6. What is abnormal Reparatory Function?
7. How is repletion made abnormal?
8. What is a' ormal Expansive Function?
9. In what ect way may abnormal Primary Function be produced?

10. What is abnormal Reproductive Function?
11. Physiologically, what organs are abnormal in abnormal Reproductive Function?

Art. 281. SPECIE AND PHYSIOLOGY.

A Specie is an incoordination having the characteristics and causes of a family of dis-eases.

A subdivision of a family; one of the type or class which characterizes a family.

Each of the Nine Primary Functions when abnormal produces two Species.

Hybrid Species have more than one function involved, and therefore are indicated by more than one letter.

Species can be indicated by spoken words, written words, symbols or groups of symbols, or any other mode of expression; but a very adequate system of symbols has been made to use for this purpose. (Art. 269.) Hence, the use of one or more symbols with their signs, will indicate the abnormal physiological processes which are involved in the dis-ease. The student should study Chiropractic Physiology in order to analyze efficiently by the equational method. For example, if Secretory Function is at fault, it is necessary to reason deductively, which secretory organ is abnormal, apply the Generic Table and find its place in the spine, then proceed to look for the subluxation in that place and list its direction of displacement.

Art. 282. FAMILY.

A Family is a group or class of incoordinations, having the same characteristics and causes.

A group or class of things, having the same characteristics and origin.

If General Function is under consideration, and if it contains any degree of abnormality, there is but one Family, namely, Paralysis. (Art. 264.)

The symbols of abnormal General Function are, O+ and O— The species of all the dis-eases, from any of the functions, may be placed in this general classification. Also, if any tissue is abnormally functioning and there is no specific classification in which it can be placed, and no symbol for it, it should be placed in the General Paralysis Family with the symbols, O+ or O—, as the case may be.

Art. 283. EQUATIONS.

An expression showing relation between cause and effect.
An expression showing equality.

Words, symbols or other expressions showing the specie and family of dis-eases; may be used to indicate normality.

In Chiropractic, instead of naming an incoordination we indicate it by equations. By means of symbols a shorthand method is given, so to speak, of writing down the Chiropractic "name" for any dis-ease, which shows at a glance which physiological functions are involved and what family they are in; and these facts tell in what Place in the spine we may expect to find the subluxations; and about how many subluxations one may expect, but remember, no rule can be made in regard to this. The true equation is written out in full in order to show equality, as, $a^2+b^2=25$. Some Chiropractic equations when written out in full, appear as semi-diagnostic, as C+E—=catarrh. Since the formula for analysis is Family plus Location equals Major, we can make the equation just given, a genuine Chiropractic equation by substituting all-Chiropractic values in the formula. Then we have: (C+E—) + M.C.P.=Major. As in grammar, we often use sentences without subjects or without verbs, these parts of speech being "understood," so in Chiropractic it is common to use merely the symbols with the rest understood. The student should learn to use the entire equation before he abbreviates it, so he will fully understand what an equation is.

Art. 284. THE NINE PRIMARY FUNCTIONS AND THE NINE PRIMARY FAMILIES, with the most common species.

Function, Family	Species
O. General Function, Paralysis,	O+, O—, M+, M—, C+, C—, S+, S—, T+, T—, E+, E—, N+, N—, R+, R—, X+, X—, Y+, Y—; also combinations
M. Motor, Motor Paralysis,	M+, M—.
C. Calorific, Prolapsis,	M—, T—, C+.
S. Sensory, Contractures,	M+, T+, C—, E—.
T. Secretory, Spasms,	M+ and M—.
E. Excretory, Fever,	C+, C—, E+, E—.
N. Nutritive, Poison,	E+, E—, T+, T—, N+, N—, Y+, Y—.
R. Reparative, Anemia,	N—, T—, R—.
X. Expansive. Tumor,	X+, R+, T+, E—.
Y. Reproductive, Degeneration,	N—C+R—, and sometimes E— is added.

The list of species after each Family can be increased, going from the direct to least direct until all eighteen species are in each Family. That brings each Family "home" to Paralysis and all the Functions involved, (which are all of them) "home" to General Function. Thus it is seen that all the Functions are General Function (service) and all dis-eases are Paralysis (lack of service). Nevertheless, in order to pin a disorder down specifically, to find its specific cause, it is necessary to have specific classification.

Art. 285. PARALYSIS FAMILIES.

Paralysis is any dis-ease; any incoordination; and any subdivision or classification of the same.

All the Primary Families are forms of Paralysis, and so are all the Species.

The tissue involved may be any tissue, or practically all the tissues.

The species of Paralysis are O+ and O—, and all the others including the combinations, such as, (C+E—) or N—C+R—). A single specie, as C+, is said to be "squarely within" a family, as, the Fever Family; while (C+E—), a hybrid specie, being a combination of two families, is said to be in the Fever-Poison Family.

REVIEW QUESTIONS FOR ARTICLES 281 to 285, inclusive.

1. What is a specie?
2. What is a hybrid specie?
3. How are species expressed in Chiropractic?
4. What physiological information do species give?
5. What is a family?
6. What is an equation?
7. What is a Chiropractic equation?
8. Give an example of a genuine Chiropractic equation.
9. What species, including all the direct and indirect can be named in any family?
10. What does the correct answer to Question 9 prove?
11. What tissue may be involved in Paralysis?
12. In what family is a hybrid specie placed?
13. When is a specie "squarely" within a family?

Art. 286. MOTOR PARALYSIS FAMILY.

A form of paralysis in which motor control is abnormal, via relational nerves.

Some species of Motor Paralysis:

M+, due to abnormal motor control, in which voluntary and involuntary muscles are unable to function; as, spastic paralysis. Direct effect.

M−, due to abnormal motor control, in which voluntary and involuntary muscles are unable to function; as, flaccid paralysis. Direct effect.

M+, due to T+, excess tonicity, as in contractures. Indirect.

M−, due to T−, lack of tonicity, as in prolapses. Indirect.

M+, due to C−, coldness producing contractures. Indirect.

M−, due to C+, relaxation produced by too much heat. Indirect.

M+, due to E−, coldness resulting from toxins, producing contractures. Indirect.

Other abnormal functions may be concerned indirectly. All of these species of course are the abnormal functioning of motor tissues.

Art. 287. Sensory Paralysis.

A form of paralysis in which there is incoordination of the special sense organs.

This does not pertain to General Sense, which is never abnormal.

Some species:

S+, direct, as in hyperesthesia.

S−, direct, as in anesthesia.

S+, and S−, due to many indirect species, as E+, E−, T+, T−, N+, N−, in which the sensory organs are poisoned by an imperfect Serous Circulation. (See Fig. 18 and 27)

S+, due to inflammation, C+.

S−, due to introduced poisons.

Art. 288. Contracture Family.

A form of paralysis in which there is excess contractility in tissues, with special reference to motor tissues.

Some species:

M+, direct, in motor tissue (muscle) due to abnormal motor control. In which the motor tissue is too often in the contracted state; or remains contracted when it should relax; or contracts in unexpected ways and at unexpected times as in Voluntary Muscular Incoordination. In this incoordination the patient sometimes appears mentally deficient but most certainly is not, but has an extraordinary developed will power to manage muscle which will not pull coordinately.

M+, indirect, in motor tissue, due to T+, in which there is too much tonicity, because of excess adrenalin.

M+, indirect, in motor tissue, due to E−, coldness from toxins.

M+, indirect, due to C−, general or local coldness.

O+, direct excessive contractility in any tissue.

Art. 289. Proplapsis Family.

A form of paralysis in which there is lack of Connective Function in any tissue.

Some species:

O—, direct, lack of Connective Function in any tissue.

M—, direct, lack of contractility in muscle tissue, as in flaccid paralysis.

M—, indirect, due to T—, lack of tonicity in motor tissue, as in some kinds of hernia.

O—, indirect, due to T—, lack of Connective Function in connective tissue; ex., weak ligaments in prolapsed uterus.

Other species may be involved indirectly.

Art. 290. Spasms Family.

A form of paralysis in which there is lack of functional or relational control; with special reference to muscles.

Some species:

M+ and M—, direct, due to abnormal motor control, in which muscles are unable to coordinate, producing sudden or extreme contractures with alternate relaxations; or simultaneous contracture in the members of paired muscles.

M+ and M—, indirect, due to C— or E—, resulting in coldness which causes muscle to contract spasmodically. Thermogenesis is due mostly to oxidation of carbon. In some kinds of toxins, as when there is cyanosis, there are not materials in the blood or serum to produce heat.

Art. 291. Fever Family.

A form of paralysis in which there is lack of proper thermogenesis or thermolysis or both.

C+, direct, in calorific organs, as in febrile dis-eases. (Art. 193)

C+, direct locally, as in inflammation.

C—, direct, in calorific organs, as in chills, or chronic coldness.

C—, direct, locally, as in a cold hand or foot, etc.

C+, indirect, due to E—, as in febrile dis-eases. (Art. 193)

Other species may be involved, as N+, N—, T+ T—, etc.

Art. 292. Poison Family.

A form of paralysis in which there is lack of proper elimination, secretion or both.

E—, as in febrile dis-eases. (Art. 193)

E+, as in Dry Man. (Art. 160)

E—, as in Wet Man. (Art. 159)

T+, E—, or Y+, as in epilepsy. (Art. 192)

N+, as in Seredema. (Art. 161)

E—, as in Uredema. (Art. 162)

Other species that produce poisons in the body, or introduce them into the body may be said to be species of this family.

Art. 293. Anemia Family.

A form of paralysis in which there is abnormal nutrition, reparation, or lack of repletion.

Some species:

N—, due to lack of nutrition, as in emaciation. Either because food has not been supplied to the body or because it has not been prepared for assimilation properly by digestion and secretion.

N—, or T—, as in acromegaly. In which cells do not have the proper food for assimilation, either because they are lacking in food supply or because they are not supplied by secretory organs, or prepared by secretory organs.

R—, direct, as in a withered limb. Cells are depleted from direct or indirect subluxations. Also the said organ, as a muscle, may be depleted from lack of use and until brought to normal by normal exercise, (Art. 176) is anemic.

N—, as in atrophy, direct, depletion because of lack of metabolistic mental impulses.

Art. 294. Tumor Family.

A form of paralysis in which there is a growth of cells not physiologically used by Innate; cells not required in the body for coordination.

Some species:

X+, as in osteoma.

R+, as in goitre.

N+, as in fatty tumors. (See Seredema, Art. 161)

T+, as in cystic tumors.

E—, as in wens, etc.

Chiropractically, one cell too many is a tumor. But where there is one, there are apt to be more, and these generally are encysted. Real tumors are due to hyperactivity of expansional centers, hence X+ or R+. It represents lack of control of the birth of cells, consequently new cells are made not according to Innate's plan. (See Arts. 69 to 78) Then such cells are present in the body, using the good serum that is intended for the other cells—in fact, drones. Since they have no coordinate connection they are functionless. If Innate has a chance, she will "kick them out," but is prevented by subluxations which caused them in the first place. Therefore Innate does the next best thing, and that is, to "fence them off," segregate them from the useful parts of the body, over which she does have full control. As long as these cells can "steal" nutrition and other benefits of "good society," they thrive as benign tumors; but if they should be subjected to the hardships of N—, C+, and R—, then they become malignant tumors. If with the constant degeneration of the tumor cells, new cells of the same kind are

constantly being made to die and decay, then it is what is called a cancer.

Art. 295. DEGENERATION FAMILY.

A form of paralysis in which there is decomposition of tissue; decay.

Its only specie is (N—C+R—) to which E— is sometimes added.

The term is not used exactly as it is in the dictionary or in medical books but is used in a specific sense, meaning decay or decomposition. N—, the tissue cell dies (actually) from lack of nutrition; C+, the cell decomposes because of the heat; R—, it is not removed promptly if at all. Owing to interference with transmission, the only attention that Innate can give to this condition is by means of her little soldiers, the leucocytes and lymphocytes, who die bravely in combating the impurities of the necrosis, and their dead bodies form pus. The cells of tumors may be subject to the same process and in that case are called malignant tumors. Such a dis-ease as Degeneration, as well as Anemia, etc., is likely due to impingement on metabolistic (vegetative) nerves.

REVIEW QUESTIONS FOR ARTICLES 286 to 295, inclusive.

1. What is Paralysis?
2. What is Motor Paralysis?
3. Give its direct species. Its indirect species.
4. What is Sensory Paralysis?
5. Is General Sense ever paralyzed?
6. Give the direct species. The indirect species.
7. What is Contracture Family?
8. Give direct species. Indirect species.
9. What is Prolapsis Family?
10. In what tissue may prolapsis, according to the Chiropractic idea, occur?
11. What is Spasms Family?
12. Give direct species. Indirect species.
13. What is Fever Family?
14. Give direct species. Indirect species.

15. Give a common example of general C+ condition.
16. What is Poison Family?
17. What is Anemia Family?
18. What is Tumor Family?
19. According to Chiropractic, what constitutes a tumor?
20. What is the character of tumor cells?
21. What is Degeneration Family?
22. What is its only specie?
23. When "benign" tumor cells are subjected to "NCR" what do they become?
24. Give the Philosophy of cancer.

Art. 296. Analysis.

Chiropractic Analysis is the process of finding which subluxation or subluxations to adjust, according to Major Methods.

The classification of effects with the view of finding the cause.

Or finding the cause without the formality of classification of effects.

Methods: the art of using palpation, nerve tracing, taut and tender fibers, spinograph, meric system, equations, and the Neurocalometer.

Since the use of the N.C.M. has an art and a technic all its own, and is taken care of by another department, we will have to leave this very direct method, and explain the older round-about method, which Chiropractic has used for many years.

Art. 297. The Philosophy of Major Work.

Major Methods is the concentration of the material resources of the body on one abnormal condition at a time.

"Shot-gun" adjusting lowers the Constructive Survival Value in the body. It has long been observed, clincally, that adjusting too many subluxations or adjusting too often makes the patient very weak and if carried to excess is very harmful. The reparation required in getting well is just as exhaustive as any other form of extreme adaptation; as getting acclimated, spring fever, extreme physical exertions, extreme mental work, mental shock, worry and the like. (Arts. 133, 134, 195, 196.)

It is not a question of forces, Innate can get plenty of them to supply the body in general. It is not a question of "scattering" Innate's forces, but a scattering of reparatory materials to too many places, calling upon all well tissue cells which are in the business of rendering reparatory service, tiring them and using the available materials which they have on hand and not giving them sufficient time to prepare more. By adjusting one Local and its attendant Conditions, the material resources of the body can be directed to one place at a time and this will be no great drain upon Reparatory function. The other subluxations, which are the causes of less severe incoordinations can wait until the Major Condition is well cleared and then the worst of them can be attended to next. In this way the Reparatory organs have sufficient time to prepare reparatory materials; time is given to bring into the body, new food materials, digest them, prepare them and use them. If this is not done, the extreme adaptation will cause Innate to deprive other cells of the body, which are in no way connected with the disorder, of their constructive values; make them give up some of the things which they have and which they should retain, to "make up a relief for the sufferers." This weakens and depletes all body cells, and therefore the whole body. This must be restored. The appetite of a convalescent is well known. Sometimes this extreme use of constructive values and "terrific" appetite is observed in growing children.

Art. 298. Major Condition.

The major Condition of a case is that which is most vital to the health or life of the patient.

It has reference to effects which usually are indicated by the symptoms of dis-ease.

It is the effects of a cause or causes; a subluxation or subluxations.

A case can have only one Major Condition at a time.

Art. 299. MAJOR.

A Major is the subluxation or subluxations causing the Major Condition.

It refers to the cause of the effects; the cause of dis-ease.

A case can have only one Major at a time.

A Major which usually has both Local and Condition, has one or more subluxations. Usually one for the Local and one or more for Condition. (Art. 130)

Art. 300. MINOR CONDITION.

A Minor Condition of a case is an abnormal condition which is not so vital to the health or life of the patient as the Major Condition.

When the Major Condition has been restored to normal the worst Minor Condition becomes major, automatically.

A case can have more than one Minor condition at a time.

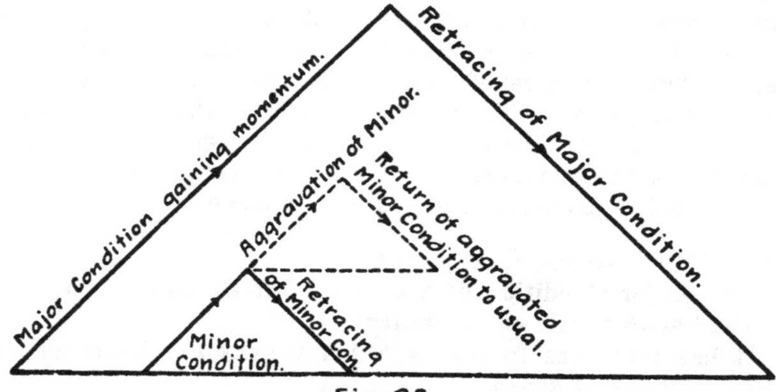

Fig. 28.

A minor condition is not adaptative (compensatory) to a Major Condition, though it may be aggravated by the Major Condition. (See Fig. 28)

A Minor Condition has its own causes in the spine, and adjusting the Major does not remove the Minor.

Art. 301. MINORS.

A Minor is the subluxation or subluxations causing the Minor Condition.

It refers to the cause or causes of effects; the cause or causes of dis-ease.

A case can have more than one Minor at a time.

A Minor, also, has Local and Condition, and therefore has one or more subluxations. One for Local, usually, and one or more for Condition.

Art. 302. THE FACTORS OF MAJORS AND MINORS.

A Major has direct and indirect effects. The direct effects are due to interference on the local nerve supply. The indirect conditions are generally due to interference with transmission affecting the Serous Circulation. Therefore a Major usually has one, two or more subluxations. Sometimes one subluxation makes both direct and indirect effects. The subluxation causing the direct effect is called Local, or Location. The subluxation or subluxations, causing the indirect conditions, is called Condition.

A Major having local and Condition is a Combination Major, and most Majors are of that kind.

Adaptative (Compensatory) conditions are indirect, and should never be adjusted for, directly.

Some indirect conditions are caused by indirect impingements, (as pressure upon a nerve by tumor) but the cause of the pressure is itself caused by a subluxation in the spine (Prin. 31)

Conditions	Direct	....	Majors have them. Minors have them.
	Indirect	Adaptative	Majors have them. Minors have them.
		Not adaptative..	Majors have them. Minors have them.

Art. 303. Rules of Major Methods. (Page 50, Majors and Minors)

If the patient is feeling better but getting weaker, he is over-adjusted. (Art. 297)

If the patient is feeling worse but getting stronger, he is retracing. (Art. 297)

Never adjust a chronic case oftener than once every twenty-four hours. (Art. 297)

The rule of acuteness or chronicity (as to time) is determined by the palpable "hot box" in the spine, (See The Art of Chiropractic) or by the tenderness of Taut Fibers.

The rule of degree of effect is determined by the tenderness of nerves emitting from the subluxation.

The rule of area (place of) is ascertained by the use of the Meric System.

The rule of the major and minor subluxations is proven by the equational system.

"The less you adjust the oftener you can. The more you adjust the less you should." That is, if your combination contains three subluxations or more you should not adjust oftener than every other day, or three times a week, and in some cases only once or twice a week. If your Major has only one or two places, then you may adjust every day for a time.

If your Major has only one or two places, then you may include a Minor, if it does not have too many subluxations.

The location of a headache will determine the inferior zone in which coordination exists. (Arts. 222, 223)

The degree of the headache determines the degree of effect which determines the degree or acuteness of incoordination in the inferior zone.

Review Questions for Articles 296 to 303, inclusive.

1. What is Chiropractic Analysis?
2. What two ways are there of finding the cause?
3. Give the Philosophy of Major Work.
4. What is a Major Condition?
5. What is a Major?
6. What is a Minor Condition?
7. What is a Minor?
8. What is a Combination Major or a Combination Minor?
9. What is a direct condition?
10. What is an indirect condition?
11. What is a Compensatory (adaptative) Condition?
12. Is a Minor Condition adaptative or compensatory to a Major Condition?
13. When does a Minor Condition become a Major Condition?
14. What indirect conditions may be produced by pressures in the tissues instead of in the spine?
15. What is the cause of such indirect pressures?
16. Give and explain each of the Rules of Major Methods.

Note:—The student is advised to read the Article on Etiology in the back of this book. It is a practical continuation of the discussion of analysis begun in Junior Text.

Senior Text

The Senior Textbook is an elaboration of the Principles of Chiropractic, and advanced work in theory and practical phases.

Art. 304. Dates.

The history of Chiropractic is really the history of adjustments. Quotation from Volume IV:

"Although Chiropractic was not so named until 1896, yet the naming of 'Chiropractic' was much like the naming of a baby; it was nine months old before it was named. Chiropractic, in the beginning of the thoughts upon which it was named, dates back at least five years previous to 1895. During those five years, as I review many of these writings, I find they talk about various phases of that which now constitutes some of the phases of our present day philosophy, showing that my father was thinking along and towards those lines which eventually, suddenly crystallized in the accidental case of Harvey Lillard, after which it sprung suddenly into fire and produced the white hot blaze." (B. J. Palmer)

As Chiropractic grew, other important things useful in Chiropractic were discovered: Palpation, between 1898 and 1900; Nerve Tracing, 1905; Meric System, 1909; Spinograph, 1910, Taut and Tender Fibers, 1922; Neurocalometer, 1924. (Note—I heard B. J. explain Taut Fibers in 1920 in his classes, as if it were then old to him. But no one seemed to pay much attention to it until in 1922, when he began to emphasize it; so, 1922 is the date usually mentioned. R. W. S.)

Art. 305. History of Adjusting.

I prefer to quote B. J. Palmer in "Majors and Minors," page 7, in order to tell the History of Adjustments:

"The first patient who received a Chiropractic adjustment

was Harvey Lillard, a colored man. The incident, in brief, follows. He had been deaf 17 years, so much so that from the Fourth Floor of the building where he was janitor he could not hear wagons moving or street cars rolling on the streets below. When asked how he became deaf, his explanation follows: 'While in a cramped, stooped position, I felt and heard something pop in my back. Immediately, I went deaf.' To one who was observant, a student, that would be an accidental eye-opener, and it was to D. D. Palmer who asked, 'What is the connection between the back and hearing in the ears?' He examined the back. By good fortune, the first case in which a spine was examined with that thought in view, a LARGE bump was found. It was not one of the common bumps we see today in palpation, but so prominent it could be seen with the eye.

"The following consequential reasoning occurred. If there was no bump when the hearing was good, and the production of this bump destroyed hearing, why don't the reduction of the bump restore hearing? The first attempt to correct, what is now a subluxation, was then made. The patient was put upon the floor, face down, and a shove-like movement given. The "bump" was reduced by the first three shoves, and in three days hearing was restored. Harvey could hear a watch tick at the average distance you and I can today.

"The next question was, if the reduction of one bump in one man restores hearing, why won't a similar bump, in other people, produce deafness, and if it does, why wouldn't the reduction of these bumps, in the same way, restore their hearing? It was tried on others. By a peculiar series of circumstances, the results did not come as readily in their cases, but eventually they came.

"Then the third question arose: If a bump in the back caused deafness, why not other parts of the spine produce other dis-ease? So our question has gradually enlarged until by a systematic systemic series of investigations, covering years, you have your Chiropractic of today.

"Education advanced. After a period we ceased calling them 'bumps.' They became 'dislocations.' We, at a later time, were impressed with the idea that this bump was not a dislocation. It was, in reality, not a dislocation but partial, more assuming the character of a luxation, yet not a luxation. It was a subluxation.

"When we had assumed, as a matter of education, that breadth of ideals where they became subluxations, we no longer assumed to shove. We developed the 'push and pull principle,' which was of various forms and methods.

"We began, at a following period, to study the spine from a **MECHANICAL** point of view. Until this time the only people who attempted to study the spine, as a machine, were osteopaths, although pathologically they still regarded man as chemistry and physics.

"We confined our observations of mechanical ideas to the spine, so much so that we brought out the 'Knowledge of the Kinematics of the Spine'; both normal and abnormal, as to position, appósition, and subluxations. We then began the study of the pathological, traumatic and anomalous conditions of the spine. At that time began the gathering of the osteological collection which we now possess, for the purpose of elucidating the theories then held and propagation of others.

"It became necessary that we know the human spine. That was the keynote of the study of **CAUSES** of diseases of man. We studied spines of all characters; thousands of other bones that we might better reach a new thought or idea in progress. How well that has been done you know today. Hours, months, and years were spent in the study of 'dead bones' to be able to give thoughts that may be taught in a few minutes. Yet it took years to reach the conclusions given in a few minutes.

"When we studied the spine, mechanically speaking, we

realized that 'treatment' was far-fetched in its application, as describing the thing we attemped to do. Being a machine, mechanically constructed, mechanically subluxated, it should be mechanically **ADJUSTED.** Then came the word 'adjustment.'

"Approximately six years ago we began a series of clinical tests or investigations from a new viewpoint. I refer to the **Spinograph.** Until that period the X-Ray had not been used in its application to human spines in living individuals for the purpose of ascertaining the approximate detailed apposition of the vertebrae, normal, abnormal and traumatic. When we made our first series of **Spinographs** we were the first to touch this vital question. There existed no previous technique for our observations or work. It became necessary to develop a system of taking spinographs to prove that subluxations existed, where and of what character.

"We began tabulating these observations, which today we are ready to say makes another step. These conclusions are based on the readings and studies of over 50,000 spinographs, all of which were taken in our laboratory with this definite end in view.

"It is no longer sufficient to say that we adjust with the recoil. We are ready for our next step, which you may call '206,' altho I prefer the 'Toggle-Recoil' because of its application by the new series of observations made from the spinographic facts.

"History is 'his-story.' The 'his' in this case being the author who has lived it, been the cause for a large majority of it, therefore the source of the facts here recorded could not be improved." (B. J. Palmer)

Art. 306. Four Viewpoints of Area Adjusted. (From Maj. and Min., page 9.)

"From the question of area of the spine worked upon, there have been four viewpoints in adjusting work:

"1. Ordinarily we shoved but one of the back-bones and our patient got well. All of which was pure accident for we did not know why this place should, neither was there a rule for application. Ask where to shove for this or that and we didn't know. The spine was unexplored territory.

"2. Being unexplored territory, wishing to get our cases well irrespective of what he had, knowing that it came from the spine somewhere, we shoved every back bone at each 'sitting' each day. We began at the 7th cervical and went clear down to the sacrum—we did not shove cervical vertebrae in those days, we were afraid to. We shoved them all, one by one, on the ground that (a) we didn't know where to shove for any one particular trouble; (b) we had no meric system, the spine was not mapped out; (c) therefore hit them all to be sure to hit the one involved. It was not a hit-or-miss proposition, it was a hit-'em-all method, so we couldn't help but get the one involved. It was a case of the lazy man's load; being too indolent to think or reason, we made a shot-gun series of shoves. Much like 'Uncle Howard' Nutting says he 'got the burglar in his house.' He 'started at the garret, went clean down to the cellar, shooting into every corner where a burglar could hide,' therefore 'he was sure he got the burglar.'

"Notwithstanding, this extreme shot-gun method was in vogue in the Chiropractic styles of 1896-7; notwithstanding, a major application of our meric system began in 1898, and the major application went out of style and has been ever since; yet, inconsistent as it now appears, there is one lone advocate in our ranks who insists upon the every-vertebra-adjustment idea today. Not being taught today in any Chiropractic school, not being known by the largest majority of our ranks, it is not known except to the oldest Chiropractors, hence when it is sprung at some meeting, it awakens a bit of interest not because of its reason or logic or brilliancy of deduction, but because of its startling contrasting nature.

"3. The third viewpoint came following the deduction of the radiation of nerves from specific parts of the spine to specific organs of the body. The meric system being the basis, the 'specific system' of adjustment came into vogue. We now adjusted only those subluxations for which the patient had a dis-ease. For example: our case has heart, stomach, liver and bowel troubles. The subluxations—a la meric system—were H. P., S. P., K. P., and P. P. This man instead of getting 17 shoves on the back got but 4, one for each. It eliminated the useless and concentrated on the useful. It was direct, a subluxation for a dis-ease. Thus its title—'specific.'

"4. The fourth viewpoint is our present 'Major and Minors' wherein we even make the 'specific system' a major and minor one in reality. Under this system we classify the symptoms of the four given troubles above and possibly find that two or three of the dis-eases this case has, are adaptative to the one or two subluxations, hence are minors of the major; the adjustment of the latter taking care of the former. (More of this appears later.)

"There have been in reality four periods in the history of Chiropractic 'moves.' **First,** the shove, with its variations from Nos. 1 to 78; **second,** the push and pull, with its changes from Nos. 70 to 200; **third,** the recoil, with its modes from Nos. 201 to 205; **fourth,** the period of the toggle-recoil or '206'." (B. J. Palmer)

Art. 307. The Palmer Toggle Recoil.

The Palmer Toggle Recoil, No. 206, is still being used as the one specific and best "move" which accomplishes the greatest percentage of adjustments. However, since the time the above was written by B. J., the New Posture, or Knee Posture, or Palmer Posture, came into use as a new phase, about 1922. It is Dr. Palmer's opinion, supported by the Faculty of The

P. S. C., that it is the best posture for the patient, which, used with No. 206, is the best combination to date. (See The Art of Chiropractic, textbook of The Palmer School of Chiropractic.)

Art. 308. HOW CHIROPRACTIC WAS NAMED.

Chiropractic was named by Dr. Samuel H. Weed, a minister well versed in ancient languages. Chiropractic is a word composed for the Greek; *cheir* meaning the hand, and *praktos* meaning done; hence, done by hand. Chiropractic has always run true to its name. The chiropractor adjusts subluxations, with his hands only, and therefore must have dexterity and skill. This is art.

Art. 309.. THE MAJOR PREMISE. **Principle No. 1** (Art. 24)

Universal Intelligence is in all matter and continually gives to it all its properties and actions.

Since it is universal it is common to every locality. Therefore, it is in anything and everything that is in the same locality. In the beginning it created matter; it did not, then, abandon matter but creates or unfolds thoughts for it every moment. This solicitude maintains matter in existence. The physical "properties" which matter has, are but force (energy) continually given to it by intelligence. In a like manner, the quality that matter is said to possess, is what intelligence is giving it. Life, as Chiropractic sees it, is a quality or character that matter may have, occasioned by the presence of, or attention of intelligence, having continuation or duration, involving time. (See Webster). No lesser agency than Universal Intelligence can prevent any of these things but the perfect expression of intelligence, according to what man wants, may be prevented by the limitations of matter. Even this is a universal law and is a phase of the Universal Cycle.

Life is combination of intelligence, force, and matter. Matter makes up the material universe—intelligence is the immaterial universe, and force is what binds them together. We perceive force as forms of energy.

Matter is that which fills space and its function is to express force. It does not fill all space, but there is no limit to the places you may find it. You may travel in space (if you could) for an unlimited time, and no matter how far you got, you would find material. The amount of it is infinite. "Infinite" means having no limit—no boundaries. "Universal" means everywhere—common to every locality. Therefore, being infinite and everywhere, we use the term Universe. If you subtract from the material universe, any amount you wish to name—no matter how large—it would not diminish the total amount. That is what infinity means.

The Immaterial Universe is the Intelligence that made all this. It, too, is everywhere, and therefore it is in all matter. It created everything, so it must have "known how" infinitely, and is all-wise. It is stronger than the strongest thing it made; and older, for it was there first. It is omnipotent, and unlimited. It fills all time, space, and distance.

The definitions of Chiropractic give it plenty of latitude in the realm of things universal. Therefore we are able to go back to the most fundamental principle of all; to "get our backs against the wall," so to speak, and know that we are starting at the beginning. To question this fundamental is to be like the child who turns a picture over to see it from the back, or asks who made God.

Art. 310. The Chiropractic Meaning of Life.
Principle No. 2.

The expression of intelligence through matter is the Chiropractic meaning of life.

The meaning of the term *life* has many interpretations. It is usually accepted to mean existence, or duration, or a vague idea of both. To Chiropractic, it is definitely the expression of intelligence; the manifestation of intelligence. Then in this broad sense the meaning is not limited to mere organic matter, but includes all matter. Therefore, we will be obliged to make a deductive classification, going from the general to the specific, (Art. 12) and deal with the specific; viz., universal life and organic life.

Art. 311. The Union of Intelligence and Matter. Principle No. 3.

Life is necessarily the union of intelligence and matter.

Without intelligence, matter could not even exist. Without matter, intelligence could not be expressed. We are never aware of motion unless we perceive matter moving. The study of physics shows us that some form of energy gets into matter to make it move. Without this energy, matter is inert. The study of physics also shows us that no matter is totally inert; therefore it always has some energy in it. Energy must have an origin. From its character of precision and accuracy, we deduce that its origin is intelligence—nothing less. These facts from which we derive our conclusions are axioms—can be perceived everywhere. Our recognition of the intelligence of life or of motion in matter depends upon our ability to recognize law.

Art. 312. The Triunity of Life.

Life is a Triunity having three necessary united factors; viz., intelligence, force, and matter.

Without intelligence, matter could not even exist. Without matter, intelligence could not be expressed. Then there is a bond between intelligence and matter that cannot be dispensed with. These three factors; intelligence, matter, and the bond between them, are inseparable. The bond is called force. It is sometimes called "The Missing Link." Unlike other sciences, which study them separately, Chiropractic studies them all together. From this fundamental arises Dr. Palmer's comparison and his epigram. (See Art. 20.)

Art. 313. The Perfection of the Triunity. **Principle No. 5.**

In order to have one hundred per cent life, there must be one hundred per cent of intelligence, one hundred per cent of force, one hundred per cent of matter.

It is obvious that the three factors of the triunity are inseparable; they are not separable in part, if one hundred per cent perfection is to be maintained. Since intelligence is always one hundred per cent perfect, and always creates one hundred per cent of force, **it is certain that if any imperfections of the triunity exist,** (clinical findings show that they do exist) **that matter is the only part of the triunity that can be imperfect.** Since matter cannot be destroyed by any lesser agency than the Creator, it is obvious that this imperfection is not in matter itself, but in the quantity, quality, and arrangement of matter. Hence, **there are limitations in structures of matter;** in its imperfect building; its imperfect arrangements; the wrong kind of matter for the purpose or even the lack of matter which should be in that structure but is not. From this fact arises the expression so often used fundamentally in Chiropractic. **The expression of intelligence may be hindered by the limitations of matter.**

Art. 314. The Principle of Time. **Principle No. 6.**

There is no process which does not require time.

Since action of matter implies a procession of events, a continuity, naturally time enters into the triunity as an element. Time is an element necessary to the bond between intelligence and matter. Force is a word implying action; action is process. Action implies one event after another. One event after another, forming a series, implies time. No happening, even though it takes only a moment, but happens in a unit of time, or a fraction of a unit of time.

Art. 315. The Amount of Intelligence in Matter. Principle No. 7.

The amount of intelligence for any given unit of matter is always one hundred per cent, and is always proportional to its requirements.

There are any number of instances in the existence of matter which prove that it has the requisite amount of attention from the Creator. That requisite amount is enough and no more. It is, therefore, the perfect amount—one hundred per cent. "Amount" means perfection, and that is what is needed for the maintenance of the unit as it is. No power less than the Creator could deprive a unit of matter of its share of intelligence; but the limitations of matter may prevent the expression of that intelligence. The "amount" that one unit has, may be less than that which another unit has, but is always one hundred per cent for that particular unit. This holds true in both organic and inorganic matter.

Art. 316. The Function of Intelligence. Principle No. 8

The Function of Intelligence is to create force.

Everything in the universe has a purpose; that purpose is its function. Intelligence is in the universe, therefore it has a function. It is evident that the function of intelligence is to think. Thinking is the origin of force. Creating is the thinking or unfolding of thoughts. The force of thought is the greatest of all forces, for it is really the fundamental of all energies; of all dynamics.

Art. 317. Mind. (116 to 125 V)

Mind is the activity of Innate Intelligence in the brain as an organ.

The introduction of thought into matter via the brain. (Prin. 3, 8, 10, 13.)

Chiropractic maintains that Innate Intelligence is the power which governs the body; is the ego itself. You are your Innate Intelligence, and your Innate Intelligence is you. If you claim that you are master of your Innate, that is a mistaken assumption of values and is the same as Innate belittling herself. Surely, Innate would never do this; but when it appears that she does, it is a mis-expression. (Prin. 24)

Mind is the term applied to what intelligence does when it is at work.

Innate Mind and Educated Mind are terms used to indicate the kind of work being done.

When Innate does not work, there is no mind.

Let us compare a musician to the Power; his instrument to the brain, and music to mind. When the musician plays on his instrument, as an organ of expression, there is music. When the musician ceases playing, there is no music expressed.

In Chiropractic, the term *mind* is considered a little differently than it is in psychology. In psychology, one mind is considered in two divisions—conscious and subconscious, with no definite division between them. Psychology considers that this mind is the governing intellect and implies that while the subconscious mind may govern metabolism and the like, the conscious mind is your ego; is really the master. We gather from the teachings of psychology, which is based upon a materialistic view, that one can willfully govern his own destinies, even to the extent of healing.

Chiropractic does not use the terms *conscious mind* and *subconscious mind* at all, for there is absolutely no application of these terms to anything Chiropractic. Chiropractic Philosophy is not a study of psychology, any more than it is of chemistry or physics. Chiropractic recognizes and honors all the *findings* of the psychologist as it does that of the physicist. It makes use of these findings as it does those of the physicist and agrees with psychology as long as it is consistent with Chiropractic. In other words, there is a Chiropractic psychology, which is the study of the mind.

All the psychology that is considered in Chiropractic can be studied under the division called "Mental," the third step of the Cycle.

Art. 318. Innate Mind. (125 V)

Innate Mind is the activity of Innate Intelligence in the innate brain as an organ.

The product of this activity is Innate thoughts or mental force.

The act or business of assembling forces in Innate brain.

Even when "she" uses educated brain, she first uses innate brain. (See Fig. 4.)

If Innate ceased giving attention to a tissue cell one single instant, that tissue cell would either act incoordinately, be poisoned, or be bodily injured.

All of these dangers being made are by the unadapted universal forces present in all matter. (Prin. 1, 11.)

This attention is given in the form of mental impulses, which are adapted forces, to cause the tissue cell to act in an adaptative manner and thus escape or overcome the dangers, however slight. Therefore, the innate brain must be used every instant by Innate and consequently, Innate mind is in existence all the time. (If the musician plays all the time, there will be music all the time.)

Art. 319. Educated Mind.

Educated Mind is the activity of Innate Intelligence in the educated brain as an organ.

The product of this activity is educated thoughts; such as, **reasoning, will, memory, etc.**

Innate controls the functions of the "voluntary" organs via the educated brain. (*See diagram, Fig. 4.*)

Educated thoughts are mostly for adaptation to things external to the body.

Educated thoughts are never outwardly expressed until Innate does it through Innate brain; for instance, one may have a thought, but be unable to express it vocally, if Innate is unable to operate the organs of speech owing to interference with transmission of mental impulses. In any case, we should not know how to operate the organs of speech even though we can will them to act. The educated thoughts may be kept within the brain and as Chiropractic says, expressed there, but which psychologists say make a physiological change in the tissue of the brain. We see no reason why we should not agree with this theory.

In the last analysis, all educated thoughts; education, will, memory, reasoning, etc., are for adaptation to things external to the body.

They are for welfare, comfort, betterment and safety to the body. Though we sit down in an easy chair and read a book, go to a show, these, after all, are processes of education which are for a more competent adaptation to environment. The fact that it may give us pleasure, does not detract from the fact, for successful adaptations always give pleasure; it is a natural psychological law.

The reason that man ranks the highest among living things is because he possesses an organ for that class of adaptations more highly developed than those of others.

"Voluntary" movements are those caused by Innate which conform to or are influenced by the number of times that movement has been made before. In other words, it is an educated movement; and its efficiency is dependent upon experience in doing that thing.

The term *voluntary* has reference to the will.

Voluntary movements are those we educationally will to do.

Analyzation shows us that this is Innate adapting a move to "synthetic" environment; to a group of "stored-up" percepts; instead of immediately fresh ones. For example, we decide to take a walk. The decision came from no outside influence, but it was born of a group of feelings or thoughts which we had experienced before.

We do not use the terms *voluntary* and *involuntary* because they imply that something might be involuntary to Innate Intelligence, which is impossible.

Art. 320. The Philosophy of Education. (*See Webster for education and percept.*)

The Philosophy of Education is that every experience and percept is stored away in the brain, in a manner not well understood by any science.

Education is the term applied to the amount of stored-up experiences and percepts.

Reasoning is the present comparisons and classifications of stored-up experiences together with present percepts and experiences.

Memory is a new mental adaptation to old percepts and experiences.

Will is mental or physical adaptation to a new grouping of old percepts and experiences, usually influenced by the present.

Knowledge is the term applied to stored-up educational values when they are so classified and grouped as to be readily useful.

Wisdom is the term applied to mental skill in classification and comparison of educational values together with present percepts; "common sense."

Instinct is the initial small amount of experience recorded

in the brain for a "nest-egg." Living things blessed with very much of this have little ability to accumulate anything new.

A genius is one who has an unusually augmented group of educational values centered around one phase of human activity; or has this group instinctively developed to start with.

The usefulness of educated mind to Innate depends upon the amount of experiences stored away and present ability to group these experiences. An old man may have gone through many experiences, but stored few percepts. In that case, he has small education. Again, an old man may have stored away many percepts, but owing to illness, childishness, or other incoordinations, may be unable to make adequate present comparisons. A feeble minded person, being born that way, would be unable to store many percepts, so experience would avail him but little. In that case, it is probable that the brain tissue is defective or deficient, so that Innate has not adequate material to work with. (Prin. 24.)

Innate does not record in the brain all that she knows, or all that she does in the body. In fact, only a small portion is recorded. The amount that Innate can record is limited by the brain tissue, even in the best of brains. Thus, Innate's expression is limited by the limitations of matter. (Prin. 5, 24.) To express infinite wisdom, Innate would require infinite brain tissue. Therefore the educated mind is finite and also limited to a lifetime, at the end of which the material records are "returned to dust."

Educated minds probably have very few entirely original thoughts. They are so bound by instinct, habit, precedent, and the limitations of matter, the influences of environment containing thousands of similar influences and combinations of circumstances, that few minds are peculiar enough (literally they *are* peculiar), to lead off into untrammelled pathways, What they do is new to them and new to contemporaneous minds and so it is said to be entirely new. Perhaps it is; perhaps no human mind ever thought of it before, but it is certain that it is not new to any Innate. Universal Intelligence knows it, and Innate as a part of Universal knows anything that is and will be pertaining to the matter in her care. Therefore, what man invents is well known to Intelligence and would likely have been expressed before, had the same happy physical and circumstantial combinations existed before.

Art. 321. Consciousness. (127, 314 V) (Webster.)

Consciousness means awareness.

The present process of classification and comparison of percepts by Innate Intelligence.

Innate mind is active and aware all the time and receives all impressions.

(Note—a percept is an educational impression.)

Educated mind is aware part of the time; Innate records and compares percepts there during waking moments.

The term "awareness" or "consciousness" is better understood when applied to educated mind.

Innate receives impressions in innate brain all the time, but while we sleep, these, even the ones from the special senses, are not recorded. When we are awake, the reports from the special senses, and many others, are recorded, more or less definitely, and we are able to recall most of them, if the occasion and combination of circumstances are favorable.

For example, if we commit to memory a piece of poetry, and then "forget it," and twenty years later commit it to memory again, it will seem vaguely familiar, and "learning it by heart" is easier than it was the first time.

Again: if we hear a band play a certain piece of music, and if we notice the strains at all, even without interest, the same strains will sound familiar years afterward, and may even call back a visualization of the place where it was heard.

Art. 322. Unconsciousness. (314 V)

Unconsciousness is the lack or absence of functional activity in educated brain.

Metabolistic activity, however, is not necessarily lacking.

Normal unconsciousness is the normal withdrawal of functional activity by Innate; as, in sleep.

Abnormal unconsciousness is the condition when there is a lack or absence of functional activity, not brought about by Innate, but due to interference with transmission of mental impulses, trauma, or poisoning.

There is no unconsciousness in innate brain as long as there is life in the body.

Normal unconsciousness, as sleep, is necessary and beneficial. It is the natural method of Innate to relax the body and brain and relieve them from all educated function which is very wearing and productive of waste materials. It is a sort of "moratorium" allowing time for tissues to be cleansed, repaired, and brought up to their full status of construction.

Abnormal unconsciousness, as abnormal sleep or coma, is not natural; is not beneficial, and is not brought about by Innate. It is not in any way desirable to Innate, and while in that state the tissues of the body and brain are being deprived of Innate's ministrations and sometimes are damaged beyond repair.

Art. 323. Specific Phases of Unconsciousness. (313 to 320 V)

Sleep is a normal unconsciousness as an adaptive act for bodily reparation.

Dreaming is an abnormal activity of some educated brain cells during sleep.

Sleep, if it is normal, is accompanied by perfect relaxation and is a complete resting of the educated brain. If, however, there is some interference with transmission, and perhaps poisons in the Serous Circulation due to poor elimination, indigestion, or other incoordinations, some of the educated brain cells are not resting as they should be and are acting when Innate does not wish them to do so. This pseudo-functioning is not caused by Innate, but by poisons keeping the cells awake. (229, 317 V)

Since all the brain is not awake and there is not perfect intercommunication between all cells, perfect ideation is not obtained, and their concepts are apt to be sketchy and erratic, hence the fantasy of dreams. From this it can be seen that dreams are mild mental insanity. (316 V)

If a large enough section of the educated brain is awake, with the rest of the educated brain asleep, it is possible to get a connected train of thought on one line; consequently, some remarkably clear thinking sometimes is accomplished in dreams. As, when a student who has been worrying about a mathematical problem, easily solves it in a dream. The working section is not bothered by other influences and is able to be used in concentrated thinking.

Sleep talking is a form of dreaming in which the center from which the organs of speech are governed is awake.

If no reasoning centers are awake at the same time the "talking" is apt to be mere gibberish, there being no thoughts to utter.

Sleep walking is a form of dreaming in which the centers from which the locomotive organs are governed are awake.

This may or may not be accompanied by wakefulness of some reasoning or talking centers.

Fainting is a form of unconsciousness due to sudden anemia of the brain; sometimes adaptive and sometimes not.

If it is adaptative, it is a protective measure by Innate to rescue from sudden or violent physical or mental stress. If it is not adaptive, it is not a condition desired by Innate, and is in no way beneficial and may even be dangerous.

Coma is a form of unconsciousness, strictly abnormal, and is often a symptom of approaching death.

In a profound coma it is impossible to wake the patient and death soon ensues. There are other forms of coma not fatal but always serious, in which it is possible to wake the patient, but with considerable effort. (See Symptomatology.)

Narcotic sleep is an abnormal sleep due to paralysis of educated brain tissues by poisons. (315, 308, V)

Hypnotic sleep is a state of unconsciousness induced by relaxation. (315 V)

Normal sleep is accompanied by relaxation. Profound sleep—perfect relaxation. No educated thought—no educated expression. To reverse this process, as we can see many such reversals in nature, perfect relaxation is accompanied by sleep. No need for educated expression, therefore there are no educated thoughts; a law of cause and effect and adaptation. The will is the first to succumb. Hypnotism is accomplished by monotony. Monotony, by its sameness, calling forth a long succession of identical adaptations, induces relaxation and sleep follows. This is accomplished usually through the sense of hearing and of sight. To gaze fixedly for a long time will induce hypnotism. A monotonous sound, as the hum of a dynamo will also act the same. The hypnotist makes use of both of these, also of suggestion.

Art. 324. Mental Insanity. (316 V)

Mental insanity is unsound mind due to unsound educated brain cells.

Incoordination in educated brain.

"Dreaming in greater degree" (Palmer).

"Just as the different tissues of the body are dependent upon nutrition for the proper performance of their functions, so is the educated brain." (Palmer)

The educated brain tissues can be made unsound by interference with transmission of metabolistic impulses (*see vegetative impulses in* 317 V; 286 *Morat*; 281 *Pottenger*) which make them susceptible to poisons in the Serous Circulation. If these cells are unsound they cannot function properly and coordinately, hence their product, thought, will be unsound.

The term *insane* is used synonymously with *unsound* in Chiropractic. To speak of insanity does not mean mental insanity, necessarily, in Chiropractic. When it is necessary to indicate the latter, the two words, *mental insanity* are used. We also speak of *physical insanity* meaning unsoundness of any tissue cell. The common, or medical usage of the term insanity is to indicate mental insanity only. The student is cautioned to be sure to learn this difference in the use of terminology.

Art. 325. The Amount of Force Created by Intelligence. Principle No. 9.

The Amount of Force Created by Intelligence is always one hundred per cent.

Force is an immaterial thing; there is nothing to prevent intelligence from creating all it wants of it. But intelligence being perfect, therefore incapable of incorrect action, creates the requisite amount—no more, no less. The amount of force created by Innate in the brain cell is the proper amount to perform a specific act—no more, no less—hence one hundred per cent. The amount created a moment later for the same tissue cell, may not be as much or the same quality, but would be exactly suitable for the occasion. This shows the law of adaptation.

Art. 326. The Function of Force. Principle No. 10.

The Function of Force is to unite intelligence and matter.

We would never know there is such a thing as intelligence, since it is abstract, unless it is shown to us by matter; that is, expressed. Matter cannot exist without the attention of intelligence. Structures of matter cannot exist without the building forces of intelligence. Structures of matter cannot continue to exist without the maintenance by intelligence. This is accomplished by the application of force by intelligence. Thus force is the connecting link or bond between intelligence and matter.

Art. 327. The Character of Universal Forces. Principle No. 11.

The forces of Universal Intelligence are manifested as physical laws; are unswerving and unadapted and have no solicitude for structures of matter.

Bodies actuated by physical forces will not go one iota out of their way to dodge anything in their paths. Things actuated by these forces may be injured or destroyed by their rigor. There is not the slightest variation of their amounts, qualities, or direction in order to protect a single thing. They are antipodal to adapted forces. However, the student must not conclude from this, that Universal Intelligence is maliciously destructive. It is but the working of the great cycle; the plan of Universal Intelligence that this be so, in order to maintain life. Universal Intelligence, by putting localized portions of itself in matter, builds up structures in order that there may be something to tear down. What would happen eventually, if no structure was ever torn down? It is clear that creation would cease and there could be no further life; for structures must be destroyed in order that living things continue to live. A little thought will show us that every bit of food we eat or have eaten is organic matter, vegetable or animal, it matters not which, both have had Innates and have been deprived of their lives in order that we might live! Another thought; suppose all the people who have lived in all the thousands of years were living now, is it not possible that the entire surface of the earth would be covered several layers deep with their bodies?

Let us compare your watch to one of Innate's structures for an analogy. This watch is made of molecules and atoms which are just as valuable to Universal Intelligence in the elemental state as they are in a structural state. The structure, however, was of value to the factory which made it, and is to you, who possess it. In the hands of both, it gets extreme care. You do not trust it to the tender (?) mercies of universal laws by leaving it outdoors in all kinds of weather; by putting it in water or letting it fall. You keep it carefully in your pocket, suspended on a chain, or in its case. At every instant of its structural existence, you keep it in a safe place and see that it is repaired when it needs it. To be convinced of what universal laws will do to a tissue cell, a structure valued by Innate, you should take your watch, a structure valued by you, and hold it over a hard floor or stone and let the law of gravity have it for a fraction of a second.

Art. 328. INTERFERENCE WITH TRANSMISSION OF UNIVERSAL FORCE. **Principle No. 12.**

There can be interference with the transmission of universal forces.

The phenomena of Universal Forces are common, and its interference is too common to be discussed at great length. A tree makes shade when the sun shines; lead plates interfere with X-rays; brass stops magnetism; rubber and glass interfere with the passage of electricity, etc., etc. Whether these forces be radiant or conducted, there is a way to interfere with them. If they are being conducted through material, a gap in the conductor will stop their flow; and a diminishing of the size of the conductor will diminish the amount which gets through. As swiftly as the energies travel in the radiant form and with apparent ease, they all prefer to pause, enter, and be conducted by matter. If this were not true, we could have no electricity for use, no compasses, no radio sets, no shade for comfort, and no sunburns. Each of these energies has a preference for certain kinds of matter. Having these well established facts about natural phenomena, then is it not reasonable to suppose Innate's forces might be radiant, but like other forms of energy, prefer a conductor and have a preference for the kind of conductor, which is nerve tissue? And, if this is true, is it not reasonable to suppose, though we cannot see this mental energy, that the impingement of this living conductor will interfere with the flow? It is true; it is no longer in the realm of theory; it has been proven time and again, when adjustments have gotten sick people well.

Art. 329. THE FUNCTION OF MATTER. **Principle No. 13.**

The Function of Matter is to express force.

Nowhere in the Universe can there be matter that does not receive the caretaking of Universal Intelligence. The Great Intelligence keeps it up to date every moment and no bit of material is without its share of vibration for the creative thinking of Universal Power is transformed into what we know as forms of energy. We are never aware of these forces until they are expressed by matter. You cannot perceive a motion unless matter does it, and matter will not move, unless a form of energy gets into it. The same may be said of other forms of energy that we know in our study of physics; such as, heat, light, and electricity. These forms are all interchangeable, hence life is but vibration in degree. The forms, of which we have spoken, are according to the unchangeable laws of physics, therefore unadaptable. It applies to inorganic matter.

Though structures of matter may have many varied functions, all of them are primarily to express force. It is impossible to conceive matter without force or force without matter, and we know that force originates in intelligence.

NOTE:—The term *force* is used in Chiropractic as *energy* is in physics.

Art. 330. Universal Life in All Matter. Principle No. 14.

Force is manifested by motion in matter; all matter has motion, therefore there is universal life in all matter.

This is a principle derived from, and really belonging to No. 2. Life is necessarily the union of intelligence and matter. Intelligence is an entity. Matter is entity. The character of matter when intelligence is present, is what we called *life.* It is made known to us by matter expressing the force which intelligence creates. "Life is manifested by vibrations, according to degree." Molecules have vibrations—manifesting force. Nothing but intelligence could issue the force. Tissue cells have vibrations—a greater degree of life, manifesting force. Bodies of "animate" things have more movement (from within); still more life. It requires intelligent creative forces to cause such movements. Therefore, an organism, with signs of life, has more intelligence united with it than the molecule. (See Fig. 6) The vibrations of molecules and atoms are manifestations of universal life. Our ability to perceive life is exactly proportional to our ability to recognize Universal Intelligence all about us. Every structure of matter from a lump of clay to the tiger has intelligence in it, exactly proportional to its state of organization. The higher the grade of structure, the higher the grade of intelligence present, to make it and keep it that way.

"Degree" in Chiropractic terminology is taken to mean "degree of perfection"; therefore, it involves quality as well as quantity.

Art. 331. There Can Be No Motion in Matter without the Effort of Force. Principle No. 15.

Matter can have no motion without the application of force by intelligence.

This is a fact that is so obvious that it is easy to overlook.

No one ever saw motion, but everyone has perceived matter moving. It was the matter which was seen; and when it possessed motion it was perceived that it changed location, or was changing location. An act is an intangible thing and it is never perceptible to us, unless matter makes it so. If no force were applied to matter, it would be totally inert. Of course no one has ever seen matter, which was in that condition. It is the writer's opinion that if such were the case, it would cease to exist. It is a proposition reduced to the absurd. All matter has motion and therefore has what Chiropractic calls universal life. The origin of force being intelligence, then any motion is indicative of intelligence, if one cares to note it. But how about matter which has a force applied to it and does not change location? We know such to be true. The answer to that is, we must apply the Laws of Motion and realize there are greater forces than the applied one, which cause the matter to remain stationary. A given portion of matter has molecular motion which we cannot see, and may apparently be at rest.

Art. 332. Universal Force in All Kinds of Matter. **Principle No. 16.**

Universal Intelligence gives force to both organic and inorganic matter.

If Universal Force is universal, which it is, it is impossible for any matter to be where Universal Force is not. Organic matter is but inorganic matter built (organized) into structures, and has its full quota of Universal Forces. It should be kept in mind, however, that they are fully under the control of Innate Intelligence; that is to say, adapted. If the student has followed the subject closely through the book, he will see, easily, that Innate does not lack for forces to adapt and assemble for her use, and all without a cable from Universal Intelligence for conduction. (See Fig. 6)

Art. 333. Cause and Effect. **Principle No. 17.**

Every Effect has a Cause, and every Cause has Effects.

It is evident that one could not exist without the other. There could be no reason for the existence of a cause, if it did not have effects. It is an axiom, that there could not be an effect without a cause causing it. The study of Chiropractic is largely a study of the relations between Cause and Effect, and Effect and Cause.

Art. 334. The Signs of Life. **Principle No. 18.**

The Signs of Life are evidence of the intelligence of life.

They are motions of the adaptive kind which show the presence and government of a localized intelligence. They differ from the motions of universal forces, in that they show selection and the judgment of local intelligence in every phase. They meet, use, or oppose every environmental circumstance, if it is within the range of their limitations. There are five principal signs of life. Their names in order of importance are: assimilation, excretion, adaptability, growth, and reproduction. An organism may have these signs so latent that it is difficult to tell whether the organism is alive or not. Yet this low organism has its share, its quota, the requisite amount of intelligence for its state of organization.

Art. 335. Organized Matter. **Principle No. 19.**

The material of the body of a "living thing" is organic matter.

Organized matter is structures of molecules and atoms which have been assembled for the purpose of functioning adaptively. They are structures that have been built by their innates to house them (the innates). They are, therefore, under the solicitous care of those intelligences, the same as any house would be under the care of its owner. The house of an innate intelligence is built and "kept in repair" by its owner. The structure is precious to the intelligence that built it, but it is not precious as a structure to Universal Intelligence, except insofar as it is a part of the Universal scheme to have structures built in order to tear them down.

Art. 336. Innate Intelligence. Principle No. 20.

A "living thing" has an inborn intelligence within its body, called Innate Intelligence.

It is the local intelligence which has built a house for itself and keeps that house in repair, and is the intelligence to which the condition of the structure is of supreme importance.

No one will deny that it requires intelligence to build a body. It cannot be denied that it takes intelligence to build even a tissue cell. No scientist, however clever, has been able to do it and never will, for it is a task for The Infinite. It must be remembered that infinity is in a tissue cell just as much as in stellar space. It cannot be done by man, no matter how efficient his laboratories are. Moreover, man cannot even repair one of these tissue cells if it is damaged. The cells and the bodies are built according to a plan. It takes an infinitely wise Architect to make those plans. Though scientists have studied anatomy and histology for centuries, their knowledge of the body leaves as much unexplored as Darkest Africa before it was explored. Sugar is organic matter having the formula $C_{12} H_{22} O_{11}$. It is made by the innate intelligence of plants. Let chemists take the same elements in the same proportions, combine them chemically, and they will have a compound of C, H, and O, but it will not be real sugar. Why? Because the infinite wisdom of an innate intelligence was necessary.

Let us, in this step of our study, look upon Innate Intelligence less romantically and more scientifically. Not as a little god coldly aloof somewhere in our bodies; whom we personify with a capitalized name and whom the more conceited of us think we must chastise occasionally; but as a mathematical law of nature.

Art. 337. The Mission of Innate Intelligence. Principle No. 21.

The Mission of Innate Intelligence is to maintain the material of the body of a living thing in active organization.

It is the ambition of Innate Intelligence to build the body and then keep it actively organic. The Universe would not be complete without everything; hence a universe could not be complete with only unadapted forces and universal laws of the destructive kind. In order to complete the cycle, there must be construction. In order to complete the cycle, a local and specific application of intelligence is necessary.

Art. 338. Evolution Values.

A series of similar adaptations repeated a number of times results in a change of shape and texture of a tissue.

If there is a failure of such adaptations there will be no adaptive improvements in the tissue. The failure is due to interference with transmission.

If no need arises calling for adaptive improvement, such changes will not be made and the specie settles into a type.

If there is not a constant use of the adaptive improvements of tissue, it will be removed or reduced to the rudimentary, by Innate.

If the change in tissue, due to successful adaptation, becomes permanent through use, it will be transmitted to posterity.

If the descendants continue to use improvements which were inherited, they become permanently established as property of the race.

The unsuccessful adaptations are not transmitted to posterity for in that case there are no values to transmit.

Dis-ease is a failure to adapt, therefore is not inherited.

(Art. 207.)

Whenever there is adaptation made in a tissue cell by Innate, there is perfect physical personification of Innate—her plans perfected. The organism successfully has passed the Xth. milestone in the history of the universe. Innate knows that all the tissue cells of that structure are adequate for the present; but Innate knows that there are other "milestones" to pass and that the circumstances of the future occasions may be different. If the tissue cells have not passed the present milestone successfully and made adaptation, they certainly will not be any better prepared for the next one. The value that the organism accumulates by experience, in this manner, is Accumulative Constructive Survival Value. The organism now is ready to do easily what it did the first time and to withstand a greater adversity the next time. The "essence" of these values is inherited by succeeding generations of that organism. Note, we do not say, if a workman has calloused hands, that his son is bound to have calloused hands. No, the change is slower than that. If several generations of workmen have calloused hands, the offspring of that line will have tougher skin on the hands. However, even in the life of one animal or plant, we easily can perceive the structural strengthening (within limits of course). The action for the moment of stress, that we spoke of, was adaptation and so was the structural strengthening that followed. (See foregoing definition.) From this arises the statement mentioned before. Adversity is the mold that the Creator uses to shape the forms and destinies of living things. "Great pilots were made on deep seas and rough waters." The living things that we perceive about us today have the forms and structures they possess, because every cell in them is the result of intellectual adaptation sometime in the past. From this we can see from whence came the expression "the survival of the fittest."

"The tree that never had to fight
For sun and sky and air and light,
That stood out on the open plain,
And always got its share of rain,
Never became a forest king
But lived and died a scrubby thing.
The man who never had to toil,
Who never had to win his share
Of sun and sky and light and air,
Never became a manly man,
But lived and died as he began.
Good timber does not grow in ease."
(Better Homes and Gardens, April 1927.)

The successful adaptations were inherited, that is, the survival value of it was. Obviously, the unsuccessful adaptations cannot be passed on to posterity, for in that case there is no survival value. There is nothing to inherit. Also, if there is no occasion for; no call for intellectual adaptation; no adversity to be met, there will be no adaptation, hence no survival value. Therefore, if a race of beings is called upon to face the ever-changing conditions of the universe with its evolution, that race will fall into a type that has gotten behind the advance of the world, and will find it harder to adapt when the necessity for it comes. That is what happened to the dinosaurus.

Therefore, step by step, physical personification advances with the changing institutions of the universe. On that basis, the next tissue cells expanded are better equipped. This also is the explanation of acclimatization. Not only does it pertain to the expansion of better cells in the present body, but that perfection of plans is given to succeeding bodies of the race.

Should there be a failure of adaptation for any reason—because there was no call for it or because subluxations prevented it, there will be no survival value for inheritance. Since we use a unit system in our work, as explained in the Normal

Complete Cycle in Freshman work, likewise we might say that survival value is the unit of evolutionary value; positive values transmitted to posterity as a foundation to build better.

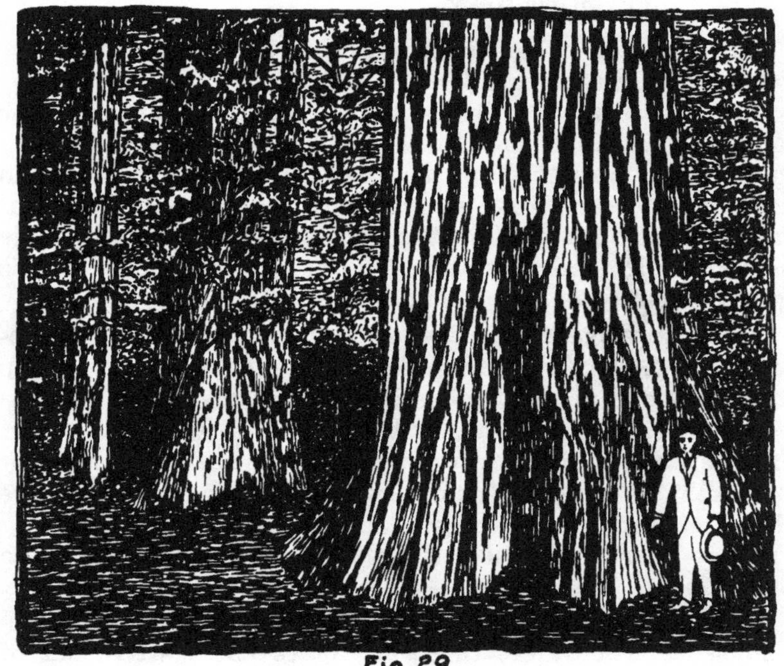

Fig. 29.

Art. 339. THE QUALITY OF INNATE INTELLIGENCE.
Principle No. 22.

There is one hundred per cent of Innate Intelligence in every living thing.

The "Quantity" of Innate Intelligence in one thing *may* not be as much as the "Quantity" in another living thing, but it is the requisite amount, hence one hundred per cent for that thing. (See Principle No. 7.)

Art. 340. The Function of Innate Intelligence. **Principle No. 23.**

The Function of Innate Intelligence is to create adaptive forces to be used in and for the body.

Everything in the universe has a purpose and that purpose is its function. Obviously, Innate Intelligence, being in the universe, has a purpose. Objects of inorganic matter do not need adaptation, so they have no *special* attention from Universal Intelligence. This special attention is given to certain units of matter, by Universal Intelligence, and the name of this *special attention* is Innate Intelligence.

Innate Intelligence, the law of organization, continually coordinates the forces and materials within the organism to keep it actively organized. That is to say, creating. "Act of making, producing, fashioning, or bringing into existence." "Act of constituting or investing with a new character, title or the like." (Webster.) Innate takes elements of no adaptive character, puts them together, "investing with new character," and now a new structure is brought into being, and is so maintained.

Nothing less than intelligence could do this. It is all accomplished, not by creating new forces and matter "out of nothing," but "investing" what is already existing with new character. Thus the natural energies within the body are assembled and made to do the work of organization. In this light, then **Innate Intelligence** is the intelligence within the organism, which systematizes the forces already there; it is, **scientifically speaking, the principle of organization.** Its creations are forces systematized adaptively, and materials built into intelligently planned forms.

Art. 341. The Limits of Adaptation. Principle No. 24.

Innate Intelligence adapts forces and matter for the body as long as it can do so without breaking a universal law.

It is evident that extreme adaptation cannot be made for the body. Adaptation of matter can only be to the point where molecules and atoms *must* obey physical and chemical laws. Innate can manage these laws up to a certain point by manipulation, but cannot change or destroy them. She can only use them to the limits of matter. Therefore, Principle No. 5 applies to this one. Man can adapt universal forces for his use and convenience, so it should not be so difficult for Innate to do it. Should Innate fail in these adaptations for any cause, these forces will injure or destroy her tissues.

Art. 342. The Character of Innate Forces. Principle No. 25.

The forces of Innate never injure or destroy the tissues in which they work.

The forces of Innate are constructive—not destructive. While there is wear on the part that functions at the bidding of Innate, these parts are just as rapidly repaired. On the contrary, the forces of universal, while they may cause an organ to act in a manner which resembles its function, and which causes wear, do absolutely nothing to repair it. The action of universal forces upon organisms may be so violent as to destroy them directly. The forces of universal, as for instance electricity, will cause the muscles of a dead frog's leg to act like function, but it does nothing for repair. When the wearing has wasted the muscle tissue, it will not be in condition to be called a good organic structure, and will soon cease to act.

That something which travels over the nerves, which is arranged in cyclic form, is really an intelligent current of life.

People used to think it was a physical force, or a chemical force that acted according to the laws of physics and chemistry, and caused natural phenomena in the tissues of the body in a mechanical way, as gravity does in falling bodies. They thought it might be electricity that flowed out over the nerves as it does over wires from the power house, and that it might act upon tissue cells in a chemical way, as it does in a bath for silver plating. Now we find that none of these are true for the following reasons: If a body were governed by a law as invariable as the law of falling bodies, and as inadaptable, it would be an automaton. If electricity, which is only a form of energy, were a power that governed the actions of organs, it would be as apt to destroy the nerves and tissues as it does the wires from the power house, and the lamps and motors unless it too, is governed by an intelligence. For electricity does not exhibit any solicitous concern for the material through which it works; neither does chemical action do so. Besides, if these facts were true, it would be possible for man to create man in a laboratory, as he creates physical and chemical phenomena. Man cannot build even one tissue cell or repair the same if it is damaged. He may be able to keep a tissue cell alive for a time in artificial surroundings, but the tissue cell merely exists; does not function or do the thing for which it was created, any more than a bear in hibernation shows activity. No, this life shows that it is an adaptable law, able to make instantaneous changes according to environmental conditions of a tissue cell. None but the Creator can change a law, make laws, or circumvent physical laws, so the life current must be a force directly from Law itself. It is not hard to see this, for the manifestations of the intelligence of life are everywhere about us; in man, animals, insects, plants, and lower organisms. It builds all these, provides all their needs, circumvents adversity, repairs them when damaged, and maintains them until death. Then, this power leaves them and they rapidly return to their elemental state—molecules and atoms.

What is in the living, which a moment after, is not in the dead? What has gone that has kept these molecules and atoms together in a unit of life, which is able to show manifestations of intelligence, sensibility, and signs of life? Mental force, that which flows over nerves to their peripheral ending. This force or message is specific for the momentary needs of a tissue cell. It must therefore be a more highly organized force than that given to molecules and atoms.

A lump of clay may be said to have some organization, for it is a lump, but Universal did not endow it with a special warden to see that it stays a lump. It has no power to remove it from danger of disintegration, but must take whatever fate brings it, without any attempt to circumvent it.

Art. 343. Comparison of Universal and Innate Forces. **Principle No. 26.**

In order to carry on the universal cycle of life, Universal Forces are destructive, and Innate Forces are constructive, as regards structural matter.

From our study of physics, we know that the universe is full of energy. We see it manifested in every bit of matter. There seems to be no limit to the amount of energy that may be in the space occupied by matter, but there seems to be a limit as to how much of it a given bit of matter can express. Yet that limit may be of astonishing proportions. Just what may be the electrical potential in, say, a pint of water or a marble? Like matter, energy cannot be destroyed, but we see its manifestations reappearing in many different forms.

We observe that energy seems to travel; or at least it can express itself in matter at a distance from its source. We say that it travels by radiation and conduction. When it radiates, it travels swiftly—approximately at the rate of one hundred and eighty-six thousand miles a second. As well as it travels by radiation, however, it seems to like to pause and "play around" in matter. If this were not true, we could not have radio receiving sets for the radio would scorn our aerials. So, though it must travel much slower in matter, it seems that it really prefers that mode.

With many forms of radiant energy, there can be interference with its transference. We will not say all forms, for we do not know, but we do know that an umbrella interferes with the sun's rays considerably. Lead hinders X-rays; brass hinders magnetic rays, etc.

In matter, energy travels at a widely variable rate of speed depending upon the form of energy and upon the kind of material and the shape of the material. Through some materials, a given form of energy will scarcely travel at all. Thus we find that electricity prefers some metals, such as gold, silver, copper, iron, and the like, but does not pass readily through glass or rubber. Heat will pass through silver, copper, and gold readily, but not glass, asbestos, etc. Magnetism passes through soft iron easily, but not brass or copper or gold and the like. Also, we find that since these forms are radiant, they will easily be caught by the kind of matter they prefer.

There can be interference with the conduction of these energies, as when the conductor has a gap or when its thickness is diminished. When interference with conduction is thus offered to a conducted form of energy, it will be transformed, partly or wholly, back into the radiant form or into some other form. As in a conductor of electricity, we find that electricity, when it suffers interference, transforms into heat and radiates.

Mental energy in the body seems to obey the same laws. As to its radiation, that is another story and is too lengthy and entirely too theoretical to be within the scope of this article. In the conducted form of mental energy, we have more data and plenty of its manifestations. We find that it, too, prefers a conductor and uses nerve tissue for its conveyance. About what mental energy *is*, we are just as much in the dark as electricians are about electricity, but as electricians can do practical work, nevertheless, so chiropractors are not hindered by that lack of knowledge. Theories are a help and are progressive if they are based upon soundly established facts; and as the electrician bases his practical work upon a theory, so can the chiropractor.

Like other conducted forces, mental energy can suffer interference by interoosing a gap, by impinging the conductor, or by deranging its substance.

Let us study another phase of the universal energies. Universal Intelligence, with its universal energies, fills all the space in the universe, and every spot in the universe. Any place without it would be outside of the universe, which is impossible and absurd. The body, then, is no exception. Universal energies permeate every cell. But there is this difference: in the body, normally, Innate keeps these forces all balanced, controlled, adapted to her uses at all times—every moment. In fact, that is how "she" does her work—by using the universal energies she finds at hand. There are always plenty of them. Interference with her balancing forces, which she has assembled (from universal supply of course) prevents balancing and controlling the forces resident at the tissue cell. Interference with transmission causes the universal forces, in that given spot, to be instantly unbalanced and therefore not behaving as Innate wants them to. Of course, these universal forces must be expressed by matter, as any kind of force must be. That is a Chiropractic fundamental; but what material have these universal forces at hand to express them? Anyone can see that it is the tissue cell, for that is the spot we are talking about. Then, this cell is expressing some physical or chemical forces, without the management of Innate Intelligence.

All the energies of the body must be controlled by Innate by balancing, restraining, and augmenting them by the transmission of other forces from the universal source. This is Innate's job; her mission in the body; her function. She can break no universal laws; create nothing new; but can "juggle" the existing forces to build existing matter into structures to house her, and then continually "juggle" more forces to maintain that house. Let her vigilance be interfered with one moment, and the universal forces play pranks; that is, they are pranks according to Innate's estimation.

For organic matter, there are adaptable forms of force. These forces show that intelligence has originated them or managed them, and they are for the building and maintenance of living organisms. Should these forces be withdrawn, the living organisms revert to the elemental state wherein their molecules act according to the unswerving laws of physics and chemistry. A living organism has signs of life, which is evidence that it is under the care of intelligence; evidence of special care.

Having these forms of adaptability, sensibility, and the forces which govern the organism, it can respond to any new set of circumstances—not unswerving action but changing action, according to the demands of the moment. In a collection of living cells, as a living unit (for instance, an animal) these forces come from a central point. This points out that intelligence in a well-organized unit has a headquarters.

If we use the hypothesis that mental impulses are energies, then it must be a very carefully composed unit of energies, prepared (created) by Innate in order to impel the cell to proper action, which must be coordinative. Mere action is not sufficient, that would be "stimulation"; it must be right action in quantity, quality, direction, and time. We might conceive of this mental impulse as being composed of certain kinds of physical energies, in proper proportions, which will balance other such forces in the Tissue Cell; as electricity, valency, magnetism, cohesion, etc., etc. Perhaps some of these energies are not known to us in physics. What right have we to assume that we have found them all? The writer presents this as a hypothesis or theory in order to get a working basis. In other places in this book, other theories for the same thing have been offered, for the same purpose.

Art. 344. THE NORMALITY OF INNATE INTELLIGENCE. Principle No. 27.

Innate Intelligence is always normal and its function is always normal.

This is a principle from the Triune of Life (Prin. 4) for more specific application. Intelligence is always perfect—always one hundred per cent. The forces which it assembles are always correct. They are not correct when they reach Tissue Cell if there is interference with transmission, but that is not because of imperfection in Innate's work, but because of the limitations of matter (Prin. 24). It is because the conducting tissue is imperfect or the receiving tissue (Tissue Cell) is imperfect. Both the conducting tissue and the receiving tissues are matter which is the third factor of the Triune of Life, and the only member of it which can be imperfect. The imperfection, of course, is in structure. The molecules of a wrecked locomotive are just as good as those in a locomotive in running order, but the wrecked locomotive is imperfect in structure and therefore is not a good organ to express man's wishes.

Here again we see embodied in a principle, Local and Condition; Local, referring to the conducting material, and Condition referring to the functioning—or receiving material.

Art. 345. The Conductor of Mental Force.

Principle No. 28.

The forces of Innate Intelligence operate through or over the nervous system.

Nearly all of us have read or studied some physiology. We learned the bones, muscles, and organs and the chief functions of the various parts of the body. We have always known that there is a spinal cord in the human body. We learned, in a general way, "that the brain controlled our movements" and the actions of our organs, and that sensation depended upon the system of nerves. The fact that this system might go wrong did not occur to us, or if it did, we were apt to think it not important.

Since most laymen have gone this far in physiology, when the chiropractor explains how incoordination can and does occur through this wonderful system of nerve tissue, it looks reasonable to them. But at first the layman is apt to get the idea that the chiropractor stimulates these nerves, thinking of the effects only. Therefore, it is necessary to explain that stimulation is not the same as the natural current which is being delivered to all parts of the body. If every living thing depended upon stimulation from the outside in order to have its organs function every one of them would have to have a doctor attending to them day and night, continually sending in stimuli, which shows the absurdity of such a belief. **The chiropractor aims only to restore**—to bring about restoration. He adds no more current but removes the obstacles to the normal flow of that which should be supplied to the tissues from the inside. He is able to show how pressure upon nerves can hinder the normal flow and the manner in which he removes the pressure, so that Innate, who is able to attend this body of tissue day and night may deliver that which is necessary to the organs. The doctor could not give this continuous service, but Innate can. The service of Innate is not stimulation, for stimulation is addition—not restoration. Stimuli are unadapted universal forces, not messages of control. Stimuli only add more uncontrolled universal forces to tissues which are already in the grip of such forces.

The brain is the headquarters of Innate's control—the seat of the mind. It is very delicate tissue and is kept in a bony cavity, well padded and protected. The manner of its function is, and has always been, a mystery. But for that matter, the manner of functioning of any tissue is still a mystery—that is Innate's business. Since the brain is tissue and composed of tissue cells much like any tissue cell, except in form and purpose, it is probable that they function as other tissue cells, merely responding with their signs of life—adaptability—to the forces which Innate delivers to them to use or to transmit.

The brain is in two parts and each part has two lobes. It is composed of soft gray matter on the outside portions, called the cortice; and of white matter in the inner or medullary portion. The gray matter is masses of nerve cell bodies which are much the same as other cells, in that they have bodies, nucleii, protoplasm, etc., but they differ from other cells in that they have exceptionally long white branches. Masses of these white branches are the white portions of the brain. The cell is called a neuron, the long single branches are called axons. The branches of the axons at their distal ends are called terminal arborizations. The short branches on the bodies are called dendrites. (See Fig. 8.)

The brain might be likened to an electric power station. In it is generated a current of some kind. From the brain, leads the Spinal Cord. It is composed of bundles of Axons which form the white matter surrounding the gray matter of the cord. The gray matter of the spinal cord is made up of nerve cell bodies that are similar to those of the brain. The bundles of nerve axons, and the column of gray matter in the center, may be likened to an electric cable which leads from the power station. (See Fig. 34.)

There are thirty-one pair of spinal nerves which branch from the spinal cord. This branching from the spinal cord is inside the canal which transmits it, and the branches emit through openings in the protecting wall of bone; that is to say, through openings between the segments of the spine. They again divide and subdivide and pass to every part of the body—called the periphery.

After leaving the spinal cord, the nerves divide and ramify to certain parts of the body. That is, the bundles of axons separate and the fibers go to different parts, just as electric wires branch from the cables into buildings and dwellings. These, in turn, branch and pass to the cells in organs and tissues, as electric wires run to lights, motors, heaters, and many other things in buildings. (Of course this analogy cannot be exact—analogies only show *similarity.*)

Every tissue cell in the periphery has its nerve supply. That means that every tissue cell has nerves which carry to it mental impulses. This we might liken to the current from the power house. If all the flesh of the body could be removed and leave only the nervous tissue—nerves and all their branches—the body would be completely and visibly represented by the thousands and thousands of nerves which reach every tissue cell.

Thus it is seen that there are nerves distributed from the brain to the tissue cells, and collected from the tissue cells to the brain. Nerves from the brain are called Efferent nerves, and the nerves to the brain are called the Afferent nerves. The bundles of afferent fibers enter into the spinal cord at the back or posterior, and the efferent fibers leave the spinal cord at the front or anterior. These terms and facts are not new, but have been used for some time by physiologists and psychologists. (See Fig. 34.)

We will now call your attention again to the fact that this is a *cyclic* arrangement. We want you to compare these nerves to the like arrangement of arteries and veins. Arteries are efferent in relation to the heart, and veins afferent in relation to the heart. It is not hard to perceive, for blood is visible, and it is evident that there is no haphazard arrangement. It is a cyclic arrangement and the blood flows in a cycle.

Since the *nerves* are in cyclic arrangement, this also is not a haphazard arrangement, and they were intended to carry something. Though invisible, that "something" is more vital than blood.

Art. 346. Nervous Tissue.

After having had this general survey, let us study these tissues and their purposes a little more in detail. Nervous tissue comprises all of the nervous system; the brain, the spinal cord, spinal nerves and their branches, ganglia, and plexuses. It is the material connection between Innate Intelligence and the tissue cells in the various parts of the body. It also, in the brain, serves as the material through which Innate introduces her forces into material. So thorough is the nerve distribution ("nerve supply") of nerve fibers that there is not a single portion of the body (except cuticle and keratinous appendages) into which a needle can be thrust without striking some of them. For a detailed study of nerve tissue and structures of it, the student is referred to any standard anatomical work on the subject.

In Chiropractic, nerve tissue structures are divided as follows:

The Central Nervous System, consisting of the brain tissue in the cranium. The Peripheral Nervous System, consisting of the Spinal Cord, Cranial Nerves, Superficial System, and Visceral System. The Superficial System consists of the Spinal Nerves and their branches. The Visceral System consists of the gangliated system (the so-called sympathetic system), the internal plexuses, and communications with the Spinal Nerves and with the Cranial Nerves. In anatomy, the Spinal Cord is included with the Central Nervous System, because of its meninges being continuous with that of the brain. If that classification holds throughout, the eye is also a part of the Central Nervous System, since the posterior five-sixths of the eyeball is enclosed by meninges continuous with that of the brain. But, Chiropractic makes a different classification, regarding all nervous tissue, which is *conveying* mental impulses to and from the tissue cells, as Peripheral Nerves, since they supply tissues. Even the nerves in the Cranium, which supply tissues, come under this classification. (See Interbrain Cycle, Art. 112.) (See Fig. 8.)

Art. 347. Brain Cells.

A Brain Cell is a cell of nervous tissue—one of the four primary tissues. It has many of the characteristics of other tissue cells, having a body and a nucleus. Its widest difference from other cells is its branches. It has many branches; in fact it has so many of them that a drawing or photograph of a brain cell looks like a map of the Amazon River. The shorter body branches are called Dendrites, and a single, long, thread-like branch, extremely long in proportion to the cell body, is called the Axis-cylinder, Central Process or Axone. These axons, where they are medulated or covered by a white sheath, form the fibrous-appearing or medullary portion of the brain, as the corpus callosum, pons, medulla oblongata, etc. The axons pass from brain cell to brain cell, from lobe to lobe, from hemisphere to hemisphere, from brain to brain (cerebrum to cerebellum). They offer perfect inter-communication between all brain cells and between the brain cells and body cells. The axons of a nerve or brain cell are supposed to be its most important part. The drawing in Fig. 8 would have to be several yards long to show them in proper relation. Brain cell axons are not always long, but many of them are long enough to pass from the medulla far down the spinal cord or out into the periphery. The axons of nerve cells of the Peripheral System are usually much longer than those of the brain cells. There is much more to be said about brain cells, but this is sufficient for our purpose in this book.

Art. 348. Peripheral Nerve Cells.

As with Central Nerve Cells, for our purpose, a brief description of Peripheral Nerve Cells is all that is necessary. They are tissue cells (nerve tissue) having a body, nucleus, protoplasm, etc., as any other tissue cell. They are living organisms having adaptability; requiring mental impulses and nutrition as any other tissue cell. The writer is emphasizing these points, for it is the curse of Chiropractic, one of the things that have done much to corrupt the science, that students of Chiropractic *will persistently* forget that the nerve cell is a living thing, very sensitive and delicate, and mental impulses are immaterial messages and not a material something which can be dammed back in the nerve by an interference, as by the flood gate. The nerve cell's function is to convey mental forces by the "wriggling" of its protoplasm. It "wriggles" or "squirms" obediently at Innate's bidding, responding by its Adaptability (see Signs of Life) and by its behavior, informs Tissue Cell what Innate's demands are. In other words, it gives the Tissue Cell something to respond to by the use of *its* adaptability. **The student is urged to remember that mental means mental, and Mental Impulse is an urge; a thought in motion, going somewhere.** From this necessary digression, we will return to histology.

The branches of a peripheral nerve cell are not so numerous as those of brain cells, for the brain cell usually has many dendrites. The axons are extremely long, running long distances in the spinal cord or through the plexuses. The brain cells usually have arborizations in the medulla which communicate, in ganglia, with the dendrites of nerve cells there, whose long axons extend down the spinal cord in the "white columns," (see Fig. 34) thus emitting from the cranium through the foramen magnum. At the meric level in the spinal cord, Efferent Nerve is about to emit, the descending axon enters the gray column in the center of the cord where it arborizes (terminates) and communicates with a cell whose body, with other similar cell bodies, form the gray matter of the cord. This new cell also has a long axon which then emits from the spinal cord on the anterior (front) side of the spinal cord, in company with many others, in the conduits called anterior roots. The anterior root joins with the posterior root (see Fig. 34) inside the spinal canal, forming the spinal nerve. The axon then passes through the intervertebral foramen in the conduit, called the spinal nerve; thence to the tissues or to the Visceral System. Thus by many relays of histological structures is Efferent Nerve made. Efferent Nerve, remember, is the name applied to the route from Brain Cell to Tissue Cell.

The terminal arborizations of the nerve cells are closely intermingled with the short body branches of the next cells. The terminal twigs of the arborizations come within an almost imperceptible distance of the tip ends of the dendrites, leaving a gap, apparently. These gaps are called synapses. While anatomy does not show any visible connection between these nerve fibers, nerve physiology laboratory experimentation shows that there is communication between them, nevertheless. These synapses are the basis for a very pretty theory of education of the psychology (see Philosophy of Education, Art. 320).

This laboratorical finding does no harm to our "brain cell to tissue cell" idea, as has been stated by some Chiropractors. On the other hand, it is most excellent proof of that Chiropractic tenet. In telephoning from Davenport to New York, one does not use one continuous wire with no breaks in continuity, but a relay of wires. The connections between these different wires are very definite and **the route of the message is continuous.** Efferent Nerve is the route of the message in the body. Also, it supports the statements made so often in this book that each nerve cell is a living organism with adaptability, which accounts for their ability to carry messages. The arborizations do not connect with the dendrites by anatomical continuity, but the arborizations create a "field" to which the sensitive dendrites of the next cell respond, picking up the message and acting accordingly. All through the body in other ways, we see this law in effect. For instance, in the uterus during pregnancy, the foetus has no nerve or blood connection with the mother's body. It is an independent unit, in that it picks up its own nutriment from the serum in the placenta and responds with its own Adaptability to the environment which the uterus offers.

The chiropractor's fear of this idea is because it is the basis of the arguments of medicine in favor of reflex action. But this fear is ungrounded. The physicist argues that impressions from the periphery (he calls them stimuli) will, in a ganglion where the synapses are, offer forces to which efferent nerves from the ganglia respond and thus send back stimuli to the periphery. The writer can see no sense to this argument. If the Tissue Cell had stimuli, why should it ship it around in this senseless manner only to receive stimuli again? Stimuli are stimuli, and one stimulus is as good as another, being physical energy in some form. Chiropractic fundamentals point out that universal forces are already in the tissue cell to furnish dynamic action, and all that they need is management to furnish functional movement. Just mere movement is not function. The only reason that can possibly exist for having something come over a nerve cell to Tissue Cell is harmonizing management. If Tissue Cell shipped its stimuli over an afferent nerve to a ganglion, and got nothing but stimuli in return, it seems to the writer that it must be a sadly disappointed cell. Chiropractic does not see any good ethics in each cell working "for itself and the devil take the hindmost." Chiropractic recognizes the fact that the human body is a too highly organized unit to have its control scattered about in numerous ganglia. The body is an organism; an organism is an organization; an organization is a—well, see Webster's Dictionary, or Art. 230, if it's more convenient. In an organism so highly centralized as the human body or any other animal activity, there can be only one commander; captains, colonels, lieutenants, etc., would be out of place. Besides, the physicist does not mention any adaptative management, he merely states that the stimuli leaves the cell, goes up to the ganglion, and bounces back (reflex). What fun would there be in that? Such an explanation leaves an "awful" unsatisfied feeling like a story that does not end.

In this book, Chiropractic explanations are based upon laboratorical findings where necessary. It is foolish to deny them; better to make use of them.

The findings are not at fault. It is the human reasoning upon them which may be at fault. The writer believes that the Chiropractic reasoning upon laboratorical findings is the better. (See Art. 10 to 13, incl.)

Art. 349. Efferent and Afferent Nerve Cells.

The Efferent and Afferent Nerve Cells have a definite and significant arrangement. The Efferent Cells have their axons extending toward the Periphery, and their dendrites branching toward the Center. Conduction is evidently through the cell from dendrites to cell body, thence through the axon to the arborizations, then to the dentrites of the next cell. (Gray 751). (See Fig. 33)

The Afferent Nerve Cells (sensory nerves) are arranged with their axons extending from the cell body toward the Center and away from the periphery. Sensory nerves frequently have their cell bodies in or near the special sense organs with the axons gathering together in conduits leading toward the brain. For example, the retina of the eye has eleven layers, most of them being alternate layers of nerve cell bodies, and of arborizations. The axons extend toward the brain. Of course these structures being tissues are supplied with Efferent Nerves, some of them coming all the way from the Visceral System in the trunk, via the cavernous plexus.

Art. 350. The Brain. (Palmer Vol. IX)

The student is advised to look up the pictures in the anatomy textbook. A few brief statements about the anatomy of the brain will suffice for our needs.

Anatomically, there are two brains, the cerebrum and cerebellum. The cerebrum is in hemispheres which rest upon the corpus callosum and these structures together weigh about forty-three ounces. The hemispheres are largely gray matter, especially on the outside, but the corpus callosum is all white matter, being bundles of bridging fibers from one hemisphere to the other. The cerebellum, the small brain, is not in hemisheres, but in lobes, being gray on the outside and white on the inside. The cerebellum weighs about five ounces. These two brains are connected with each other, and the spinal cord, by bundles of white fibers called the pons and the medulla oblongata, both structures, together, weighing about one ounce. The brain (or brains) is covered by a strong membrane consisting of three layers called the meninges.

By referring to the anatomy textbook, it can easily be seen that the cells of the brain are connected with each other, and all communicating with the cells of the body by the numerous branches.

The brain is said to be the seat of the mind. In Chiropractic we not only consider it the seat of mind, but the headquarters of control by the inborn intelligence which governs the body, whether it is resident there or not.

Art. 351. The Spinal Cord. (Craven, p. 40 Vol. XV) (Palmer Vol. IX.)

As with the brain, a few brief statements about the anatomy of the spinal cord will serve our purpose, supplemented by study of orthopedy and anatomy.

The Spinal Cord is a long cylinder of nerve fibers, surrounding a core or column of gray matter. It is from one-fourth to one-half inch in diameter; about one and one-half ounces in weight, and about eighteen inches in length. It extends from the foramen magnum to the second lumbar vertebra. It has a covering called the meninges which is identical in structure with that of the brain, but differing from that of the brain in that it is not close to the bone. The spinal cord is suspended in two places by the meninges. At the foramen magnum, it is supported by the upper end, and its lower end is anchored by the filum terminale to the coccyx. Sometimes there are fibers attaching the meninges to the body of the axis vertebra or to the body of the third or fourth cervical vertebra. The meninges is thus suspended inside of the neural canal without touching the bony walls, but is well padded by connective tissue and fat to protect it. The cord proper, inside the meninges, is suspended by two rows of minute ligaments called dentate ligaments. Pictures and descriptions of these can be found in Palmer's anatomy textbook.

Art. 352. Anterior and Posterior Horns. (Craven, p. 421 Vol. XV) (Palmer, Vol. IX)

The cross section of the spinal cord shows the column of gray matter as an "H" shape or "butterfly shape." The four ends of the H are called cornua or horns. From the horns, nerve roots emit from nerve cells in the gray matter of the cord which are in turn connected to the nerve fibers in the white columns. In Chiropractic terminology, the roots emitting from the anterior horns are said to be efferent nerves, and those entering the spinal cord at the posterior horns are said to be afferent nerves. (See Figs. 34 and 35)

Art. 353. Spinal Nerves. (Palmer Vol. IX.)

The Spinal Nerves are formed by the union of the anterior and posterior roots, mentioned in the foregoing paragraph. There is a ganglion on each posterior root, just before it unites with the anterior root. The union of the roots, and the ganglia are on the inside of the neural canal. The united roots form a spinal nerve on each side—a pair. These emit from the neural canal through the intervertebral foramina, superior to each vertebra, or rather between the vertebrae.

Art. 354. The Superficial Nervous System.

The Superficial Nervous System is that division of peripheral nerves which supplies the superficial tissues of the body; such as muscles, bones, skin, limbs, etc. It consists of the spinal nerves, their branches, and plexuses.

This is the Chiropractic classification. The nervous tissue is divided into Central and Peripheral divisions. The Central System consists of the brain. The Peripheral System (Chiropractically) consists of the spinal cord, spinal nerves, plexuses (of spinal nerves) the cranial nerves, and the Visceral System. The Peripheral System is divided (Chiropractically) into the Superficial System, Cranial System, and Visceral System.

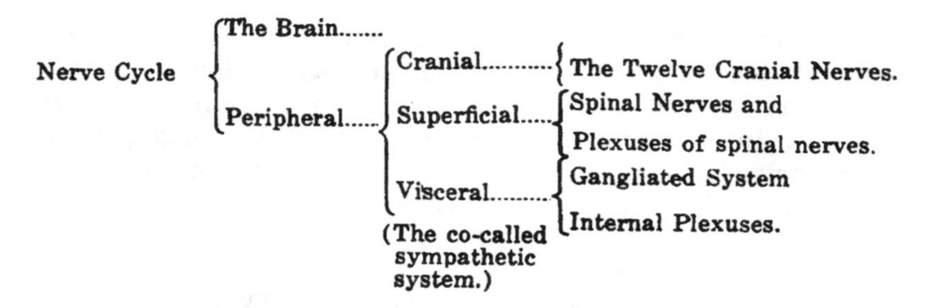

Art. 355. The Visceral System.

The Visceral System consists of the gangliated cords, and other ganglia as well as the plexuses of the trunk, including cranial communications, and the rami communicantes of the spinal nerves.

This system is what is known in surgical and medical anatomies as the sympathetic system. It consists of the numerous ganglia in the neck, thorax and abdomen and pelvic cavity. Perhaps the main parts of this system are the two gangliated cords which are parallel to the spine, anterior and lateral to it, one on each side. Axons from the spinal nerves enter these gangliated cords (conduits) through the rami communicantes, and arborize around the Visceral Nerve Cells, thus forming Efferent Nerves to the various viscera through this system. The gangliated cords might be called (analogously) the "stair cases" by which Efferent Nerve descends to certain preganglionic levels to pass to viscera; or ascends to do the same, or to climb still farther, back into the cranium through the carotid and cavernous sinuses, there to join the conduits of cranial nerves, and thence to the tissues supplied by the cranial nerves. These climbing axons also join with the lower cranial nerves through communicating nerves from the upper ends of the gangliated cords. The Visceral System is a very important part of the system of nerve distribution from the spinal cord,

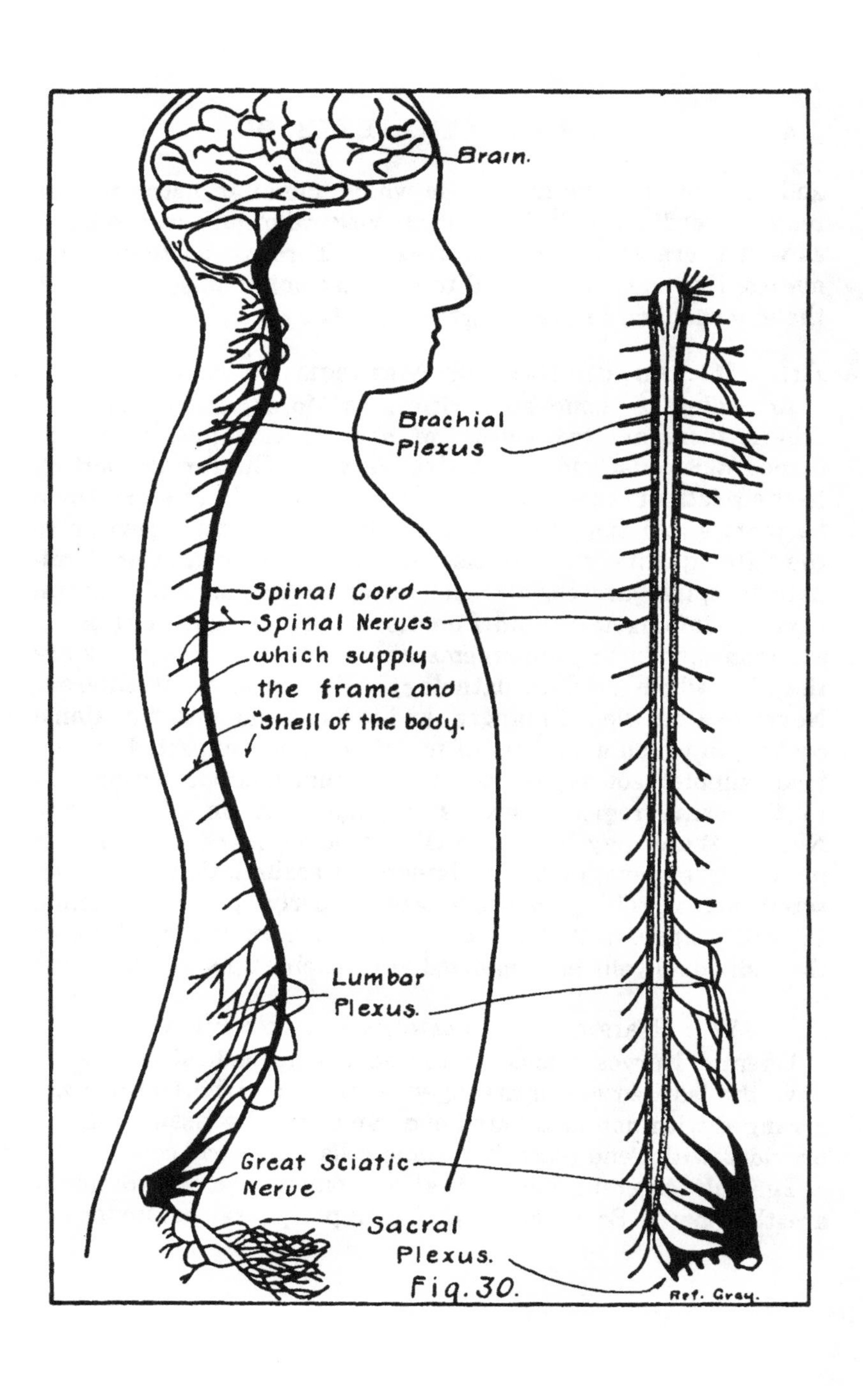
Brain.
Brachial Plexus
Spinal Cord
Spinal Nerves which supply the frame and "shell of the body.
Lumbar Plexus.
Great Sciatic Nerve
Sacral Plexus.
Ref. Gray.
Fig. 30.

and accounts for the manner in which spinal adjustments can restore coordination in the various visceral organs of the body, as well as cranial organs and viscera. Through postganglionic nerves, Efferent Nerves lead to the vasomotor muscles of both the external and internal parts of the body.

Art. 356. Functional and Metabolistic Nerves.

According to some authorities, as Morat, Pottenger, and others, there are two classes of nerves, as named above, or named Relational and Vegetative Nerves. The former pertain to the relational control of the parts of the body to make them harmonize in action, hence coordination. The latter pertain to the "life" quality given to tissues. The former kind predominate in spinal nerves, and the latter in cranial and visceral nerves. Impingements on Functional Nerves cause organs to act inharmoniously; impingements on metabolistic nerves are the kind which produce pathology. For instance, if Efferent Nerve to a muscle is impinged, and it has to do with functional control, in which a phalanx of muscle cells are expected to contract simultaneously, there will be inharmonious action. If to the same region there is impingement on Metabolistic Nerves, there may be abnormal reproduction of muscle cells producing myoma, or bad judgment in assimilation producing seredema, or failing to assimilate properly, produce anemia. In fact, it appears that it has to do with normal caretaking of the individual cells as connected with their signs of life.

Art. 357. Peripheral Arrangements of Nerves.

Efferent Nerves (called motor nerves in medical language) have the last nerve cell arranged so that its arborizations are arranged with non-medulated ends amongst the tissue cells, or provided with "end plates" in some cells as muscle cells.

The only Afferent Nerves that anatomists are certain about are the Special Sense Nerves. Their peripheral equipment is

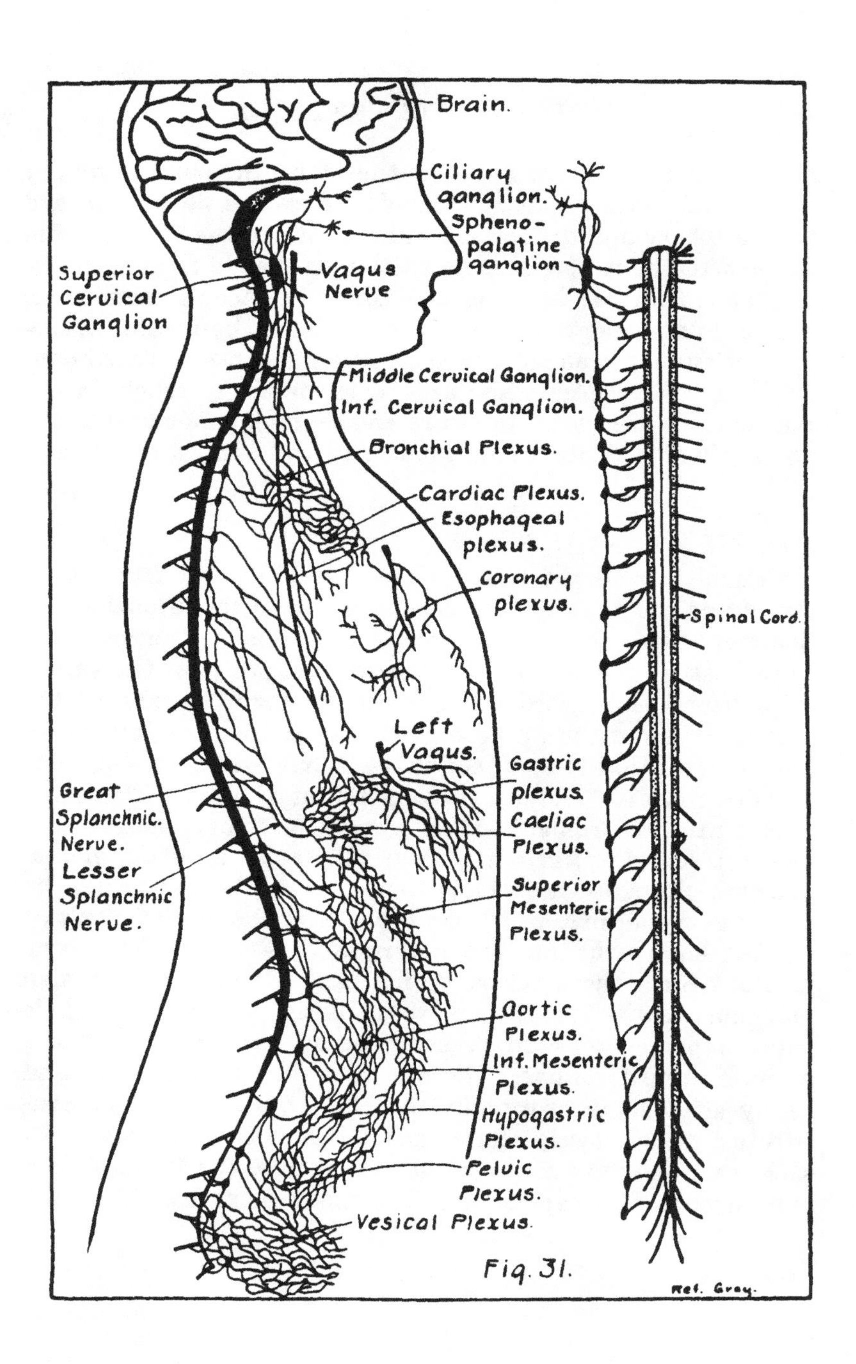
Brain.
Ciliary ganglion.
Spheno-palatine ganglion
Superior Cervical Ganglion
Vagus Nerve
Middle Cervical Ganglion.
Inf. Cervical Ganglion.
Bronchial Plexus.
Cardiac Plexus.
Esophageal plexus.
Coronary plexus.
Spinal Cord.
Left Vagus.
Gastric plexus.
Caeliac Plexus.
Great Splanchnic. Nerve.
Lesser Splanchnic Nerve.
Superior Mesenteric Plexus.
Aortic Plexus.
Inf. Mesenteric Plexus.
Hypogastric Plexus.
Pelvic Plexus.
Vesical Plexus.
Ref. Gray.
Fig. 31.

easier to study in anatomy, since they form the parenchyma of the special sense organs. Their dendrites are always toward the Periphery and their axons extend toward the Center. The axons often have special construction as receptors of environmental vibrations; as, rods and cones in Jacob's membrane, non-medulated dentrites in the taste buds, hair cells in the Sneiderian membrane of the nose, and the non-medulated dendrites in the corpuscles and around vibrissae for touch, in the Pacinian corpuscles for pressure and muscular movement, and non-medulated dentrites in papillae of the skin, for heat and cold.

Art. 358. CRANIAL NERVES.

Cranial Nerves are those which emit in pairs from braih structures and the medulla oblongata within the cranial vault. Some of them pass through small foramina in the cranium, to the tissues and viscera of the head; and one pair, the vagus, is prolonged downward so as to supply many organs of the trunk. It is not the purpose of this book to enter into nerve anatomy, for that is a subject by itself, but to show the student possible routes of Efferent and Afferent Nerves. There are twelve pairs of Cranial Nerves, namely, olfactory, optic, oculomotor, trochlear, trigeminal, abducent, facial, acoustic, glossopharyngeal, vagus, accessory, hypoglossal. There is one, the acoustic or auditory, which does not leave the cranial vault at all, but enters the inner ear through the internal auditory meatus. Since these nerves do not pass through the foramen magnum via the spinal cord, there is no possibility of their being impinged by cord pressure or by impingement in the intervertebral foramina. These nerves are partly efferent and partly afferent (sensory kind). The first (upper) six constitute a rather closely related group, which communicate with each other and have axons joining them from the Visceral System through the carotid and cavernous plexuses. The last

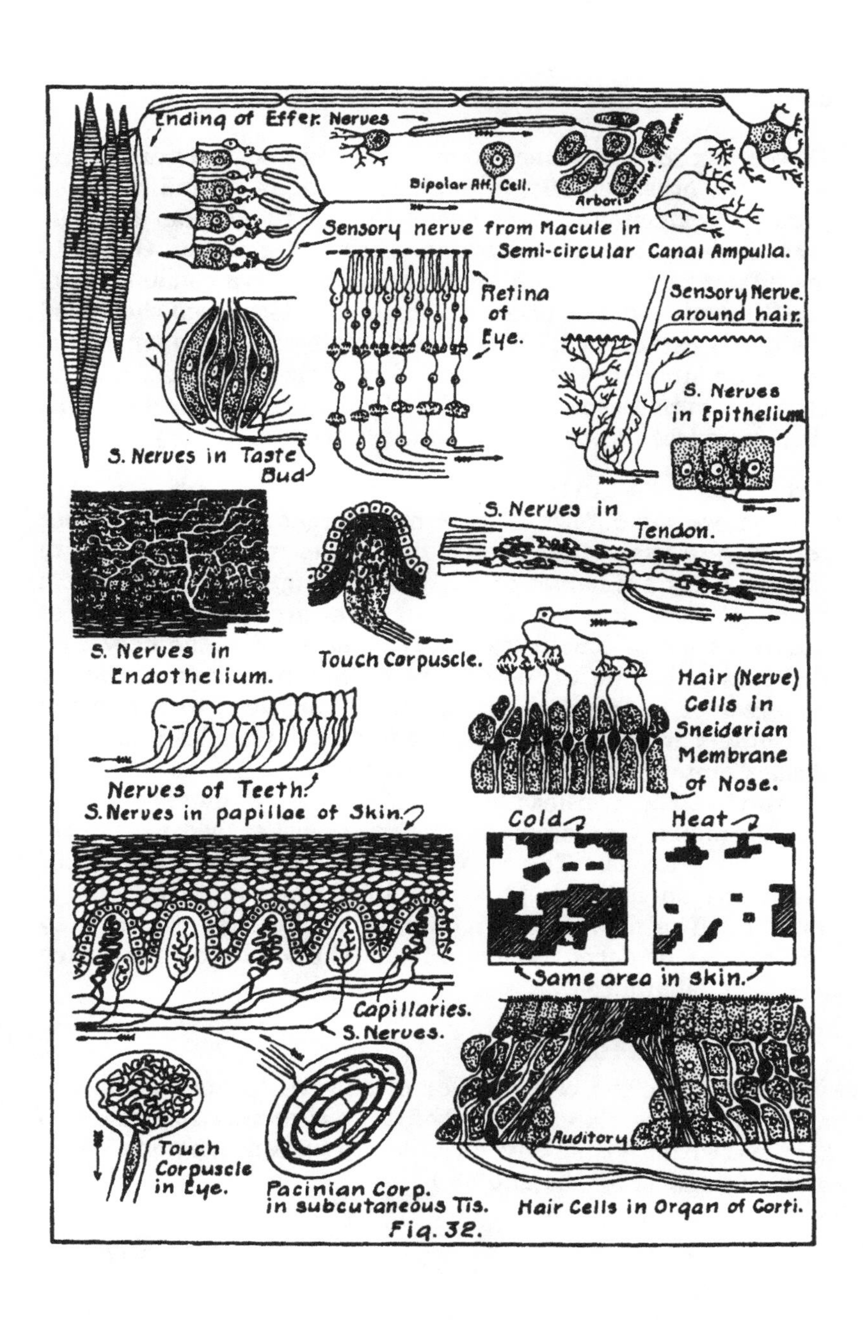

Ending of Effer. Nerves
Bipolar Aff. Cell.
Sensory nerve from Macule in Semi-circular Canal Ampulla.
Retina of Eye.
Sensory Nerve around hair.
S. Nerves in Epithelium
S. Nerves in Taste Bud
S. Nerves in Tendon.
S. Nerves in Endothelium.
Touch Corpuscle.
Hair (Nerve) Cells in Sneiderian Membrane of Nose.
Nerves of Teeth.
S. Nerves in papillae of Skin.
Cold
Heat
Same area in skin.
Capillaries.
S. Nerves.
Touch Corpuscle in Eye.
Pacinian Corp. in subcutaneous Tis.
Auditory
Hair Cells in Organ of Corti.

Fig. 32.

(lower) six form another group closely related, communicating with each other, chiefly through the ganglia in and near the jugular foramen, and have axons joining them from the Visceral System, through the superior cervical ganglia. Owing to the efferent nerves which join the cranial nerve conduits from the Visceral System, functional communication from the spinal system is established. Therefore, impingements upon spinal nerves do interfere with transmission of mental impulses to exactly the same tissue regions supplied by cranial nerves. This, then, produces incoordination in those tissues.

Art. 359. Conduits.

When we say Efferent Nerve or Afferent Nerve, we are not referring to anatomical nerves, but to the route from brain to tissue. They are names of particular things. The route from brain to tissue does not consist of an entire nerve, but one of the axons which constitute a very small part of the nerve. A nerve is a bundle of nerve axons and may contain many hundreds of them. Some of the axons may lead to one region and others in the same sheath or conduit may lead to other tissues quite distant from the first mentioned. As in a city, the lead cable overhead contains a large number of wires leading to many different points, so an ensheathed nerve contains many axons. The nerves branch very many times, but the axons do not, except where they have arborizations in ganglia. The nerves as conduits, or ensheathed cables, may anastamose or form meshwork, but the axons do not; they pursue a definite course.

Art. 360. Plexuses.

Plexuses are the crossings or meshwork of nerves, or conduits in various places in the body. It is merely Innate's system of "wiring" the body, in order to obtain adequate nerve distribution. (Figs. 34 and 35.)

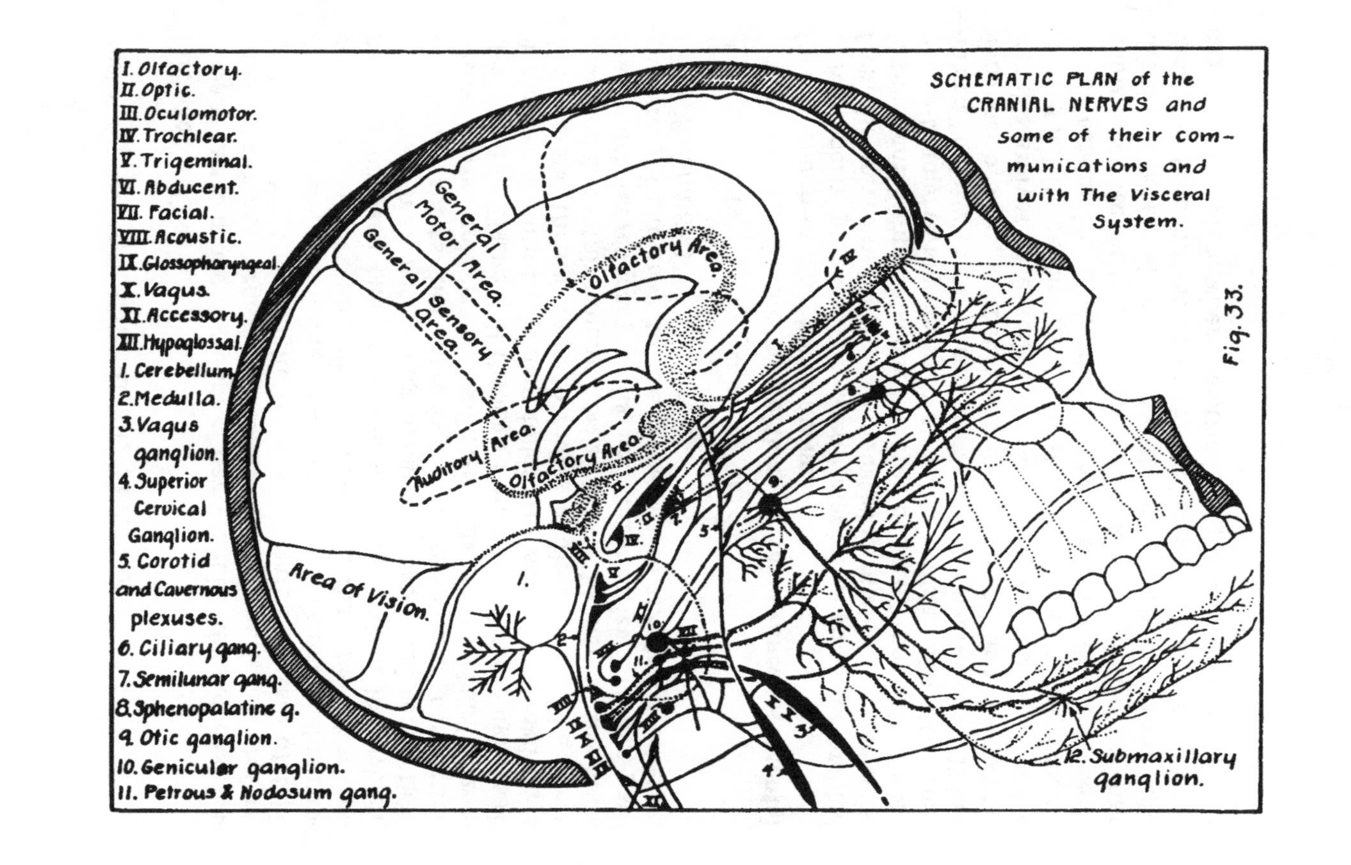

SCHEMATIC PLAN of the CRANIAL NERVES and some of their communications and with The Visceral System.

Fig. 33.

Art. 361. Ganglia.

Ganglia are nodes or groups of nerve cell bodies and arborizations. They are formed principally of gray matter, therefore. In Philosophy, they might be called Innate's system of telephone centrals, containing what nerve physiologists call synapses. The Chiropractic idea of synapses is that they offer connections between one nerve cell and the next in line which, while there may not be any apparent anatomical connection, physiology shows that there is a real "telephonic" connection between arborizations and dendrites. The route is definite from Brain Cell to Tissue Cell through a number of these synapses. A number of auto trails may follow the same state road for a distance and then diverge to routes of their own. The nerve axon which contains many fibrils may be likened to the state road which serves many trails, and the arborizations in a ganglion may be likened to the place where the trails diverge. (Figs. 34 and 35.)

Art. 362. Transmission.

Transmission is the conduction or conveyance of mental force through or over nerve axons.

A properly prepared (created) mental impulse, assembled from the universal supply, is conducted normally by nerve cells. If the mental impulse is one hundred per cent (normal) it does not do the nerve any harm at any time. (Prin. 25.) It is conducted "quietly" with normal action of the nerve cells. There is no loss of energy (if it is energy) in transit and the mental impulse arrives in exactly the same proportions that Innate started it. It does not matter that we do not know the manner of the conduction of the mental force; neither do electricians know how electricity is conducted by a wire. Some say that there is a potential represented through the wire. Some say that it is by polarization of the molecules of the wire. Some say there is a place where electricity is present in quantity and

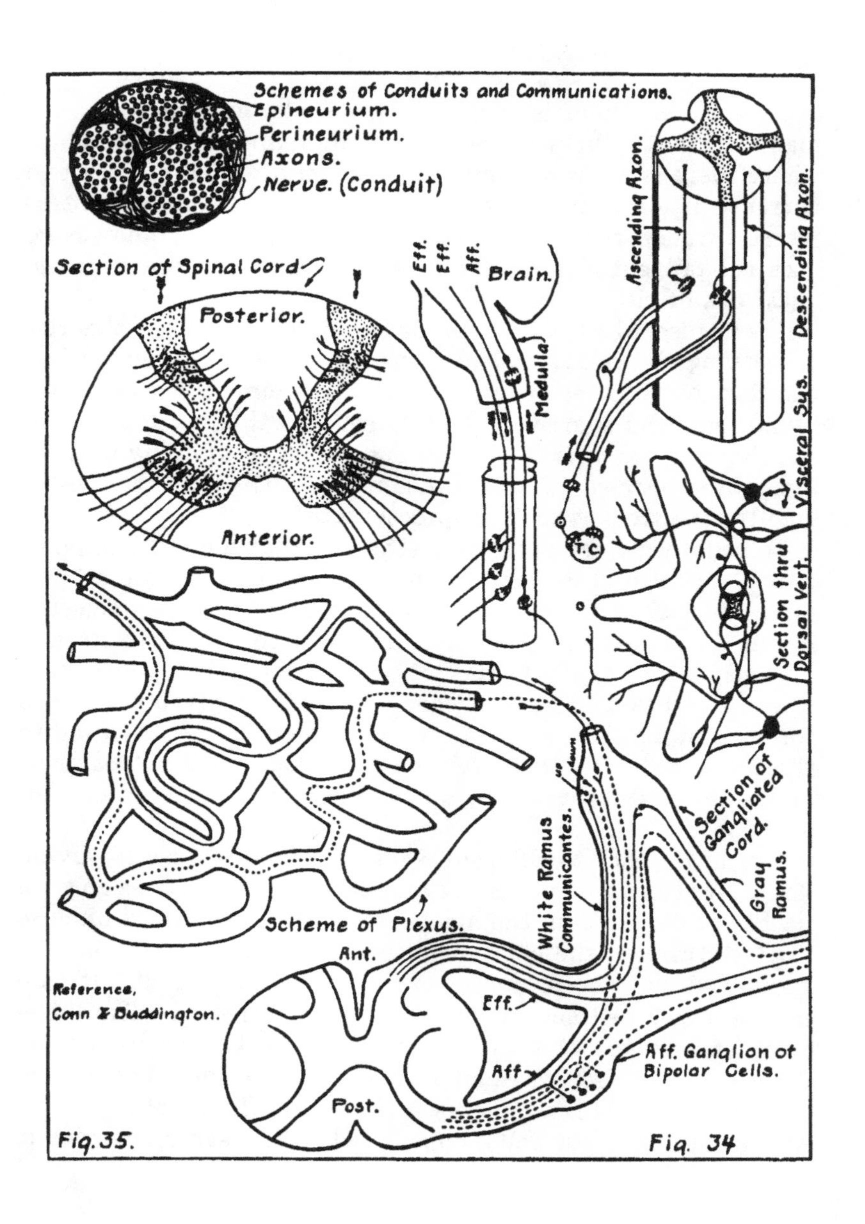

Schemes of Conduits and Communications.
Epineurium.
Perineurium.
Axons.
Nerve. (Conduit)
Section of Spinal Cord
Posterior.
Anterior.
Eff.
Eff.
Aff.
Brain.
Medulla
T.C.
Ascending Axon.
Descending Axon.
Visceral Sys.
Section thru Dorsal Vert.
Section of Gangliated Cord.
Gray Ramus.
White Ramus Communicantes.
Scheme of Plexus.
Reference,
Conn & Buddington.
Ant.
Eff.
Aff.
Post.
Aff. Ganglion of Bipolar Cells.

Fig. 35.

Fig. 34

a place where there is none or very little, and the dynamic manifestation is the movement from high amounts to the place where there is a low amount. Others claim that there are two currents of electricity, negative and positive, running contrariwise through the wire. Yet this positive lack of knowledge does not prevent electricians from making many practical applications of electricity.

It is no discredit to Chiropractic that it also must use theories concerning the transmission of mental forces. The writer has heard many theories about this subject. Some are good, some indifferent, and some very bad indeed. In this book, a few of the theories are offered but the ones selected are only such as are well supported by the Fundamental Principles, and thoroughly consistent with Chiropractic tenets.

To begin with, let us assume (theory) that a mental impulse is really a form of energy. If this is true, then the mental impulse must be composed of various kinds of energies selected by Innate to balance or annul or augment the energies already present there. (Prin 1, 16.) Then the mental impulse must have correct percentages of each energy for a given tissue cell for a given moment, and this composition must be delivered to the tissue cell with absolutely no loss, else it will not balance, as Innate expects it to do, according to her Intellectual Adaptation.

Let us get back to Efferent Nerve. It is a tissue cell—living flesh. Its function is to convey mental energy. It does so with no loss of values from the mental current. The mental impulse "slides" through the nerve axon ideally, with no loss. But the tissue cell must be in good working order to do that. It cannot be a sick cell and perform its duty perfectly. The molecules of the normal nerve vibrate in accordance with proper function. A perfectly assembled material, the nerve has perfect polarity and wastes no energy. Therefore, the mental impulse arrives at the tissue cell compounded of the same energies in the same proportions with which it started out. A perfectly assembled force of this kind balances or governs the forces in the tissue cell.

Here is another theory. Let us assume that in Efferent Nerve there is a current of energy which is the vehicle of the mental impulse, assuming that it is a message instead of a physical energy. This current energy is conducted by the nerve. According to that, then, the nerve can be compared to a telephone wire which is kept energized by electricity, to make it sensible to variations caused by the vibrations of the voice. With no steady current the wire would be "dead"; with an unsteady current there would be "static" noises. Therefore, the wire is kept "alive" by a steady electric current which, because it does not vary, allows the diaphragm in your receivers to remain quiet until someone speaks into the transmitter. Then the vibrations of the voice, by means of the magnet in the transmitter, produce variations in the electric current so that it is no longer constant, and its variations cause the diaphragm in your receiver to vibrate. In this manner the voice of the speaker is reproduced in your telephone. The vibrations of the speaker's voice never leave the telephone booth, but they are reproduced in your telephone, perhaps a thousand miles away.

In a like manner, we may say, according to this theory, that there is a steady flow of energy in the nervous system which conveys the message much as the telephone does. The mental impulse is entirely a mental thing; a thought in motion; a thought being conveyed by an energy, as in the telephone the thought is conveyed by energies. The energies may suffer interference and the message becomes damaged if that is the case, and is unintelligible to the tissue cell, wholly or in part.

The writer offers another theory which he likes best of all, because it fits the Fundamental Principles in every particular.

The mental impulse is not an energy at all. It is a message. A message is not a material, an energy, or a thing physical in any sense. It is a thing mental. It can be made by a mentality only, and be received by a thing mental, only. Mentality makes it and sends it to an object of matter. The matter is incapable of doing anything with it; incapable of receiving it. If matter alone could receive a mental impulse and act upon it, you could fill your body with buttons, silver spoons, safety pins, knives, corks, or any other inanimate objects you care to name, send them mental impulses and causes them to function. Of course that is absurd. Mentality must hail mentality. The tissue cell is not an inanimate object but a living organism with adaptability. Intelligence is there to greet the message (Reception). It is clear that Innate must have living cells to carry on correspondence with. The nerve cell is the messenger. Innate Intelligence gives it an "urge" which is for Tissue Cell. The Nerve Cell is a living thing with adaptability. It behaves in a certain manner through its whole length and breadth proportional in every way to this mental urge which Innate has intrusted to it. At its terminals the "urge" appears in an unmistakable manner, and Tissue Cell receives it. Having adaptability, Tissue Cell responds just as readily as Nerve Cell did, and in a manner exactly proportional to the intent of the "urge." In a nation of people, the Law of Demand and Supply is not operated by huge currents of dynamic forces of millions of watts, but by an intangible thing much more powerful. Neither is it by command of government; it is much more powerful than government. A little thinking will show that the urge which sets in motion the great movements of commerce and industry is **not analogy but actually mental impulses.** In this manner, Innate represents the Law of Demand and Supply in the body, and the whole procedure of Coordination in the body is entirely mental, else the body would be as any other lump of clay.

Art. 363. Interference With the Transmission of Innate Forces. **Principle No. 29.**

There can be Interference with the Transmission of Innate Forces.

We have seen that universal forces can suffer interference with transmission (Prin. 12) whether they are radiant or conducted. Innate forces are no exception to the rule and so there can be interference with their transmission through or over the nervous system.

The most delicate tissue in the body, nerve tissue, is so sensitive to injury or annoyance that it cannot "put up" with any rough treatment. It cannot stand pinching or crowding or rough "shouldering." Impingement annoys it very much, so that its molecular or its protoplasmic activity is not correct in that case and it does not pass the mental impulse along the length of its axon smoothly—does not let it "slide through" without loss. No, along its angry or unsound length the mental impulse loses percentage; perhaps greatest at the point of impingement, for farther along there is less to lose, and when the mental impulse arrives at the tissue cell, it is no longer a true mental impulse but perhaps just another "pranking" universal force. This view will apply no matter which of the three theories is used.

There are as many theories about interference with transmission as there are about Transmission itself. Let us pursue the subject, using the three theories which were offered in explanation of Transmission.

If a nerve is made abnormal in any part (as by impingement) there cannot be normal function of that nerve cell, which is a living organism. The mental impulse is robbed of some of its values and henceforth is (partially or wholly) not a perfectly assembled unit of energies as Innate sent it, but a somewhat dis-sembled unit. It no longer passes through the nerve "quietly," but "jangles" all the way. It is not entirely harmless to the nerve, and the nerve cell is not "vibrating" normally as it should, as any cell should, when normally functioning. When the pseudo mental impulse arrives at the tissue cell, it is not the perfectly assembled unit that Innate started out on the journey to the cell. It has a proportion of quality which is nothing less than mere unadapted universal forces, unable to balance properly the universal forces, already in the Tissue Cell (Prin. 1, 14).

Let us now examine an electrical analogy supporting this theory. Even with electricity, the energy is not all transferred at the beginning of the resistance. The energy which is lost by difficult transmission takes another form, becoming radiant heat. In an electric wire giving resistance, heat is lost along its entire length. The electric lamp has approximately twelve inches of filament in it, to give resistance so as to produce light. If all the heat and light this arrangement could give were at the point of union of the incoming wire with the filament — just a mere point — we would not have very much light. The entire twelve inches wastes electricity—deprives the current by its imperfect conduction—so that it changes form, becoming radiant, thus we get light and heat.

In the nerve the same thing takes place practically. Mental energy is wasted along the entire abnormal part of the nerve. Heat comes from the entire deranged length. If the interference is high in the cervical region, the angry nerve axon wastes mental energy all along through the spinal cord and on out to the periphery. Where it comes out at the foramen we are able to feel its heat; sometimes with the hand by comparative palpating; always with the Neurocalometer. Farther along, the nerve usually enters the flesh deeper and its heat diminishes, as has been mentioned before. Sometimes this nerve axon is impinged high in the cervical region, goes out into the Visceral System (the so-called sympathetic system) and runs its course in the gangliated cord and plexuses. Other times the

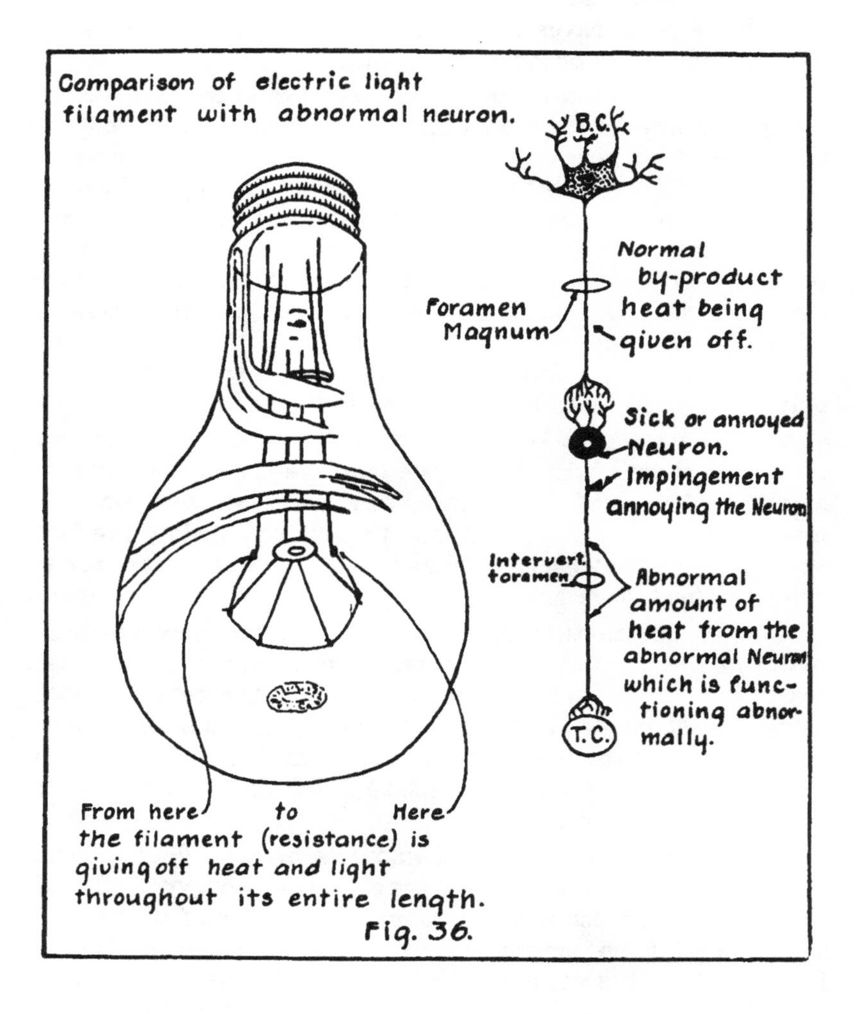
Comparison of electric light filament with abnormal neuron.
B.C.
Normal by-product heat being given off.
Foramen Magnum
Sick or annoyed Neuron.
Impingement annoying the Neuron
Intervert. foramen
Abnormal amount of heat from the abnormal Neuron which is functioning abnormally.
T.C.
From here to Here the filament (resistance) is giving off heat and light throughout its entire length.

Fig. 36.

nerve axon is undisturbed through the spinal cord and is impinged where it leaves the foramen. This is what is called a local subluxation or local impingement.

The question has been raised, if the nerve axon were heated along its course in the spinal cord or gangliated cord, would it affect the other nerve axons lying next to it? The answer to this is negative. The total degree of heat is only a fraction of a degree or at most not greater than one degree and that amount would not injure the neighboring axons. If it were possible that a small fraction of a degree of heat could injure the other nerve axons, then the heat of an ordinary case of febrile disease, which goes to a hundred and three degrees or more, would surely damage the nerves and spinal cord; not only in the spinal cord but anywhere in the body.

Another question: If a nerve axon is hot along the length of the spinal cord, why cannot one perceive the heat along this length of the spine? The answer to this is—because the bone intervenes and holds the heat, and this is explained by the fact that bone is always hotter than the softer wet tissue, for it holds the heat from any source.

Another question: Why is it that one can perceive heat better at the point of emission from the foramen? For these reasons: One, is that this point is the first accessible place along its hot length, and the heat rapidly diminishes farther along. Most of the nerves go deeper from this point. At the foramen there is only the soft tissue (back muscles) to hinder the radiation of the heat.

Another question: If mental impulses are an adapted form of energy, why would it do the nerve the "scurvy trick" of heating it? Because when it is robbed of some of its perfect assembling, it no longer is a perfectly considerate Innate force; besides it is not a question of what it does to the nerve, but what the nerve does to it. It must be remembered that this impulse in question was not made for the nerve in question, but for the remote Tissue Cell.

Another question: If Innate instantly knows that there is interference, why does "she" continue to send mental impulses that she knows the abnormal nerve cannot handle properly? Because that is the only thing she can do at the time, until she has made other arrangements which require time; and she dares not abandon the tissue cell entirely, meanwhile. As soon as may be, other tissue cells will compensate, giving adaptative symptoms, and the "case" becomes chronic, but Innate never has a chance to abandon the cell, so there always is some heat wasted. However, the nerve may become so depleted and so cool that the case may be very severe and the nerve give off very little heat. In such cases adjustments often violently increase the heat; or change it from a "cold box" to a very "hot box." That is because the depleted nerve of long standing has been called upon to wake up and carry on, and, as before, the element of time comes in. The nerve cell has to be repleted and built up to normal before it can carry a mental impulse without wastage.

Next, let us consider interference with transmission of the message, that is interference with the vehicle of the message. If the conductor of the current which is conveying the message goes wrong, the message becomes garbled, so that Tissue Cell does not understand it fully. Moreover, impingement introduces unadapted universal forces into the nerve current, and thus the message is full of "static" and unintelligible. Besides that, the nerve current could be wasted by the impinged nerve and become radiant heat as described in the other theory.

Perhaps these theories have some merit, but let's examine another one.

A nerve cell which is impinged is not a cell "at ease." Therefore, it will not "vibrate" normally in function. Its function is to convey the message. If it does not function properly it does not carry the "urge" properly, therefore the tissue receives a message which does not "read true." The tissue cell, having adaptability, always responds to the "urges" which come to it, whatever they are; if the signs of life are right in theory, it must. Not having the proper urge, it will perform improperly, exactly in ratio to the incorrectness of the message. This is called Equivalent Vibration. Of course this is not what Innate wants for coordinative purposes. We know from our study of physiology that when cells are active, they use carbon and oxygen producing carbon dioxide and waste matter, and a great deal of by-product heat. A sick cell which is laboring gives off more waste matter, uses more nutriment, and produces more by-product heat. It is well known that an impinged nerve axon gives off heat to the extent that it is often palpable with the back of the hand. Release of impingement reduces this heat, often in a very few minutes. The heat, which can be detected in the region of the spine, due to impingement is called "hot box." In chronic subluxations, where for a long time compensatory adaptation has been made, the amount of heat is almost negligible, and often variable, according to the variable demands of periphery made manifest. When an adjustment is given on such subluxations, the "Rip Van Winkle" nerve is awakened out of its depleted state and set into activity once more with a consequent sharp rise in temperature. "Rip Van Winkle" nerve cells do not produce as much by-product heat as the surrounding tissue cells of other kinds, which are "carrying on as usual." This condition before adjustment is known as a "chronic cold box." Other factors enter into what is known as a cold box. When a hot box has warmed up adjacent bone, which retains heat longer than soft (wet) tissue, and an adjustment is given, the heat from the impinged nerve is immediately reduced. The adjacent bone which retains heat for some time is now much warmer than the soft tissue over the formerly impinged nerve. This makes the latter seem "cold" by comparison. Given a few minutes for temperatures to equalize, it will be found (in these cases) that the cold box has disappeared. Sometimes an adjustment produces, apparently, a hot box from a chronic cold box. A "Rip Van Winkle Nerve" suddenly set to work, begins to give more by-product heat and the increase is much faster than the adjacent bone accumulates it, making the area over the formerly impinged nerve warmer by comparison. If some time is given for the bone to warm up also, the apparent hot box disappears. In actual practice many strange phenomena of comparative temperatures appear, but the writer believes that all of them can be solved by the application of a little thinking and the use of these principles. A problem in trigonometry does not solve itself—it requires thinking and the use of principles.

Art. 364. THE CAUSE OF DIS-EASE. **Principle No. 30.**

Interference with the transmission of Innate forces causes incoordination or dis-ease.

Interference with transmission prevents Innate from adaptating things universal for use in the body and from coordinating the actions of the tissue cells for the mutual benefit of all cells. Accordingly, the universal forces wear or injure the tissue cells, or cause them to act inharmoniously and thus injure other cells as well. When a cell is injured, worn down, or "out of condition," it is not "at ease." Mental force must reach organized matter to make it vibrate properly, that is, live. Matter may be vibrating, but if it is not vibrating adaptatively, it is not "living." Mental forces kept from matter cause it to revert to its elemental state. There is something in a living man that a moment after death is not in the *dead*. The absence of mental force in the body is called *death*. The partial absence of mental force in the body is *paralysis*.

Art. 365. Disease, Dis-ease, and Trauma.

***Disease* is a term used by physicians for sickness. To them it is an entity and is worthy of a name, hence diagnosis.** (55 M. & M.)

***Dis-ease* is a Chiropractic term meaning not having ease; or lack of ease. It is lack of entity. It is a condition of matter when it does not have the property of ease. Ease is the entity, and dis-ease the lack of it.**

***Trauma* is injury to tissues, which impairs or destroys tissue cells but the tissue cells are not sick.**

In Trauma, tissues are not degenerated or depleted. They are just injured; and this is proven by the fact that a wound will heal readily and healthily, if the region of injury or the body is not dis-eased. Trauma is in the field of surgery.

Dis-ease is the condition of tissue cells when there is incoordination. It is the result of coordination when the tissue cells do not do their duties coordinately. The tissue cells that fail to function are not always where the symptoms of trouble are; for example, gas and tympanites when the liver is not functioning coordinately. When there is incoordination, tissue cells are sick; not clean, as they are in Trauma. When there is coordination there is a good supply of things to make a tissue cell healthy. If it is healthy it is sound. If tissue cells are not coordinating, some tissue cells will be made unsound (insane) therefore they are sick and not at ease.

Many terms, viz., dis-ease, incoordination, paralysis, and physical insanity are used almost synonymously.

Art. 366. Foramen.

"A small opening, perforation, or orifice; fenestra." (Webster.)

In anatomy, this opening may be through any tissue or between tissues.

Art. 367. INTERVERTEBRAL FORAMEN. (105 XV) (47 IX) (94 Gray).

"Opening formed by notches in the pedicles of the neural arches of the vertebrae. They transmit the spinal nerves and blood vessels." (Webster.)

They are somewhat elliptical in shape and the longer axis of the ellipse is nearly vertical.

The spinal nerve does not completely fill the foramen, which also contains blood vessels, fat and areolar tissue.

Owing to the movability of the vertebrae and the possibility of the vertebrae becoming subluxated, an abnormal change in the size or shape of the foramen will cause the nerve to be impinged, if not actually pressed or pinched. This is because the walls, roof, or floor of the foramen may crowd in from their normal positions when the pedicles are moved out of their proper places. Since the work of the chiropractor depends so much upon this fact, it is advisable to obtain a thorough knowledge of the boundaries of the intervertebral foramina. (See Foramen in Fig. 39)

Art. 368. IMPINGEMENT.

"To strike or dash (on, upon, against) esp. clashingly or with a sharp collision; of etheric or aerial waves to come sharply (on or upon) a body; as, sound waves impinge upon the tympanum."

"To encroach or infringe (on or upon)."

"To thrust, force, or dash; to thrust or strike against; to collide with." (Webster.)

It can be seen from the above that *impingement* means simultaneous or successively rapid little taps or strokelets; as, of a handful of pebbles thrown against a window, or of raindrops. The meaning, however, that is used in Chiropractic, is also implied by the foregoing definitions; that is to encroach, infringe, or crowd upon. This latter definition implies that the crowding upon is a persistent, continuous pressure and not a single push.

The word *impinge* is used to indicate what the walls of an abnormal foramen do to a nerve in a foramen.

All impingements in the body (and there are many kinds) are due to subluxations, directly or indirectly. Impingements may be produced by fractures or dislocations also, for any abnormal position of a vertebra, relative to its neighbors, may impinge nerves. The first known, and the most common places of impingement are in the intervertebral foramina. When the body walls of the foramen are out of their normal positions, they crowd upon the contents of the foramen, which in turn crowd upon one or more axons in the spinal nerve. Since nerve cells are extremely delicate, very little pressure is necessary to disarrange its working capacity to some extent; enough to cause incoordination at the periphery of that axon. By far, the most of the interferences are caused by this type of impingement, though many times there may be actual bony pressure upon the nerve—pinching it in that case, probably.

Again it is necessary to remind the student that the nerve is not a copper wire, but a living tissue cell with signs of life—adaptability. Being very delicate, constant pressure, hourly or daily encroachments, even if not constant, will annoy this very sensitive tissue cell. Momentary pressures of even greater amounts would not so annoy it as this daily nagging encroachment. An annoyed or sick nerve cannot conduct properly. Sometimes great pressures do not annoy spinal nerves as much as little pressures, and no rule of severity can be formulated according to the amount of pressure, unless of course, it is a question of pinching. Pinching usually requires dislocation or fracture; a subluxation is not apt to pinch a nerve.

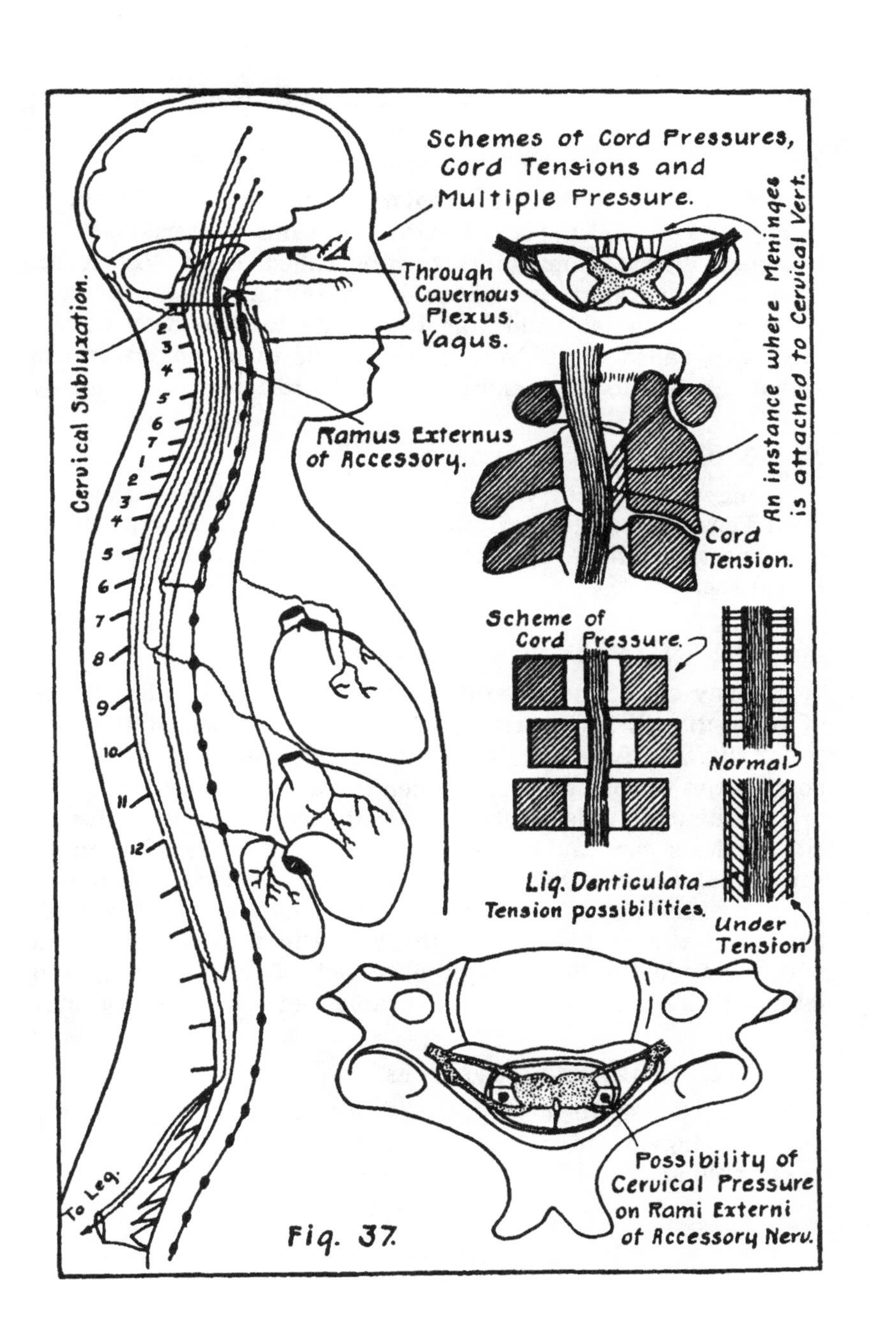

Schemes of Cord Pressures,
Cord Tensions and
Multiple Pressure.
Through
Cavernous
Plexus.
Vagus.
Ramus Externus
of Accessory.
Cervical Subluxation.
An instance where Meninges
is attached to Cervical Vert.
Cord
Tension.
Scheme of
Cord Pressure.
Normal
Lig. Denticulata
Tension possibilities.
Under
Tension
Possibility of
Cervical Pressure
on Rami Externi
of Accessory Nerv.
To Leg.

Fig. 37.

Art. 369. Cord Pressure and Cord Tension.

In much the same way, impingements can occur in the spinal canal, which is also packed with the same material as the foramen. These impingements are called Cord Pressures. There are several kinds. Those due to pressure upon the contents of the spinal canal, and those due to distortion of the meninges, called Cord Tension; those due to pathology in the spinal canal or in the meninges or the cord itself.

Art. 370. Sacral Impingements.

Inpingements occur in the spinal canal of the sacrum by Cord Tension and also by impingement upon the spinal nerves emitting through the sacrum because of distortion of the meningeal sac.

Art. 371. Cervical Cord Pressures.

In many cases, the anterior part of the meninges has fibers of connective tissue, extending to the periosteum of the posterior surface of the axis, third or fourth cervicals. This offers possibilities of cord pressures when the above named vertebrae are subluxated. Also, subluxation of any of the first five or six cervicals can cause pressures upon the external rami of the Spinal Accessory Nerve, which, emitting from the spinal cord on each side, ascend between the meninges and the cord, back into the cranial vault, through the foramen magnum where they join with the internal branch of the Accessory and later with all the lower group of cranial nerves. (See Fig. 37.)

Art. 372. Multiple Pressures.

Multiple Pressure in the case of one subluxation producing many impingements in various ways.

For this article, Fig. 37 will suffice.

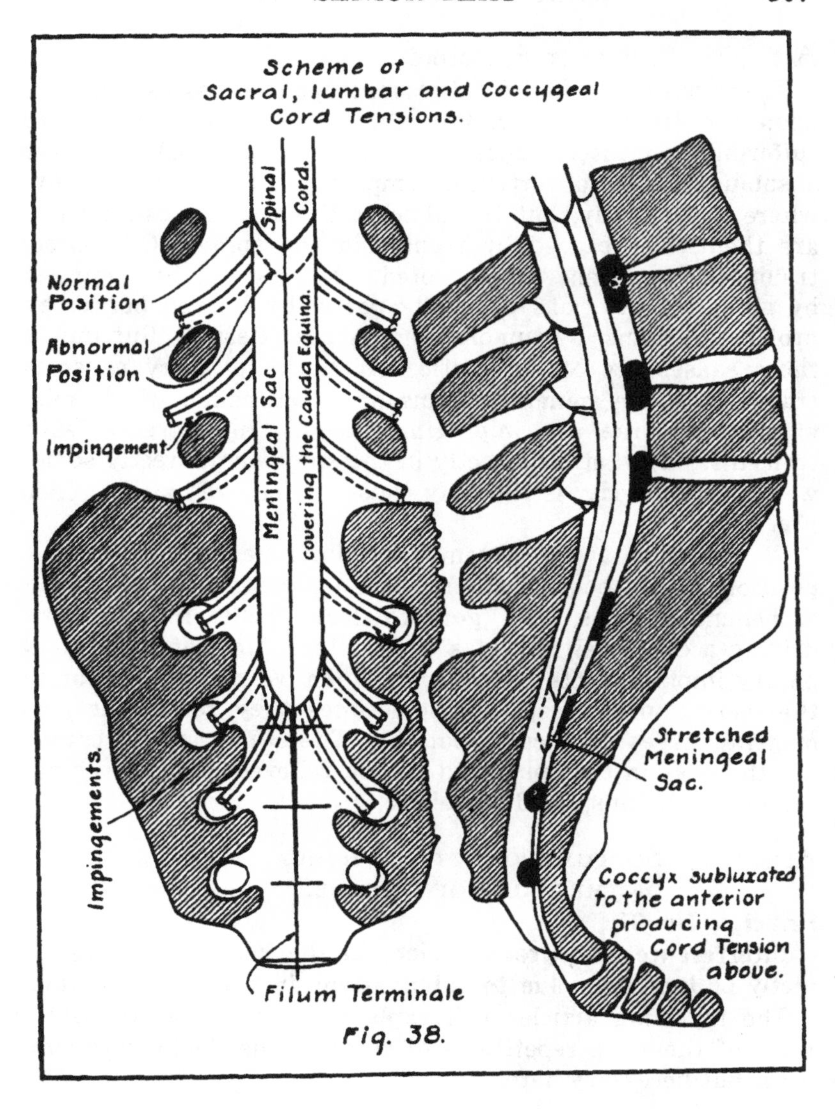
Scheme of
Sacral, lumbar and Coccygeal
Cord Tensions.
Spinal Cord.
Normal Position
Abnormal Position
Impingement
Meningeal Sac
covering the Cauda Equina.
Impingements.
Filum Terminale
Stretched
Meningeal
Sac.
Coccyx subluxated
to the anterior
producing
Cord Tension
above.

Fig. 38.

Art. 373. Indirect Pressures.

There can be an Indirect Pressure upon nerves by pressure upon the tissues surrounding them, which are themselves suffering from interference due to a fracture, a dislocation, or a subluxation of a vertebra. Impingements can occur anywhere in the body, but the abnormalities which cause them are themselves caused by trouble in the spine. Of course, traumatic conditions are excepted. Nerves can be impinged by abnormal positions of bodily parts, by broken bones, by prolapsed organs, by tumors, and by scar tissue. But unless these causes are of traumatic origin, the primary cause is traceable to the spinal foramina or spinal canal, where misplaced vertebrae are impinging fibers. Interference with transmission, whether directly in the spine or indirectly somewhere in the body, is the only cause of incoordination. (See Fig. 18)

We are often aware of temporary impingement, from some position of our bodies, which has no permanent effect, such as benumbed arms, feet "gone to sleep," aches in neck from driving a car, or sitting at a typewriter. Most of these temporary impingements are relieved when we move about or in the relaxation of sleep, but sometimes they remain as permanent causes of incoordination. These permanent causes are the ones in the spine and can be relieved only by the adjusting of the misplaced vertebrae.

Art. 374. Subluxations, the Physical Representative of the Cause of Dis-ease.

Principle No. 31.

Interference with transmission, in the body, is always directly or indirectly due to subluxations in the spinal column.

The following articles will explain this principle in detail. Some of them are repetitions of some of the Sophomore subjects, but necessary here.

Art. 375. The Normal Vertemere Cycle.

The Vertemere Cycle is the cycle from innate brain to the tissues holding in situ the vertebra in question.

A subluxation impinging a nerve from brain to organ, also impinges the nerve supplying its own tissues; that is why it exists as a subluxation. See subsequent Articles.

In the scheme in Fig. 14, the outer cycle represents the normal complete cycle from brain to organ in question; and the inner cycle represents a normal complete cycle from brain cell to "tissue cell" in the region of the vertebra itself.

Art. 376. The Vertemere Region.

The Vertemere is the vertebra in question, which is considered an important part of a zone because when it is subluxated it is the cause of disease in its zone; or is where the impinged neuromere makes its exit.

The region of the Vertemere consists of the tissues which keep the vertebrae in situ. It is important because when a subluxation exists, there is interference with transmission to this region, preventing Innate from placing or holding the vertebra in situ.

It is important, also, because when an adjustment is given, here is where the innate contraction of forces takes place.

The Vertemere Region has to do with the vertebra, intervertebral discs, the adjacent ligaments, the muscles that act upon the vertebra, subluxations, rotations, curvatures, innate contraction of forces, adjusting, etc.

(References: Vol. XV; Vol. V, p. 191, 196.)

When a person moves about during the day, bending, stooping, sitting, walking, working, etc., naturally, his vertebrae are moving continually about in relation to each other; and naturally, they will be out of alignment momentarily. Just as soon as a particular movement of the body is completed, Innate immediately replaces the vertebra to its proper place, by the functioning of the tissues holding it in its proper position. (213 V). These positions of vertebrae, while they may momentarily impinge nerves, are not subluxations. A subluxation impinges the nerves supplying the responsible tissues of a vertebra, so that when it is misplaced to the extent called a subluxation, it cannot be replaced instantly by Innate, and therefore becomes existent as a real subluxation. The action of the tissues in moving a vertebra in response to a concussion is called *innate contraction of forces.* When a vertebra has remained out of place for some time, the tissues of the vertemere become changed in form and texture; may even become pathological, and then it is said to be a *chronic subluxation.*

When a vertebra is subluxated, and Innate cannot get her forces through, to put it back to its normal position, the application of outside forces is necessary.

An analogy: Let us suppose a powerful car is stalled on an ice-covered street. The engine has plenty of power, but there is no traction. Try as it may, it cannot get away from the curb. Then a man comes to help. He intends to give a "boost" which must be in a direction that will help. His strength is puny when compared with that of the engine. Yet, if he applies it correctly, in the proper direction, the car will move out from the curb easily. The man did not push the car out; it could not do it itself, but the resultant of their combined efforts did. The man gave the car a chance to get traction; the adjustor gives Innate a chance to use her contraction of forces.

Before the advent of Chiropractic, the application of outside forces was haphazard and the chances of adjustments resulting therefrom followed the laws of chance. If you have studied *chance* in mathematics, you know the probability of adjustment was very slim. We all have read stories of miraculous accidents which restored health; particularly, paralysis being the favorite dis-ease. Accidents did adjust a few cases, and many miraculous "cures" resulted from falls, slipping down stairs, etc. It was not until the discovery of Chiropractic that adjusting became a definite and specific science.

Animals have been seen adjusting themselves. Horses, after they have been stabled a long time, or hard worked, or do not feel well, always roll upon the ground with manifest enjoyment. It is not merely to scratch the skin or to dress the hair. The writer has observed them many times. Dogs roll upon the ground also, and if one will notice, it is not smooth or soft ground that they prefer.

Many peasant peoples and primitive tribes in all parts of the world are using adjustments. The writer has been informed by natives of Poland, Syria, and Russia, and by travelers in Burma, Mexico, and from the shores of the Arctic Ocean, that tribes in those places are using and have been using adjustments for hundreds of years. The methods are interesting and various.

Art. 377. The Normal Vertebra. (See Vol. XV)

A Vertebra is one of the movable bony segments of the spinal column.

Word analysis: from *vertere*, to turn or change.

A typical Vertebra has a centrum or body; two pedicles; two laminae (forming a neural arch); two superior and two inferior articular processes, which articulate with the vertebra above and the one below, respectively, two transverse processes, arising at the union of the pedicles and laminae (one on each side extending laterally); and a spinous process, consisting of the united laminae extending toward the posterior. The two pedicles and the two laminae (the neural arch) together with the centrum, form a bony ring. The bony rings of all the vertebrae, superimposed upon each other, form the neural canal.

Between the vertebrae are pads of cartilage which separate them approximately one-fourth inch apart, and securely fasten them together. This cartilage is very elastic, owing to its laminated structure, and its consistency. It forms very flexible articulations so that the vertebrae can tip or roll in every direction, *within limits.*

The vertebrae are further secured in their positions by nine ligaments with their modifications and subdivisions. These allow the vertebrae to move in all directions, within a limited distance.

The column of segments or vertebrae, called the spinal column, is maintained in an upright position, not straight, but with a sigmoid curve, by muscles and ligaments. The muscles serve to move the segments, as well as to hold them in place.

A Vertebra is in its normal position when it is in proper juxtaposition with the vertebra above and the one below, when all its articulations are in proper apposition; and so that it does not impinge nerves and interfere with the transmission of mental impulses.

A Vertebra in this position is where Innate wants it to be, which may not be according to an "educated" ideal gained from laboratory calculations.

Art. 378. ABNORMAL VERTEBRAE. (See Vol. XV.)

A Vertebra is abnormal when it has not developed normally, is dis-eased or pathological.

Sometimes vertebrae do not grow properly. The ossification may be abnormal, as in rickets, which results in mis-shapen twisted, distorted vertebrae. If a vertebra is in an abnormal position for a length of time, that is called chronic, and subjected to unusual pressures and stresses in that position, is apt to change into a mis-shapen vertebra, especially if it is during the growing age. Vertebrae in which there is dis-ease, as in osteomalacia, Pott's dis-ease, etc., become pathological. They become squeezed out of shape, or decayed, covered with exostosis, and sometimes destroyed entirely, in which case Innate builds around them compensating bony tissue, called ankylosis, to uphold the spinal column. (See Vol. XV.)

Such vertebrae are difficult to restore to their normal positions, for they have become so fitted to the abnormal positions that they offer much resistance to adjusting. In such adjustments it is mostly the "booster's" forces that must overcome this resistance. In case of pathological vertebrae, or heavy ankylosis, or destroyed vertebrae and discs (as in Pott's disease) adjustments are impossible. We know that such cases could have been prevented if they had been adjusted before so much destruction took place.

Art. 379. Intervertebral Discs. (Ref. Vol. XV and IX)

An Intervertebral Disc is the elastic pad of cartilage between vertebrae.

An Intervertebral Disc is disc shaped and somewhat thicker in the center, like a lens. Discs average from one-eighth to five-sixteenth inch in thickness. They have a laminated structure in the center of which is a semi-fluid, pulp-like mass. The laminae (layers) give elasticity; and, although they are made of non-elastic connective tissue fibers, these fibers are kinked, which also give elasticity, within limits.

The vertebrae do not slide over the lens-like structures, but the fibers of the disc are securely imbedded in the epiphyseal plates of the adjacent vertebrae, thus attaching these strong ligaments. This structure allows the vertebra to move by stretching or squeezing the disc. The discs, acting as ligaments and as padding to sustain shocks, are very important tissues of the vertemere.

When the discs are abnormal, they are too dry or too firm, wedge-shaped, too thin, pathological, or may be entirely destroyed (as in Pott's dis-ease). The consideration of abnormal discs in adjusting is important, for they offer considerable resistance to adjustment and tend to misplace the vertebrae again, until adjustments have caused a physiological change in their texture and shape. This is accomplished both by the mechanical forces and the restoration of transmission to the vertemere.

Art. 380. Spinal Ligaments. (Ref. Vol. XV and IX.)

Ligaments are bands of fibrous connective tissue which assist in holding the segments of the spinal column in situ, allowing a limited movement of the segments.

They also assist in keeping the spinal column erect, with its normal curves. These normal curves conform to the shape that Innate desires, which may not be according to a "laboratory ideal."

There are nine principal ligaments, with their subdivisions. These ligaments embrace the vertebrae like a mesh-work tube; also having super-attachments and inter-attachments of their processes.

Abnormal ligaments are those which are pathological; too hard, too dry, prolapsed, or grown into abnormal shapes.

In chronic abnormal positions of the spine (as subluxations and curvatures) the ligaments assume abnormal forms and textures; as, being lengthened on the convex side of a curvature and shortened on the concave side.

The ligaments that concern any given vertebra, if abnormal, do much to resist adjustments (as do discs, as described before) and do not assist much in keeping the vertebrae in normal position, when they are adjusted, until enough time is allowed for them to regain their normal form and texture. This, also, is accomplished by restoration of transmission to the ligaments concerned, through the vertemere cycle.

Note: — There is an erroneous belief among laymen that Chiropractic is "good for" spinal dis-eases only. We wish to

inform both laymen and students that spinal dis-eases are only a small part of Chiropractic in the handling of peripheral causes. To the chiropractor, *all* body tissues are periphery and subject to the law of cause and effect.

Art. 381. Spinal Muscles. (Ref. XV and IX)

Spinal muscles are those attached to or which have to do with the position of vertebrae, relative to each other; and to keep the spine erect, giving to it any movement necessary in flexing or turning.

The muscles are employed constantly, especially when there is consciousness. The muscles are the means of subluxations occurring. The response to a concussion is referred to as *innate contraction of forces.* If one will try to visualize the task of keeping twenty-six blocks of bone in a correct, functioning pile, every one being moved to accommodate the different positions of the body, he can realize the importance of these muscles.

Abnormal muscles are those which are dis-eased, pathological, contracted, prolapsed, or depleted.

When dis-eased or pathological, they cannot perform their functions properly in moving or maintaining the spine in its normal position. If contracted or prolapsed, they cause rotations and curvatures. If the spinal muscles, having to do with the subluxated vertebra, are abnormal, Innate cannot restore the vertebra to its normal position; and if pathological or depleted, will offer little, if any, assistance in keeping it in its place until restored transmission gets them back to normal.

Art. 382. Curvatures. (Ref. XV)

A Curvature is a permanent, abnormal deviation from the normal contour of the spinal column; whether it augments or straightens a curve.

A Curve is the normal bending of the spinal column.

The normal spinal column is straight when viewed from the posterior or anterior, and sigmoid from a lateral view.

There are three kinds of curvatures when **classified according to direction.** A convexity toward the anterior is a *lordosis.* A convexity toward the posterior is a *kyphosis.* A convexity toward either side is a *scoliosis.* These curvatures may be combined forming *lordo-scolioses,* or *kypho-scolioses.* If a curvature is complicated by rotations, it is, for instance, a *rotatory-scoliosis.* When there is just one abnormal lateral bend in the whole spinal column, it is a *total scoliosis.* Usually, however, a curvature, which tends to throw the spinal column "out of plumb" has another curvature which tends to restore "plumb" (thus making adaptation) called a *compensatory curvature;* as *compensatory scoliosis.*

Curvatures are also classified according to cause and effect.

A curvature that is caused by a subluxation (see Vertemere Cycle) is a *primary curvature.*

Curvatures which compensate for primary curvatures are *compensatory curvatures* **and are** *secondary* **or** *adaptative.*

Curvatures caused by trauma may be classed as primary curvatures and have their compensatory (secondary or adaptative) curvatures. Curvatures caused by occupations, as hod-carrying, bookkeeping, locomotive driving, are *occupational curvatures.* They are not caused by subluxations, therefore are not primary curvatures; they are adaptative to the occupation. It would be a serious mistake to adjust for occupational curvatures, since they are not caused by subluxations, and adjustments could not abolish the patient's occupation. One could only advise him to change his occupation, or do it in a different manner. Such curvatures of very long standing have no remedy, nor are they necessarily harmful.

Chiropractic does not pretend to "straighten" curvatures by force, or to *force* an abnormal spine to an "educated ideal." That is not Chiropractic but orthopedic surgery. Neither does Chiropractic adjust with the intention of *forcing* or *driving* vertebrae into perfect alignment; for Chiropractic does not *treat effects* at all. It seeks to *remove the cause,* and the cause is always in the spine. (Prin. 30, 31.)

Primary curvatures are effects. They are the effects of interference with transmission to the muscles and other tissues which keep the spine in its proper contour. If the muscles are contracted or prolapsed, they will pull the spine out of alignment or allow it to sag out of alignment. By adjusting the cause of this, the muscles regain their tonicity and motor control, thus becoming normal muscles. These normal muscles by coordinated pulls, restore the spine to its normal shape. Absolutely, this is the only way that a primary curvature can be abolished. When the primary curvature has gone, there is no further need of compensatory curvatures (which are adaptative), so they disappear. Since occupational curvatures are adaptative, they will disappear when the patient ceases or changes his occupation.

Rule—Never adjust for adaptative conditions; adjust for the primary condition that produces them.

One should never adjust vertebrae to get them into "perfect alignment," for what one thinks is the right position "educationally," may not suit Innate—it very seldom does. That is to say, they may not be subluxations at all, and unless they are subluxations they should not be adjusted.

If in the spine of a person, the X-rays show many vertebrae "out of alignment," and if he has apparent curvatures; if he still has practically perfect health, **it is a mistake to adjust these vertebrae, for Innate has not said they are subluxations.** She has made it strongly manifest that they are not subluxations and that the spine is just as she wants it to be.

Art. 383. Rotations. (Ref. Vol. XV)

A Rotation is the condition of a vertebra when its centrum has lost its proper juxtaposition with the one above or the one

below or both, having rotated about a vertical axis, usually between the zygapophyses.

A Rotation that impinges nerves and interferes with the transmission of mental impulses is a subluxation.

The axis of a rotation is vertical and commonly near the union of the pedicles and laminae; that is to say, at the zygapophyses which act as fulcrums. When a vertebra centrum rotates to the right, or left, the tip of the spinous process usually rotates in the opposite direction. A single vertebra cannot rotate very far, owing to the limitations imposed by its ligaments; approximately to one-fourth inch or a little more sometimes.

Vertebrae rotate freely and normally with the movements of the body, but when they become permanently and abnormally rotated they are called *Rotations.* Such displacements to the right are named *Right Rotations,* and those to the left, *Left Rotations.* When a vertebra rotates more than one-fourth or three-eighths of an inch, it carries the vertebra above and the one below with it, and thus forms a *Right* (or left) *Rotatory Scoliosis.* Such a scoliosis contains three or more rotated vertebrae. (For more detail, see Vol. XV).

Art. 384. TILTED VERTEBRAE.

A Tilted Vertebra is one that has lost its proper juxtaposition with the one above and the one below, by having the centrum rotated about a horizontal axis.

This axis is not always through the center of the centrum; it may be through any part of it, so that the vertebra is tilted up on one side; down on one side; one side up and the other side down. The same may be said about the anterior and the posterior portions. When a vertebra is tilted, the disc is compressed on the side where the vertebrae are too close together, while the other side of the disc is extended, so that it is thicker than usual. Tilted vertebrae are found in an infinite

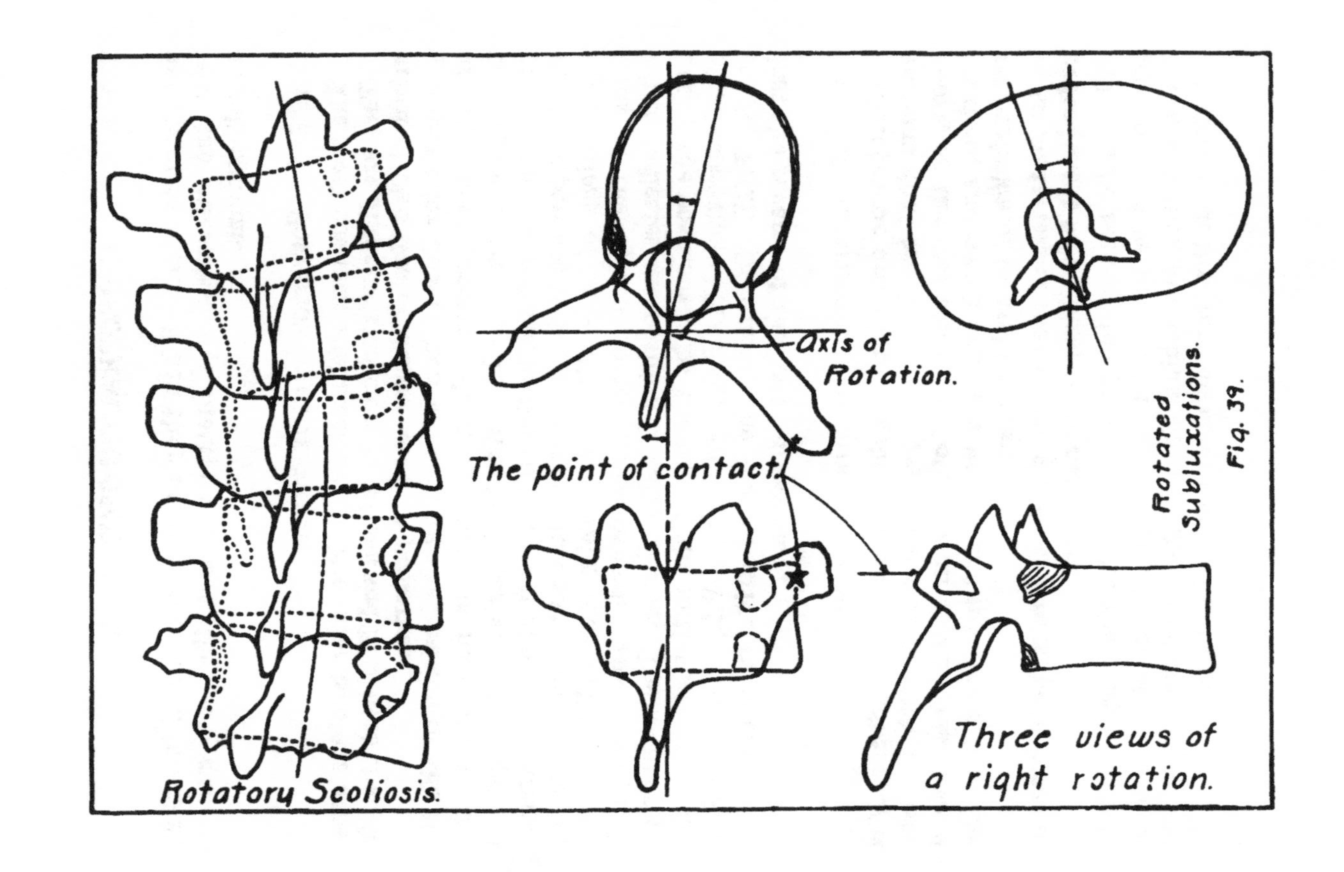
Rotatory Scoliosis.
Axis of Rotation.
The point of contact.
Three views of a right rotation.
Rotated Subluxations.

Fig. 39.

variety of positions. When they impinge nerves and interfere with the transmission of mental impulses, they are classed as subluxations.

Art. 385. Posterior Subluxations.

The most common subluxations are Posterior Subluxations. They are differentiated from Rotations and Tilts in that their principal direction of displacement is posterior.

A posterior Subluxation is listed by the position of the tip of its spinous process, which of course is posterior to the two adjacent ones. In addition to being posterior, this spinous process may be rotated to the right or left slightly ("laterality"); or perhaps to the superior or inferior. Also, there are combinations of these directions. Thus nine different positions of the spinous process are named. The description which indicates the position is called *listing*. The manner of listing the positions is by the use of the initial letters of the directions, thus: P., P.R., P.L., P.S., P.I., P.R.S., P.R.I., P.L.S., P.L.I. Of course, the line of drive in adjusting is just the reverse of the listed direction.

Art. 386. Definitions of Subluxations.

Chiropractic definition: a subluxation is the condition of a vertebra that has lost its proper juxtaposition with the one above, or the one below, or both; to an extent less than a luxation; and which impinges nerves and interferes with the transmission of mental impulses.

All the factors of the foregoing definition must be included in order that it be a Chiropractic definition.

It can be seen by the previous articles that *any* abnormal position of a vertebra, such as posteriority, rotations, curvatures, and tilts, are subluxations if they impinge nerves and interfere with the transmission of mental impulses.

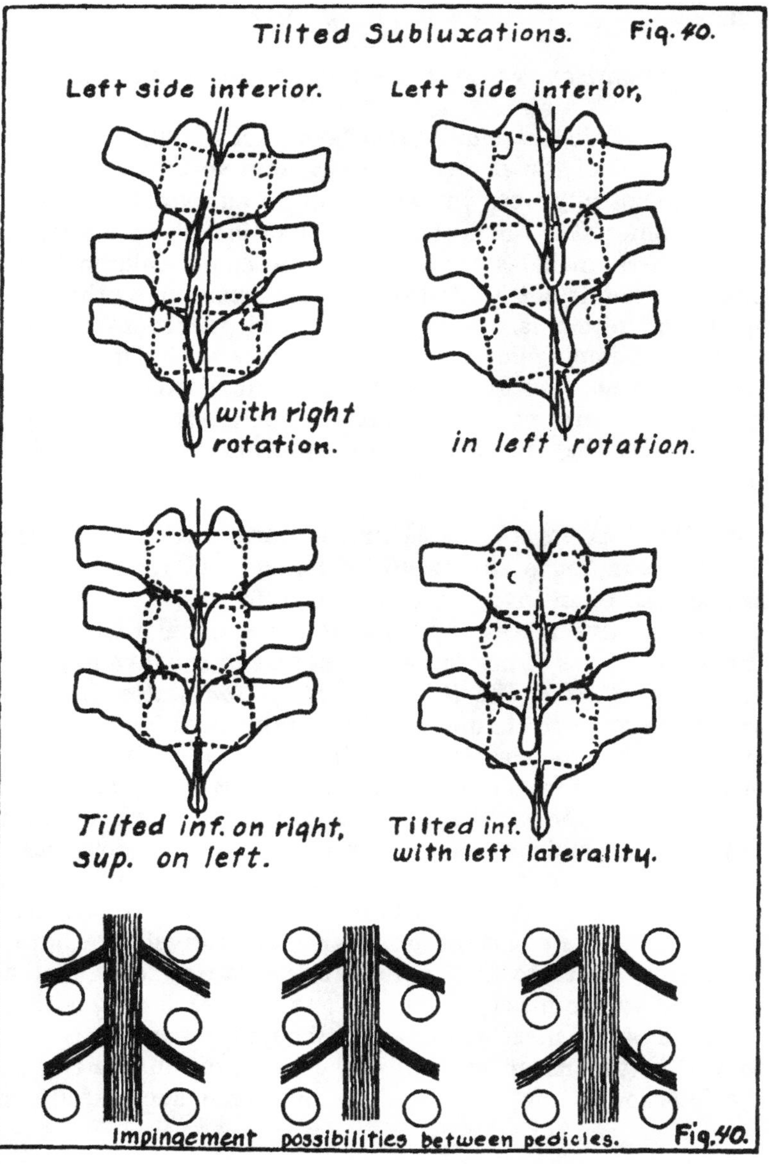

Tilted Subluxations. Fig. 40.

Left side inferior. with right rotation.

Left side inferior, in left rotation.

Tilted inf. on right, sup. on left.

Tilted inf. with left laterality.

Impingement possibilities between pedicles. Fig. 40.

For comparison, we give the anatomical or surgical definition:

"A partial dislocation." (Dorland) A subluxation is the displacement of the elements of *any* joint so that its articulations are not in proper juxtaposition, to an extent less than a dislocation. (Note—dislocation and luxation are synonymous.) It, of course, includes the joints of the spinal column though this definition is not limited to the spinal column as the Chiropractic definition is. Also, the surgical definition makes no mention of impingement and interference with transmission, for that is no part of surgery. The subluxations shown by spinography are not Chiropractic subluxations until it is proved that they interfere with transmission of mental impulses.

Art. 387. Subluxations Defined According to Cause.

A Subluxation is the result of unbalanced resistive forces in response to an invading penetrative force.

The resistive forces, in this case, are unbalanced because of the limitations of matter, or the nature of the invading force. (180-185, 187 V.) The *third law of motion* states that every action has an opposite and equal reaction. A subluxation is an abnormality produced in the body by resistive force in response to an external force. It is not produced by the direct application of the external force. A force which results in the subluxation of a vertebra very seldom strikes it. This force, of course, has a reactionary force in the opposite direction, but that does not concern us. To the invading force, Innate makes resistance, adaptively. There is reactionary force to this, which Innate causes to be met and absorbed by the mass of the body, as the recoil of shooting is absorbed by the mass of the gun. Should the penetrative force be within the range of body tissue adaptation (Prin. 24), the invasion is met, balanced or overcome successfully and

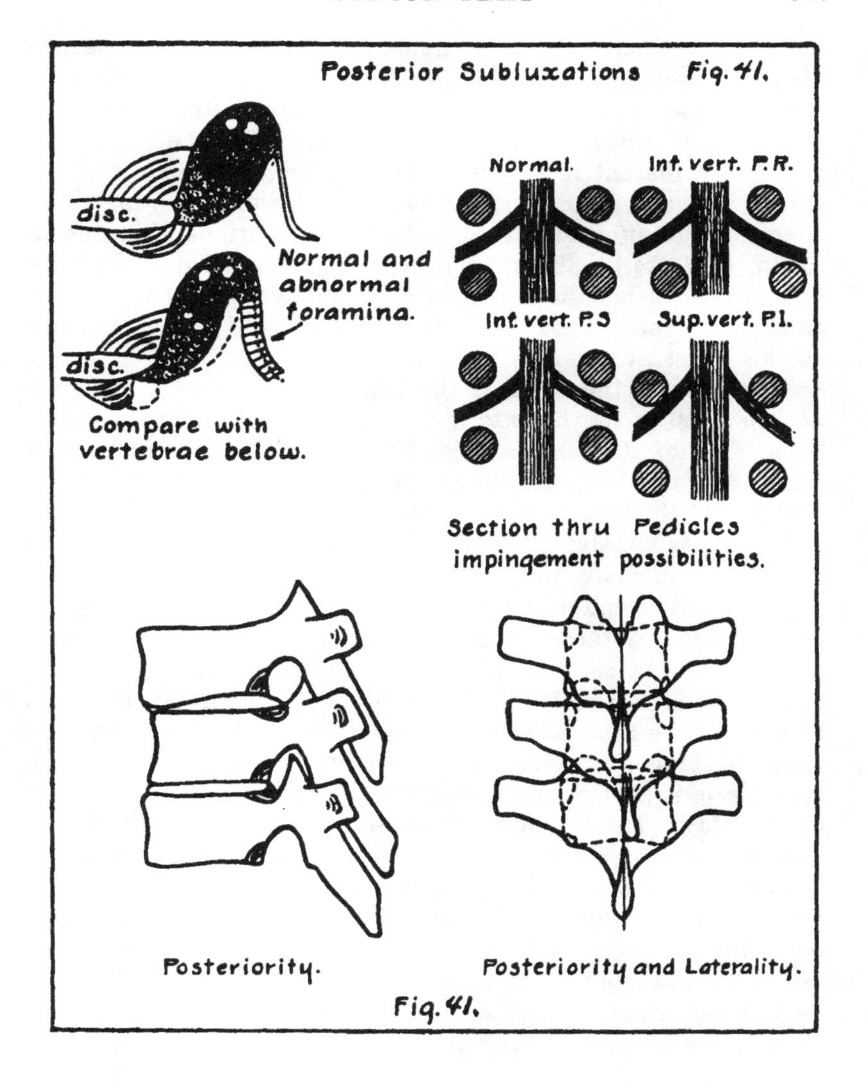
Posterior Subluxations Fig. 41.
disc.
Normal and
abnormal
foramina.
disc.
Compare with
vertebrae below.
Normal.
Inf. vert. P.R.
Inf. vert. P.S
Sup. vert. P.I.
Section thru Pedicles
impingement possibilities.
Posteriority.
Posteriority and Laterality.

Fig. 41.

nothing happens; except, perhaps, local injury to the tissues struck. Should the penetrative force act upon body tissues when they are not in a position to react readily, then the resistance will be untimely, therefore unbalanced. The student is not for an instant to suppose that Innate is too slow or that Innate is unable; but Innate always has to work with material, therefore her efforts are limited by the limitations of material. (Prin. 5, 6, 24.) She makes intellectual adaptation quickly enough and sends impulses readily enough, but the tissues cannot act readily enough when in awkward positions, and so the forces are unbalanced.

That part of the mass of the body which absorbs most reactions to such movements is the spinal column, for it is the foundation of the whole body. Naturally, the greatest strain falls upon that vertemere which is absorbing the most reaction. If the resistive force be unbalanced, the reaction to that force is unbalanced likewise, therefore the muscles of the vertemere misplace the vertebra.

The question has often arisen: why is the spine always the part affected by these unbalanced forces? The answer to this is: the spine is *not always* the part to suffer, but is the *most common* place to suffer from unbalanced resistive forces, because it is the foundation of the body. It is important to note that unbalanced resistive forces produce sprains, dislocations, torn tissues, prolapses, or fractures, in most any active part of the body. **This is the fundamental principle of jujitsu.**

Example: Suppose a person were accustomed to making a leap from a platform to the ground three feet below. He could be blindfolded and still make the leap without the slightest injury. But, if, unbeknownst to him, a deep pit were dug where he expected to land, and this pit filled with feathers or some other soft material, the blindfolded jumper would more than likely possess some subluxations after the jump. Obviously, it would be impossible for the fall to hurt him otherwise. He could receive no concussion of forces from outside his body. Yet his Innate expecting hard ground at three feet had resistive forces prepared, which having nothing to act upon were unbalanced and produced subluxations. (For another example see Poison Cycle, Art. 200.)

The first natural resistance made by Innate is mechanical. This is the first response made by Innate because it is the most ready retaliation at hand. In case of invasive chemical forces, or any other intangible (or rather a force not mechanical), it is first met by Innate by mechanical resistance. Later, Innate will produce counteractive chemicals, but that requires more time (Prin. 6). Naturally, a mechanical force matched against a chemical force is like striking at shadows, and if at all violent will result in subluxations, strains, etc.

If a person is called upon to make a sudden and strong resistance to a push or a blow when he is in an awkward relaxed posture, to receive it, he will feel the reaction in his back. (187, V) Even if he is in a prepared posture, if the strain is beyond the endurance of his tissues a subluxation will occur.

Example: If a man is lifting an object, the pull of gravity is downward, and he is trying to move it upward—so much for that pair of forces. The pull on his arms is downward and the resistance of his spine is upward—the internal pair of forces. Should he try to lift something too heavy for him, his back will withstand, for a time, the strain upward; all the muscles straining to keep those blocks of bone stacked up, under the pressure. Then as he lifts harder he reaches the limit of his tissues. The weakest place gives away first, and with traumatic suddenness, there are unbalanced forces acting in the weakest vertemere.

Art. 388. External Forces.

External Forces are environmental or universal or physical forces; forces not assembled by Innate Intelligence.

Their main characteristic is that they are not adaptive, though they can be adapted. (Prin. 11, 23.)

They may be either beneficial or harmful to the body.

They may be applied either inside or outside of the body.

Some are always inside the body (Prin. 1, 16) ; **they cannot be kept out, but if the body is normal they are always adapted when inside.**

They may affect the body in numerous forms; as, physical, chemical, and mechanical (which is also physical).

They are necessary to the body to maintain universal balance. The student should understand that they come to the body in circumstances, weather, food, drink, sunlight—myriads of ways. Because they come in from without, they are called *external,* although they may have internal application. The student should not get the idea that they *always* impinge on the surface of the body from the outside—that is not an ideal way to receive a dinner, for instance. Sometimes they are harmful.

Art. 389. Penetrative Forces.

Penetrative Forces are invasive forces; forces external which force their way into the body, and their effects upon tissue, in spite of Innate's resistance.

Or, they are forces in the body which Innate does not desire, and which she tries to expel; or to prevent their action.

They are in numerous forms; as physical, chemical, and mechanical.

These forces are well known. We fail to acknowledge some of them if they are insidious. They may enter the body as chemical forces and begin their destructive work by corrosion or calling for violent adaptation. (See poison cycle.) The forces of weather as heat , cold, etc., call for unusual adaptation sometimes. Severe exertion demands severe adaptation.

However, all the Penetrative Forces do not provoke violent rejection—some are more subtle.

Penetrative Forces, which are mechanical, are applied outside of the body usually, though not always. They may be from *any* direction. The direction of these mechanical penetrative forces has nothing to do with the direction of the subluxation they cause, if they cause subluxations. They do not strike the vertebra they subluxate, but may strike a part of the body very remote from them; for it is the unbalanced reaction of the resistive concussion that does the subluxating.

In some cases, penetrative forces result in benefit to the body; and that is when they are scientifically applied. An adjustment is that kind. However, any adjustic move that is not scientifically given (direction *does* make a difference here) is not beneficial and is likely to be harmful. The fact is often presented that some unscientific adjustments do get sick people well—but so do some accidents; but an accident is too uncertain to be a reliable doctor.

Art. 390. Internal Forces.

Forces made by Innate.

They are for use in and for the body.

They are universal forces assembled or adapted for use in the body.

They are for adaptation to other universal forces.

Internal Forces, which were spoken of before as *innate forces* have been quite fully described in many other places.

Art. 391. Resistive Forces.

Resistive Forces are Internal Forces (innate forces) called into being to oppose Penetrative Forces.

They may be in many forms; as physical, chemical, or mechanical.

Example: physical, as movements of tissue cells; chemical, as antidotes, oxidations, etc.; mechanical, as "bucking" when a patient is being adjusted; mental, as educated adaptations, will, etc.

When ill-timed or unbalanced may produce strains, sprains, torn tissues, fractures, luxations, or subluxations.

When ill-timed or unbalanced, it is not the fault of Innate, but the limitations of matter. (Prin. 5, 24.)

They oppose, or join some penetrative forces as determined by Innate; as, in adjusting.

Resistive forces have been described in the previous articles. Chemical resistance has been given in Poison Cycles.

"*Bucking*" is the term used to describe what a patient does when he is getting a poor adjustment or has had previous experience with poor adjustments.

If the body is not in an awkward posture; or if Innate is educationally aware of an impending force, the body will always successfully oppose an invading force, if it is not beyond the limits of adaptation of these tissues.

Art. 392. Innate Contraction of Forces.

Innate Contraction of Forces are the efforts made by Innate Intelligence through the tissues of the vertemere region in response to a concussion.

When a subluxation occurs, it is because the reaction to Innate's resistance (in the body) is ill-timed or unbalanced, through the limitations of matter.

When an adjustment occurs, it is because the reaction in the body to Innate's resistance is called forth, scientifically and intentionally, by the adjustor, so that the reaction is joined with the adjustic force in timeliness, amount, and direction.

Posture is an important factor in these; awkwardly relaxed or unprepared or unequaled to strain, in subluxating; scientifically relaxed in adjusting.

In other words, the first resistance that Innate makes to a mechanical blow is mechanical resistance, even though later she accepts it as "something good." The force must be delivered as a concussion, so as to call forth a resistance, that there may be a usable reaction to it in the vertemere. No matter how good an adjustor is, there is a percentage of his forces that Innate cannot accept, hence she will resist. No one can calculate to one hundred per cent what Innate wants in amount, direction, and distance. That is why Innate's forces must be called forth, to do the adjusting, for she is the only power able to do it. However, every adjustor should strive to make his percentage of acceptable forces as high as possible, for if the percentage is low, it is rejected by Innate. If the force is delivered by "brute strength" in spite of Innate's objections, it calls forth no adjustic forces by Innate, and may result in trauma. In most cases of poor "adjustments", Innate will successfully reject them, which is fortunate.

When Innate makes her resistance to a mechanical force which is "good," and she has determined that it is "good," she always disposes of a percentage of the resistance by absorption in the tissues and allows the reaction to be augmented by the "good" percentage of the adjustor's move, thus forming a *resultant* force, which restores the vertebra to its normal position. This takes place in the vertemere and has to do with the vertemere cycle.

Art. 393. Luxations. (Dislocations)

A Luxation (Chiropractic definition) is the condition of a vertebra that has lost its juxtaposition with the vertebra above or the one below, or both, to the extent that its articulations are not in apposition.

"Out of joint." Dislocated.

It may or may not impinge nerves and interfere with transmission.

When a joint is dislocated, its articulations are not partially displaced as in subluxations, but are "clear out of joint"; no longer in apposition. To allow this, the ligaments are strained and in some cases are torn loose. Dislocations are traumatic and are not in the realm of Chiropractic, professionally or legally. The practitioner should send such cases to the surgeon; or, if he does anything at all with them, work under the auspices of a surgeon.

Art. 394. Fractures.

A Fracture is a broken bone or ruptured cartilage.

"The breaking of a part, especially of a bone." (Dorland)

It may or may not impinge nerves and interfere with the transmission of mental impulses.

In the spine, fragments of broken bone or imperfectly set bones, or an irregular healing of a fractured bone may impinge nerves. There is nothing a chiropractor can do about fractures, professionally or legally.

Art. 395. B. J.'s Answer to a Medical College.

It has often been said by the medical profession that no one could move a vertebra of the spinal column and that the Chiropractic claims were all fake. They went so far as to make the following test to show that it was a fake. They forgot, or else never knew that real chiropractors do not claim they adjust vertebrae, but that Innate Intelligence does it. A chiropractor would not attempt to adjust the vertebrae of a dead man, any more than a physician would give him salts to move his bowels. The chiropractor adjusts vertebrae in the living—why? Because he expects a recoil to take place and that would be impossible in a dead man. The medical college made a mechanical experiment on a dead body, and B. J. answered with an experiment just as mechanical, showing that even in this line the medical college was mistaken, and was not obliged to show his strongest argument—that is, that Innate adjusts.

Quotation: "The College of Medical Evangelists, located at Loma Linda, California. The spine used was 'fresh'! It was placed upon a structure of wood with the vertebra that pressure was brought to bear upon, entirely free from any brace whatsoever. Pressure of eight hundred pounds was brought to bear upon the posterior surface. This crushed the spinous process and some portions of the laminae. Pressure of one thousand, one hundred ninety-five pounds reduced the vertebra to almost a powdery consistency. All this weight was exerted without any movement of the vertebra itself."

B. J.'s Test in Answer: "Two boards two inches thick, twelve inches wide, and three feet long were used. A hole was bored in one of these boards and the other one was placed upon it with the ends supported but leaving the space that was to be tested entirely free from any support whatever. Then he placed a twenty-penny spike upright in the top board and adjusted it with levels so that it could not lean to either side. Pressure was brought to bear on the spike. It required one thousand six hundred pounds for the spike to begin entering the soft wood and before the spike had gone entirely through the wood, the pressure amounted to two thousand four hundred pounds. Then it is preposterous for a carpenter, with a one pound hammer, to drive a spike."

Art. 396. COORDINATION. **Principle No. 32.**

Coordination is the principle of harmonious action of all the parts of an organism, in fulfilling their offices or purposes.

It is not fully understood what mental impulses are. That is no reflection upon Chiropractic. Chiropractors know the manifestations of mental impulses. They can make practical applications of this knowledge in getting the sick well. Whatever the force is, they know that they have named a unit of it,

Mental Impulse, with as much justification as electricians have named a unit of electrical current, *ampere.*

However, as scientists, we are privileged to theorize about mental force. Claiming to have knowledge of the fundamentals of our science, we believe our theories to have reasonable plausibility. In the first place, we give credit to Intelligence for the origin of mental force, as we do in the consideration of all forces. We know that the body is of organized materials. We know that the molecules and atoms and structures constituting the body have the same interests, else they would not be together; the same specific object in view (p. 27, V) which shows that the principle of organization is in use. (See organize, Webster.)

The actions of these component parts will always be for the welfare of other component parts, but these actions can only be beneficial to those parts, when cooperative or coordinated. The forces which make these parts coordinate must be of that character which is specific and adaptative, which can be no less than mental. Then, Innate Intelligence is the coordinating principle; necessarily mental, as intellectuality. The forces and products emanating from the actions of some cells determine what must be done by other cells, adaptatively. This interchange of forces and products is managed by Innate Intelligence.

Perhaps we can use an analogy to advantage. The Government of the United States does not direct the business of individuals. A Government that is wise does not attempt to do so for no one knows one's business as well as he does himself. (Imagine the President or a Senator telling a chiropractor when and how to adjust a P. R. I. dorsal subluxation!) To attempt it would involve the Government in a multiplicity of detail, would not be effectual because none of them would know all about every science or occupation.

What is it that bids the farmer to plant his fields; the merchant to stock his shelves, and the workman to seek a job? Not altogether his personal needs, or fundamentally to build a fortune. Surely it is not a command from the Government. It is a much more powerful urge than that. It is the principle of service ; that of cooperation or coordination. This urge is not a tangible thing; it is abstract, yet a force to be reckoned with. No government may tamper with it.

It is nothing less than mental impulses. The efficiency of these is exactly proportional to true organization and completeness of transmission; of the needs of some and the satisfying those needs by others. The Law of Demand and Supply, if you notice. Oversupply or under-supply, waste or want, would be due to incoordination due to poor transmission. This does not refer to the transmission of materials entirely, but to transmission of the urge. The demand of the needy gives the urge to the service giver. The fact that he is compensated does not detract from the analogy, for so is the tissue cell compensated. The real governing principle of the United States is not a body of men at Washington, but the great mental principle of coordination without which government would be ineffectual.

Art. 397. THE LAW OF DEMAND AND SUPPLY.
Principle No. 33.

The Law of Demand and Supply is existent in the body in its ideal state; wherein the "clearing house" is the brain, Innate the virtuous "banker," brain cells "clerks," and nerve cells "messengers."

This is not an analogy, but a fact. While we are acquainted with this law in commerce, its working out is somewhat imperfect, because of the limitations of educated minds; but in the body with an infinite intelligence in charge, it has approached the perfect very closely; the only limitations being that of matter. (Prin.24) Application of this principle will show what coordination is and how necessary Intellectual Adaptation and adaptation are. It shows the union and close relation of all these thirty-three principles and any more which we care to derive from them. It binds them all together in an unbeatable unit—and that unit is the Essence of Chiropractic. Know your principles thoroughly and no problem of Chiropractic, that is practical, will trouble you long.

In order that Innate may make demand of all the tissue cells under her jurisdiction, in harmony with the organization, she must receive the demands from all the tissue cells in order to know their needs. She must have Ideation in order to make Intellectual Adaptation. The supply of forces comes from Innate directly, and the supply of materials reaches the demanding cells through the Serous Circulation. It is evident, then, that the two most important cycles upon which the others are based are the Normal Complete Cycle, and the Serous Cycle.

Let us illustrate further by the use of an analogy. An electric generator induces electricity in its rotating armature, by swinging its coils of wires through a magnetic field and "cutting the lines of magnetic force." The amount of current generated and its strength is proportional to the number of "lines cut" per second and the strength of those lines. This magnetic field is maintained by a "shunt winding," if a direct current, and by a separate small dynamo, if alternating current. As a hypothesis, suppose that when ten thousand lines of force are cut, at a given rate of speed, the generator is supplying one thousand lamps. Then suppose that five hundred of these lamps are turned out, leaving only five hundred to be supplied. Obviously, instant adaptation will have to be made at the generator, else the remaining lamps will be burned out, if not saved by fuses. Instant adaptation *is* made; it is by the automatic "feel" of the return current by the field magnets of the generator, which instantly reduce the number of lines of force from ten thousand to five thousand, and though the generator still runs at the same rate of speed, the engine running the generator breathes much easier, for formerly it required much effort to cut those lines of force.

Another entirely different theory is offered; the vibrations of a cell create an "aura" of radiant force which constitutes environmental conditions for other cells; just as a passenger in a crowded street car creates environmental conditions for other passengers which they must adapt themselves to. This force is collected by Innate Intelligence on the afferent nerves, as we do lines of earth magnetism with a compass; or radiant electricity with our radio antennae, for the purpose of coordinating all tissue cells. These forces which are inevitable emanations of any moving bodies, cells, or anything else, will act as a factor in determining what other cells will have to do in order to balance it. The coordinating of all these struggling organisms is done through the "clearing house"—the brain, and Innate is the principle; which is the Intelligence that keeps all in harmony.

Art. 398. The Universal Cycle.

The Universal Cycle is the cycle showing intellectuality perpetuated in cycles.

The cycle which explains the trend of evolution; the ever-changing institutions of the universe.

All universal laws work in cycles; the material units of the universe, as the planets and stars move in circles. The earth itself travels in a cycle and revolves around its axis. The conditions on the surface of the earth undergo cycles, as the seasons. The ever-changing phases of life on its surface are cyclic. Living things die and new life starts up again. Inorganic material is organized to be disorganized. Organic structures are built to furnish material to tear down; that furnishes material to build again. We have seen how there is an evolutionary value (survival value). Its phases are cyclic. What is the trend of this? Dr. Palmer holds that it is the cyclic change which incorporates more intellectuality in matter, thus raising the standard of created things. A progress toward betterment; toward the ideal. We quote from Dr. Palmer (page 282, V). "All of this universal cycle shows how cycles perpetuate its intellectuality, and its intellectuality-formed products, for further cyclic productions—to the end of a higher and better standard. Quantity of foruns and quantity of matter, speed of one passing through the other, has all to do with the quality of the product. It is not for chiropractors to try to improve the basic law—this is impossible—but to remove any (negative) obstructions, brought about by perversions of that law, to the further end of a greater and freer expression of what the law of cycles demands in every phase and attribute. The law of a universal cycle is absolute. 'Have I interpreted correctly?' remains for the sages of future years to say."

Art. 399. B. J.'s Utopia.

In accordance with the hopeful idea given by the Universal Cycle, Dr. Palmer's love for the human race and solicitude for the suffering, lead him to hold that chiropractors have a great mission to perform. "Not to improve the basic law—this is impossible—but to remove any negative obstructions brought about by perversions of that law, to the further end of a greater and freer expression of what the law of cycles demands in every phase and attribute." If Chiropractic would be allowed to do this, an ideal state of affairs could be brought nearer. This state of affairs, which is not impossible for chiropractors to bring about, if they had the chance, would approach the ideal. An ideal state of sociology is a utopia.

An ideal sociological state would be a country or a world without sickness, insanity, blindness, feeble-minded people, deaf and dumb, backward children; social evils, criminality, drunkenness and its attendant evils, abnormal reproduction, etc. If Chiropractic were given a chance to do its miracles and reasonable time allowed for the results to be brought about, it *could do much;* more than any other human agency has done or can do, in reducing the above named abnormalities to a minimum. This would be a great economic saving, because there could be fewer public and charitable institutions and penal institutions.

Etiology

(For Sophomores)

Art. 400. Etiology.

Etiology is the science of the cause. In Chiropractic, it is the science of the cause and the science of finding it.

The process of finding the cause is called Analysis.

There are two methods: the old way, by the Meric System, Generic Table, and Equations, which is good, but is much more indirect than the new way. The new way, by the use of the Neurocalometer, which traces to the cause, without the examination of any effects except those in the region of the spinal column. In the latter method, the chiropractor goes immediately to the back where exists the cause of all dis-eases. Since the NCM work is a science in itself, and is taken care of by its own department, we will give the old method in this appendix.

Since Sophomores begin adjusting after having been in school six months, it is appropriate to first give some methods of procedure for them. This will be followed by more elaborate explanations.

Art. 401. Classifying Effects.

Classifying effects for the purpose of finding the cause is the Chiropractic way of using symptomatology. It is the method of deducing the location of the cause in the spine, by the study of the symptoms. After its location or "place" is found, the search for the subluxation in that place is made by palpation, nerve tracing, etc. The objective symptoms are found by observation and examination and the subjective symptoms are found by questioning the patient. The history of the case should be obtained also, in order to find the duration of the disease. The spinograph is the last word in listing a subluxation; the NCM the last word in finding it.

The Sophomore should get his clinic cards properly filled out and have an analysis book of his own. On the clinic card he should write the symptoms (not diagnosis); describe the pathology (not name it); get the age, occupation, history of the case, etc. Next he should try to "figure out" from the symptoms, which organs are involved; this exercises his knowledge of physiology. Knowing which organs are involved, he will by the use of the Meric Generic table, calculate which place the subluxation is most likely to be in. Then, knowing this, he should palpate in this "place" to find the expected subluxation. Next, he should take his case to the verifier to see if his work is correct. If the verifier changes the student's findings, the student should ask the verifier why such a major was chosen. Then the student adjustor should write the verifier's major in one of the little squares on the card; write the date, and sign his name in the place provided for it. He may also write this listing in his own case book to use when adjusting. This work should be done carefully, the card filled out neatly in its proper places, and promptly turned in to the clinic clerk. Carefulness in making case records should be part of the chiropractor's training and a student careless in such matters will be careless in his own office, which may be disastrous to him sometime. Now the student is ready to adjust his patient. While this seems to be considerable "red tape" for you to do before you may "punch the patient's back," do not be in so much haste. This is the only spine the patient will ever have, and you should not be careless with it. He does not come to you for "punches in the back," but adjustments. He wants results and not haste.

Art. 402. A Rudimentary Generic Table.

U. Cer. P.	=	**upper cervical place; atlas or axis.**
M. Cer. P.	=	**middle cervical place; 3rd, 4th, and 5th cervicals.**
L. Cer. P.	=	**lower cervical place; 5th, 6th, and 7th cervicals.**
A. P.	=	**arm place; 1st dorsal.**
V. P.	=	**vertebra prominens; 6th, 7th, 1st, for landmark for counting.**
H. P.	=	**heart place; 1st, 2nd, 3rd dorsals.**
Lu. P.	=	**lung place; 2nd, 3rd, 4th dorsals.**
Li. P.	=	**liver place; 3rd, 4th, 5th dorsals.**
C. P.	=	**center place; 4th, 5th, 6th dorsals.**
S. P.	=	**stomach place; 5th, 6th, 7th, 8th dorsals.**
Spl. P.	=	**spleen place; 7th, 8th, 9th, 10th dorsals.**
U. K. P.	=	**upper kidney place; 9th, 10th, 11th dorsals.**
L. K. P.	=	**lower kidney place; 11th, 12th dorsals and 1st lumbar.**
U. L. P.	=	**upper lumbar place; 1st, 2nd, 3rd lumbar.**
M. L. P.	=	**middle lumbar place; 2nd, 3rd, 4th lumbar.**
L. L. P.	=	**lower lumbar place; 3rd, 4th, 5th lumbar.**
Sac. P.	=	**sacrum place; sacrum.**
Coc. P.	=	**coccyx place; coccyx.**

These are for the "local" or for the direct effects. The indirect effects and "condition," and some of the roundabouts are in the following:

All true headaches of the associated type are shown by the headache chart.

K. P. for eyes.
K. P. for ears.
K. P. for toxins.

U. K. P. for blood vessels.
C. P. for spinal cord.

S. P. for eyes.
S. P. for throat and mouth and lips.
S. P. for thyroid or throat glands (meric throat).
C. P. for heat regulation.
C. P. for general "conditioner."

There are many more roundabout ones that appear in "practice."

Art. 403. Major Work.

A patient will, nearly always, have several incoordinations at the same time.

The one which is the most vital to his health or life is the Major Condition.

The subluxations causing it are the Major.

The other incoordinations of the patients are the Minor Conditions. They have very little, if any, connection with the Major Condition.

The Palmer method is to give attention to the Major Condition first and when it is restored, take up the worst minor condition which is then the new major.

Clinical findings show that if majors and minors are all adjusted at the same time, or even if the major is adjusted too frequently, it makes the patient very weak and may be harmful. (See Art. 297.)

Art. 404. THE FACTORS OF A MAJOR.

A Major has direct and indirect effects.

The direct effects (conditions) are due to impingement of local nerve supply.

The indirect effects (conditions) are generally due to impingements affecting the Serous Circulation.

Therefore, a Major usually has one, two, or three subluxations.

Sometimes one subluxation has both direct and indirect effects.

The subluxation causing the direct condition is called ***Location*** **or** ***Local.***

The subluxations causing the indirect condition are called ***Condition.***

Sometimes a Major is for only one of these, but a Major that has both Location and Condition is a combination major; and most of them are in that class.

A patient never has but one Major at a time.

Some indirect effects are not "condition," which refers to the soundness of tissue cells, but to an indirect nerve pressure: as, a subluxation which causes a tumor which in turn presses upon another nerve causing incoordination somewhere else. The true "condition" which refers to the unsoundness of tissue cells, because of abnormal Serous Circulation, is a study of the limitations of matter. (Prin. 5, 24.)

Art. 405. The Inferior Meric System.

The Inferior Meric System is a system of dividing the tissues of the body into zones and meres according to nerve supply from the spinal column.

A system comprising all the zones and their meres.

The "geography" of the body.

It is of value in getting location.

Art. 406. The Superior Meric System.

A theoretical division of the brain into zones which correspond to the inferior meric zones, showing the clinical relationship between them.

The zones number from the supraorbital ridge to the foramen magnum.

When there is incoordination in an inferior zone, there is always an associated discomfort in the corresponding superior zone.

This discomfort may amount to a headache.

Art. 407. The Clinical Division of the Superior Meric System.

This division is according to the actual, not theoretical, location of headaches.

True headaches are in the brain.

False headaches are in other tissues of the head.

Direct headaches are in the part of educated brain which is the periphery of an impinged nerve in which there is interference with transmission.

The clinical division is graphically represented by the headache chart.

Headaches are of value in finding location.

Art. 408. The Use of the Meric System.

Buy or make a generic table.

Remember that Location varies in every case and the Generic Table represents an average, not a "cast iron" rule.

"Place" means a region in the spine in which the subluxation affecting a given organ is *apt* to be found; but not always.

The student is cautioned not to use the meric generic table as a rule which is never varied; as, for example, do not think that the fifth dorsal vertebra is always C. P. and "adjust" it regardless of whether it is subluxated or not, but remember that the C. P. you are seeking may be any one of the 3rd, 4th, 5th, 6th, 7th dorsals and that it may be entirely outside of this group in some cases.

ETIOLOGY

Art. 409. Rules for Picking a Major.

Getting information. If the chiropractor must make his analysis by classification of effects, then he must learn about those effects.

Location of effects. Next, it will be necessary for him to know the location of the effects, so that by his knowledge of physiology he may deduce which organs are acting abnormally.

Application of the Meric System. Having learned which organs are involved and why, and already knowing the nerve supply (anatomically) of the organs, he is able to trace to the Place in the spine where he may expect to find the subluxations. So far, he has thus been able to find the Local but the Condition offers difficulties sometimes. It is the indirect which puzzles.

Finding Condition by Specie and Family. By knowledge of physiology and the Serous Circulation, the chiropractor can deduce which organs are making the Serous Circulation abnormal. Also, knowing that the weakest part of the body will be the part which is most aggravated by the abnormal serum, he then has a check of his local findings, for "a chain is only as strong as its weakest link." The method for such deductions is to note the symptoms and place each in its proper family, which points to the organ at fault and thus you trace to the Place through the Meric System.

Find the subluxation by Chiropractic methods. When you have ascertained the places, palpate the spine and find the subluxations; assisted by Nerve Tracing, Taut and Tender Fibers. List the subluxation as to direction of displacement. If this is difficult, or if you want to be absolutely certain of your listing, have Spinograph pictures taken of the spine or of the Place.

Art. 410. Rules of Prognosis.

Age of the patient. As a person grows older the Reparation centers have given up some of their possibilities. Also, former dis-eases have probably damaged the tissues, and there may be pathology; and in all old people there is more connective tissue than in the soft, growing tissues of youth. Therefore, the chances of recovery will be slower than in the young.

Ability of the adjustor. Of course, this is an important factor. It is not hard to see that a poor adjustor, an inefficient chiropractor, could not get patients well, except by accident.

History—length of standing of the incoordination. If the chiropractor knows that the patient has had dis-eases or accidents which have badly deranged the tissues, he may know that there will be some difficulty in getting results. It is necessary to learn what the patient has been through; whether he has had an instrumental birth which might have injured the neck. If the present incoordination has been going on for some time, the chiropractor knows that the Momentum is great.

Severity of the incoordination. If the dis-ease is very severe, which it might have become, before the chiropractor was called, there will be great Momentum and Destructive Survival Values.

The chance that the patient gives the chiropractor. This is, in real practice, the chiropractor's greatest bugbear. The chiropractor should let the patient know he is the doctor. Patients are apt to not consider chiropractors as doctors, therefore disobey their orders. The chiropractors should take a firm stand about this and take no case who will not conform to the chiropractor's directions; come to take his adjustments when needed, and so live and act that the chiropractor's efforts will not be lost through the patient's misconduct. Of course, when the latter happens, the patient nearly always blames the chiropractor or Chiropractic. Often the patient will cease taking adjustments when the chiropractor is on the verge of victory, go to a medical doctor for a prescription, gets well before the medicine gets in its work, or in spite of it, then gives the medical doctor the credit for getting him well. Sometimes when the patient quits the chiropractor in the manner described and does not go to any other doctor, he gets well **after** he quits taking adjustments. This appears bad for the chiropractor unless he knows this phase according to the Philosophy of Major work. **The patient often gets well faster after you cease giving adjustments.** For this reason, it is well, after you have given a series of adjustments for a case, to let the patient rest entirely from adjustments for a while.

Art. 411. Procedure in Analysis.

Question your patient closely for information concerning his case. Get the history of the case and all the present symptoms. Remember that patients are apt to omit the essential ones which has much to do with correct procedure on your part. Do not entirely disregard "goat feathers," for, while they are of no use to you in analysis, they may give you a clue to some pertinent (not impertinent) questions which will net you some real information. Patients are sick people and are not always responsible for some of the things they tell you—sometimes the things they tell you are not reliable, especially if they are given you a "try out." With the NCM, a patient cannot deceive you, but with the old method which we are describing, deception, either innocent or malicious, is a phase you should be especially wary of.

It is well to write down the history and symptoms on your analysis card or in your analysis book. Determine the specie of each and write its symbol or symbols. From these determine the Family by summing them up, and the Family will point out the Places in the spine. After having found the Places by this formal Chiropractic equational procedure, find and list the subluxations, by palpation, nerve tracing, taut and tender fibers, Spinograph, and your knowledge of Orthopedy. Remember that any information you can gain about these subluxations is not too much, and any real and legitimate method of gaining information about the condition of the spine is not out of order.

Let us take a suppositional case and show how the chiropractor finds his major without resorting to diagnosis. The symptoms given to you or observed by you, are the following: headache, malaise, anorexia, nausea and vomiting, cough, epistaxis, and chilliness. Pain, and aching in the "small of the back" and at first constipation or costiveness and later diarrhoea. Fever, rash on the abdomen, rapid breathing, purulent stools, tympanites, enlarged spleen, scanty high-colored urine, flushed cheeks, coated tongue and sordes of the teeth. There is great tenderness and pain over the right inguinal region in the right iliac fossa.

The following tables show the disposal of this information. It can be done "mentally," but it is well to write the process out until you are well acquainted with it. It so happens that this is a group of symptoms centered around one Major Condition without any symptoms of Minor Conditions. Later, we will complicate it with symptoms of Minor Conditions and "goat feathers."

Art. 412. ANALYSIS TABLE (an example of a Major Condition, only).

Symptoms	Explanation	Specie	Family	Places
Headache	Indirect Symptom, in front and back of head	I. A.	Loc.	U. PP.
Malaise	Adap. Symp. to enforce quietness	None	....	
Anorexia	Adap. Symp. to enforce temperance in eating	None	....	
Nausea	Adap. Symp. to enforce temperance in eating	None	....	
Vomiting	Adap. Symp. to enforce temperance in eating	None	....	
Cough	Ind. Symp. lungs and bronchi irritated by extra work in	C+	Fever	C. P.
	throwing off poisons. (Art. 193)	E—, T—	Poison	K. P.
Epistaxis	Ind. Symp. ditto the above, "nose bleed"			
Chills	Ind. Symp from the chill of poisons	C+, E—	FP. fam.	CP. KP.
Pain in back	Symp. of acute subluxation in upper lumbar	Loc.	Loc.	U. PP.
	Symp. of heavily taxed eliminating organs	E—	Poison	K. P.
Costiveness	Symp. of lack of secretions in intestines due C+	T—	Fever	C. P.
Diarrhoea	Symp. of excessive exudation	T+	Poison	U. PP.
Fever	Symp. of abnormal thermogenesis and thermolysis	C+, E—	FP. fam.	CP. KP.
Rash on abd.	Symp. of abnormal poison in abdomen	E—	Poison	K. P.
Rapid breath	Ind. Symp. of overworked respiratory organs	C+, E—	FP. fam.	CP. KP.
Purulent stool	Symp. of pathology in intestines	NCR.	Degen.	U. PP.
Tympanites	Symp. of abnormal chemical action in intestines	T+	Poison	U. PP.
Enlarged Spl.	Ind. Symp. overworked spleen	E—	Poison	K. P.
sc. hc. urine	Ind. Symp. Serous Circ. deprived of water by intes.	E—, T+	FP. fam.	KP. UPP.
Flushed cheeks	Symp. of fever	C+	Fever	C. P.
Sordes tg., tth.	Symp. of Poison in stomach, deprived secretions	T—, C+	Poison	C. P.
Pain on rt. side	Symp. of pathology in abdomen, which as it happens is NCR in the Peyers patches in the small intestine	NCR	Degen.	U. PP.
				Totals
				7—C. P.
				7—K. P.
				7—U. P. P.

A summing up of results shows that the Fever-Poison Family predominates, therefore it is one of the febrile conditions, which is not necessary to know by the way; and the fact that this group of symptoms is diagnosed as typhoid fever is also of no consequence in Chiropractic. A summing up of the places shows that we have, approximately, seven U. P. P., Seven C. P., and seven K. P. (it just happened that there were seven of each in this case and is of no consequence). There are no other Places mentioned, because, as we stated before, these are all in one Major Condition. Therefore our net Places are C. P., K. P., and U. P. P. Palpate and use other assistance if necessary, to find and list the subluxations in those Places.

Art. 413. ANALYSIS TABLE (an example containing Major and Minor Conditions)

Symptoms	Explanation	Specie	Family	Places
Headache	Indirect Symp.	I. A.	Loc.	U. P. P.
Malaise	Adap. Symp.	None		
Anorexia	Adap. Symp.	None		
Nausea	Adap. Symp.	None		
Vomiting	Adap. Symp.	None		
	"Ate cake yesterday, very sick." Foolish act. Disregards Innate's warning. Should be well guarded during illness.	O—	Loc.	U. cer. P.
Cough	Indirect Symp. of overworked lungs	C+	Fever	C. P.
	"Went downtown a week ago today." Goat feathers. "Got wet in the rain." History			
Chills	Ind. Symp.	C+, E—	FP. fam.	CP. KP.
Pain in back	Symp. of lumbar subluxation	O—	Loc.	U. PP.
	Symp. of heavily worked eliminating organs	E—	Poison	K. P.
	"Moved a dresser day before yesterday." Foolish act	Loc.	Loc.	U. cer. P.
	Pain and numbness in right hand and arm, for ten years	O—	Loc.	A. P.
Costiveness	Symp. of lack of secretions in intest. due to C+	T—	Fever	C. P.
Diarrhoea	Symp. of excessive exudation in intestines	T+	Poison	U. P. P.
Fever	Symp. of abn. thermolysis and thermogenesis	C+, E—	FP. fam.	CP. K.P.
Rash on abd.	Symp. of abnormal poison in abdomen	E—	Poison	K. P.
Rapid breath	Symp. of overworked respiratory organs	C+, E—	FP. fam.	CP. KP.
	Patient's bed in ill ventilated, close shut "sick room." Poor sanitation and hygiene			
Purulent stool	Pathology in the intestines	NCR.	Degen.	U. PP.
Tympanites	Abnormal chemical action in intestines	T+	Poison	U. PP.
Enlarged Spl.	Overworked eliminating organ	E—	Poison	K. P.
sc. hc. urine	Serous Circ. deprived of water by intestines	E—, T+	Poison	K.P., U.PP.
Flushed cheeks	Fever	C+	Fever	C. P.
Sordes tg., tth.	Poison in stomach, deprived of secretions	T—, C+	FP. fam.	CP. KP.
	Had stomach trouble for years	O—, T—	Par. Poi.	S. P.
Pain on rt. side	Pathology in pelvic cavity	NCR.	Degen.	U.PP.

By summing up we get C. P., K. P. predominating. Upper Cervical Place, Arm Place, and Stomach Place are Minors and can be attended to later.

The Ph. C.

At first the course in Chiropractic at The P. S. C. was very short. It was lengthened from time to time, until it required twelve months to acquire a D.C. degree. The degree of D.C., Doctor of Chiropractic, means learned in the science of Chiropractic, for the word doctor, is derived from the Latin word, *doctus*, meaning learned. Later, when the course was extended so that students could become more proficient in Chiropractic, the degree of Ph.C. was established. Ph.C. means Philosopher of Chiropractic. A graduate with a Ph.C., in addition to being a Doctor is also a Philosopher. That is to say, he knows much more science than the Doctor does, knowing the same as he and much more. The difference between a doctor without science and a doctor with science is the same as the difference between an electrician who is a wireman and an electrician who is an electrical engineer. They both work at electricity and both may be skillful and able to apply their art but the wireman depends upon the engineer to do the brain work and tell him what to do.

In order that the graduate might really deserve his title, saying that he is a philosopher, having knowledge of the science of Chiropractic, a later ruling was made by the Faculty of The Palmer School of Chiropractic requiring the candidate for a Ph.C. to write a thesis of fifteen thousand words.

THESIS.

Definition from Webster's International Dictionary. "A thing laid down; a statement; a proposition; specif., a position or proposition which a person advances and offers to maintain, as by a candidate for scholastic honors, or one which is actually maintained, by argument. An essay or dissertion written upon a specific or definite theme; esp., an essay presented by a candidate for a diploma or degree. An affirmation or enunciation not proved, but assumed as a premise; a postulate; also, in a hypothetical proposition, the consequent."

Thus, from the definition, it is seen that a thesis is a composition written for a specific purpose about a specific theme which is technical or not, according to the school for which it is written. As every school has its particular kind, in this case it should be all Chiropractic, all philosophy and very technical. It denotes scientific knowledge on the part of the student.

It is not the diploma of The Ph.C. that makes the scientific Chiropractor but the real knowledge behind it. If one should obtain a Ph.C. diploma fraudulently, that does not make him a scientist and he will sooner or later be found out. An incompetent person possessing such a diploma discredits the school but it is not the school's fault if he stole it, any more than it is the school's fault if a burglar enters its offices and robs its safe.

An honestly obtained diploma for a Ph.C. is of real value to the person who owns it, for he can always back it up by his knowledge and skill. There is no danger that he will have his ignorance exposed. The student who doubts the value of The P.S.C. Ph.C. should be comforted to know that diplomas are stolen in all professions and should he investigate, he will find many an M.D. who has not even the technical knowledge of an old-time self-educated horse doctor.

A student who deserves this degree should be well enough informed, in Chiropractic Philosophy, to write a thesis. It is really a fifteen thousand word examination in that subject. Considering **the real meaning of Chiropractic Philosophy** this is a fair test. Chiropractic Philosophy is the explanation of the difference between the views of Chiropractors and the views of other sciences upon a natural method of healing and all the studies involved in it. This difference is in many cases radical —a right about face. An efficient knowledge of Philosophy, then, is necessary to keep the practitioner squarely within his science, since it is so easy to lapse because of previous training and the temptations to be found in the field. It is commonly thought that Philosophy is primarily "to sell" the patient; to convince him of the merits of Chiropractic and show him the wonders of the magic that can get so many people well. That is true, but it has a greater function than that. It is of far more importance that the practitioner be able to keep checking himself to avoid slipping from the science of Chiropractic, and he is unable to do that unless he knows what the science is. He must have knowledge of what the ideal is, in order to hold it. The electrical engineer does not disdain the abstract science of his profession, because it is what differentiates him from the lineman.

The character of the student body of The P. S. C. is such, that while the majority are good students and excellent adjustors and may know their philosophy quite well, they are not all trained in expressing themselves. Other schools and colleges usually have required studies in composition, rhetoric, debating, English and literature, but The P. S. C. is not able to do this with its already full curriculum and the time at its disposal.

The writer of this article is endeavoring to partly fill the need, in presenting this exposition on how to write a thesis and at the same time state what the Department of Philosophy expects in a thesis. Needless to say, since Chiropractic is so radically different from many other sciences, it is not surprising that its thesis would be somewhat different from those of other schools. It has a definite purpose and that purpose will be explained in these pages.

CHOOSING THE SUBJECT AND TITLE

Since the thesis is to be for a degree in Chiropractic science, it should contain nothing but Chiropractic philosophy. The first thing to do is choose a phase, a subject, a branch, a basic principle or a big idea from the extremely extensive field of Chiropractic knowledge and deductions.

Philosophy is a broad subject (Art. 6 and 7). Taken in its broadest sense, it explains the "why" and "how" of everything known to man. The abstract group of principles and explanations of any one of man's numerous activities and studies are philosophies. Since these are numberless, it is obvious that the kinds of philosophy are infinite. The explanations of all of them is beyond the range of one man's lifetime; would take the lifetimes of many generations. To study philosophy one must narrow his researches to a few kinds, in order not to be confused by trying to do too many things at once.

Chiropractic Philosophy is the explanation of principles and knowledge and art of everything used in Chiropractic. It is the philosophy, science and art of everything natural. Chiropractic is based upon the fact that intelligence is responsible for everything natural. The science of Chiropractic is the study of the actions of this intelligence. The art of Chiropractic is the method of restoring the actions of intelligence to sick people, in order that they may be natural. As most sciences do, Chiropractic uses applications of other sciences, so naturally, they "come in" for a Chiropractic explanation. "Everything Chiropractic" is a field big enough for the lifetime study of any person.

Therefore, to undertake to write a thesis upon a Chiropractic Philosophy in general is undertaking to treat a subject too broad for the scope of a thesis and the writer could do no more than resort to generalities. No part of it could be technical in thus hurrying over it; no idea could be worked out to its logical conclusion. It would even be too sketchy to be entertaining.

The study of composition teaches us that it is always best to narrow our subject to one strong idea. A great deal of time is devoted to this in the teaching of composition. A rule frequently stated in composition says, "Always go from the general to the specific." This is a rule that should sound familiar to Chiropractors, for they are taught that, as the meaning of deductive reasoning, which is used so much in Chiropractic. Working from the general to the specific also applies to the art of Chiropractic, for in analysis of cases, you work from the general to the specific and "pick a major."

No general discussion of a big subject can be technical. A thesis for Ph.C. should be technical.

A few simple examples of narrowing a subject will help. Take the general subject, horses, or equine family. It is much too large a subject for fifteen thousand words. If so written, it would have to be mostly generalizations though it could be entertaining. To make it scientific you need to concentrate your attention to one specie of the horse family such as, the Shetland pony, the hippopotamus, the Percheron, etc. It is easy to see how much more specific your statements could be made.

Another example: take the Jones family. It is a large family. In describing the Jones' you could do no more than generalize in a fifteen thousand word composition; but you could make an excellent biography, description or character study of John Jones, at the same time conveying an excellent idea of the Jones family.

A fifteen thousand word composition written about roses in general could not be very scientific. In order to be scientific one must write about a specie of rose, instead of the rose family.

"Major Picking."

You will not be able to keep on the subject unless you have one. Having too many ideas at the same time or trying to develop them at the same time is like having "too many irons in the fire." It will weaken your logic. No one can do several things at the same time and do them well. Even your sentences should say one thing at a time. The definition of a sentence will show that clearly. A common fault in writing upon subjects too large or about too many subjects, is that the sentences themselves lack unity and show the hurried and unsettled state of mind of the writer. A good example of such sentences is to be found in Shakespeare, in the conversation of Hostess Quickly with her debtors (King Henry, Second Part, Scene IV, Act. 11).

To be forceful, your reasoning should pursue one idea that you are certain is an idea. Your treatment of the subject should have few branch ideas, or none at all. They are apt to decoy you into bypaths or "blind alleys"; then you are obliged to extricate yourself and make another start. This makes interruptions that destroy your continuity, sequence and transition. In the range of fifteen thousand words the development of more than one idea causes you, from necessity, to state things too superficially; trying to squeeze too many thoughts into sentences and paragraphs, resulting in ambiguity.

Let everything you say support the subject. Choose your main idea so that you know you can do this. It will worry you to try to use things which do not belong to your subject. If you have ideas that you do not know where to place, that is a pretty good indication that they do not belong.

The Size of Your Subject.

It is possible to make a pretty close estimate of the amount of material that you can apply to your subject. This estimate should be made beforehand and it can be done by outlining. If you are well founded in Chiropractic, (you should be if you deserve a Ph.C.) you will know whether a subject is a "major" or not, when it first occurs to you. If you do not, it is a confession to yourself that you do not know Chiropractic well enough. Then, if you are honest with yourself, you will "get" Chiropractic so that you do.

Do not choose a subject about which you know so little that you do not know its scope; or know so little about a big idea that you cannot tell fifteen thousand words about it. The only way for you to judge its scope is to know it. No one can do it for you, for its scope depends upon what you know about it. Who knows better than yourself how much you know?

It is possible to choose a big idea and then to proceed to inform yourself about it. This takes study and research and most of all, thinking or digesting your information. Incidentally, we might add that study and research in this subject can be done better at the P. S. C. or in the P. S. C. text books than in any other school or library, since it is the fountain head and libraries are not stocked with information on Chiropractic.

An attempt to develop a minor subject results in disaster. It will not furnish material for a scientific discussion of fifteen thousand words. The student then, must resort to "filler," which is bad, or to "goat feathers" which is worse. An attempt to prolong the thesis with additional subjects is contrary to every principle of composition.

An estimate of space which may help the writer can be done easily. By examining a few pages of typewritten material and counting the number of words per line, then counting the lines, you can find how many words are on a page. By doing this with several pages, you can get an average per page. Then by dividing fifteen thousand by this average you can calculate the probable number of pages necessary and at the same time get a "feeling" of the amount required. Then by making an outline of your subject and making a test of how much you can say on its hardest part and its easiest part, you can fit it to your estimated space.

Counting Words.

When finding out how many words you have written, or have yet to write, estimate, don't count. In making these estimates do not be stingy with your words, assuming that they are pearly gems that must be counted one at a time. One of the main principles in authorship and one that all the great authors observe, is the elimination of conceit. Great authors have been merciless in discarding a great percentage of their words as worthless; doing bits over again cheerfully, as part of the business.

It is much better to have sixteen thousand words than to have only fourteen thousand. That gives you a chance to cut out parts if necessary. If it is desired to cut down on the amount of words do not "lop" off the end of your thesis with a pair of shears but take away some topics or sub-topics here and there—the ones you can spare most. The Department of Philosophy may require that you revise your thesis by taking out objectionable parts. If you have a surplus of words, you can take some out without going below fifteen thousand. On the other hand it is very difficult to prolong an undersized composition, should the Department require revision. That would necessarily mean a change in a great many places, which, if you hire your typing done might prove expensive, not to speak of trouble.

Difficult Subjects.

One should avoid choosing a subject that is too difficult. Pick out one that is within the range of your knowledge; you know best which ones are. It is not necessary to enumerate the difficulties you would fall into with a subject too hard for you.

If you want to extend the range of your knowledge and are willing to study and think and look up references, difficult subjects will be good for you. In this case, you select a subject that you consider important or one that you like and read up on it, making notes as you read. You will find this an excellent education in the science of Chiropractic. The people, who have written theses in this manner, are always glad they did so, for the research and the thinking involved, opened to their minds an understanding that could be had in no other way.

A subject you like best is the least difficult for you. You will enjoy writing about it. It will be a pleasure to think about and to reason out and to theorize. You will be eager to explain it, for when one is enthusiastic, he finds no difficulty in knowing what to say. If there are points that are not clear to you, you will enjoy looking them up in the text books and every bit of support you find, you will enjoy classifying and expressing. Your task will progress rapidly and you will be surprised to find how rapidly it is getting done. Then, when you have finished, there is the feeling of satisfaction in a task well done. You will feel that it has not been a task but more like the pleasure of a successful "deal."

The secret of the reason that the foregoing is true, is that the subjects you know best are the ones you like best—that is, when you really understand them. Then, in order to like a subject in Philosophy, know it first. You know from your own experience that you can talk about the thing you like best and are interested in; you know and like it because of your understanding. If you like none of the subjects of Chiropractic; if you do not know them and do not believe any of them, then do not try to write about them.

You will find, if you try, that the best thesis writing is done mentally and not altogether by using a pencil. After outlining and even before, sit down with your hands idle and imagine yourself explaining a certain point. It will save writer's cramp and be much easier to revise. It all depends upon your thinking. It cannot be accomplished unthinkingly like a task automatically done with the hands, no matter how many helps and prepared aids you have.

It Must be Chiropractic Philosophy.

After choosing a subject that you like and feel confident that you can develop, look it over carefully to see that it is really Chiropractic. On account of previous training in schools and at home we are apt to be interested in subjects that sound like philosophy. They may be abstract principles of something that belong to a science or line of study that is not Chiropractic. These are continuously at the back of one's mind ready to spring forth and tincture all one's thoughts on other subjects. In thesis grading this is found to be one of the student's worst enemies. Bear in mind preparing this thesis, that no matter how many other sciences may interest you, you are now engaged in writing a thesis about Chiropractic and any foreign matter introduced will destroy unity.

Examinations in the subject of Philosophy, as given in the classroom, are given to see how many facts, theories, principles and definitions you know. In an examination you give back on your examination papers and in quizzes, the material that has been given to you. The object of this is to see if you can remember and understand them. Since these things are fundamental you are not at liberty to change them; your own opinions and inventions are not desired in examinations.

The purpose of the thesis, is also a kind of examination in philosophy. It is to show the instructor how well the student understands Philosophy **by its application.** The Dept. of Philosophy, technically, is not supposed to understand how to grade the merits of any subject but Chiropractic Philosophy. That should be the point of view used by the thesis writer. While the examination shows that the student may know the principles, the thesis shows that the student is able to apply them. He can be as original as he pleases in the explanation of their application but neither in examinations nor theses can he change the principles and expect them to still be Chiropractic. He can, however, and it is better for him to do so, theorize all he likes, as long as his theories are well founded in Chiropractic. **Not Medicine.**

Many students are tempted to discuss medical phases or medical theories in some form or other. Not that they have had medical education, but are influenced by old methods which nearly every one has used before taking up Chiropractic. These students may be fully sold to Chiropractic but they want to talk about medicine to show its fallacies. To tell about the faults of medicine does not explain Chiropractic. If you do not know much about medicine you should not discuss it in any scientific article. Your statements may be fallacies and if they are you are laying yourself open to criticism. Even if you do consider the A.M.A. a dragon, that is no reason you should twist its tail in a Chiropractic thesis.

Not Pet Hobbies.

The same thing that was said about tendencies to write about medicine applies to hobbies. Many students have pet ideas that they have accumulated for years about various sciences, religions, dieting, former experiences, etc. The electrical engineer wants to have the whole thesis electrical; the nurse wants to sandwich in a few medical ideas that she painfully absorbed in many years practice; the preacher wants to spend a few thousand words in proving that Innate could not possibly be the Soul and probably there is no Innate anyway; hypnotists are apt to want to put the whole thing upon a basis of their art. The Department is not competent to grade theses on all sciences, creeds and religions.

Not Conversation.

Do not make your thesis of conversation. Conversation is too closely related to narrative to be useful in thesis work. While it might be done, it is the experience of the Department that such theses are weak. It is better not to use such forms. Examples of this kind are such as: "doctor and patient stunts";

conversation showing a discussion with a layman; a series of letters to a friend, a diary—a record of new glories revealed daily.

Not for the Layman.

There seems to be an epidemic of desire to write theses "for the layman." It is certain that such instruction was never given by the department. A thesis should be too technical for the layman. If you make your material scientific enough to answer the purpose of a thesis the layman could only have a very hazy idea of what you are telling. In order to understand a thesis, a layman would have to take the course or part of it—then he would not be a layman.

If you write a thesis simple enough for the layman to use as an "educator," and put it on your office table, you lay yourself and Chiropractic open to underestimation. If you want a thesis to be on your office table, write the hardest, most technical one you can. He thinks you are a "regular doctor" if you could write the hard one and he thinks that any person could write the easy one—perhaps he, himself, if he had time. Remember this fundamental of pedagogy: "A teacher must know at least ten times as much as he teaches." Therefore if you do not know enough Chiropractic to write a genuine thesis, it is certain that you are unable to tell the layman much

Not Filler.

A thesis should not be filled with lists of cases or lists of Chiropractic clinical successes. While they might be interesting for some other kind of composition, they do not explain the application of Chiropractic principles. A thesis is ruined by filling it with meaningless paragraphs and sentences copied from rhetorical writings. It is just as bad to fill it with a jumble of words that mean nothing—"smoke screens." Do not use a thesis for ostentation of education. It is interesting, but if it is not Chiropractic, it can have no value as a Ph.C. winner.

Not Laboratory Subjects.

A thesis on Chiropractic philosophy should not be a discussion of a laboratory subject. To write about anatomy, physiology, chemistry, psychoanalysis, psychology, etc., is not Chiropractic, though a clever writer and a good philosopher could give a good application of Chiropractic philosophy to these subjects. These are difficult, and it is not advisable to undertake them unless you are a good philosopher and clever.

The same statement applies to a lengthy discussion of germs. It is a laboratory subject and it does not take very many words to tell the Chiropractic view of germs. A lengthy discussion of this subject is the detailed study of matter, which could not be Chiropractic. What would it avail a Chiropractor to discuss minutely each germ and family of germs? It does not apply to Chiropractic any more than the names of several hundred diseases. It is as far removed from Chiropractic as an article on the chemistry of open hearth steel would be.

Not Classic Philosophy.

Do not expect to find Chiropractic Philosophy in books of classic philosophy. The philosophy of Socrates, Plato or any other writer on such subjects is not Chiropractic Philosophy. It is out of place in a thesis. However a quotation of such may be used when it is as brief as an epigram. Do not quote copiously from ancient and modern writers on philosophy and cults.

Not Creeds.

Avoid the discussion of creeds, cults, etc. Keep religion out of theses. That is what is always taught from the platform at The P.S.C. and it also applies to P.S.C. theses. While you may make brief references to them or quote from some of them, it is not desirable to weave any of these subjects into your thesis matter. In the first place they are not Chiropractic; Chiropractic does not wish to be involved in religious discussions. You might, if you are not well informed, make wrong statements about them.

Not Politics.

This seems to be as tempting, nearly, as religion. Avoid utopias, Chiropractic legal troubles, labor problems, descriptions of Chiropractors in jail, state laws for Chiropractors, political pasts and futures. While you may discuss the legal aspects of professional phases in general, an exposition on Chiropractic laws is not telling the scientific side of Chiropractic. If you want to discuss utopias, the one mentioned in the Universal Cycle will be right in line with Chiropractic ideas.

Not History.

History is not suitable for a thesis for many reasons. First, it is narrative and narrative is not good for technical explanation. You should not weaken your thesis by lengthy narrative of the history of Chiropractic. It is not suitable material for a scientific article. Histories of early methods of healing, comparisons of such with Chiropractic are mere processes of copying and represent no reasoning on the thesis writer's part and should be very brief if used at all. History of the universe, history of medicine, the rise and fall of nations, history of mankind and lengthy references to these are entirely out of place in a thesis.

Not at the Public Library.

You will find Chiropractic philosophy in your school text books. Chiropractic is not so widely known that you will find any more than the definition in public libraries. It is a waste of time to hunt for it there. You will find nothing of Chiropractic import in medical and nurses' books. It will avail you nothing to copy paragraphs from the library books and "doctor" stilted passages by putting in Chiropractic words here and there. A "doctored" article does not "make sense."

Quoting.

The question is often asked, "How much may I quote?" and "If I write philosophy as it is in the books, won't it be copying?" In answer to these questions we offer the following: you may quote definitions, rules, principles, fundamentals, epigrams, and many concise statements of authors which in your estimation are "better put" than you can do it, to help an explanation you are making. But these quotations should never be lengthy and not too numerous. A paragraph is a long enough quotation. If it is longer than that, it is not concise and you had better say it yourself. If it happens too often, it shows that you are getting mentally lazy and if you are using other people's thoughts you should not get the credit for it.

If you do use someone's concise statements, you should enclose it in quotation marks. If it is from any author that you can name or even from a friend, you should enclose it in quotation marks and give the name of the person you got it from. Neglect to do this is called plagiarism, a kind of theft. If the article you copied it from is copyrighted, you are liable to damage suit.

In giving short extracts from The P.S.C. text books you should tell where you got it, but it will not always be necessary to use quotation marks. It is not necessary to give credit for authorship in quoting definitions, principles, rules, etc., since you are expected to know those of Chiropractic which were taught you, therefore you are entitled to use them.

To make "book reviews" and put in conglomeration of copyings, quotations, and garbled versions of The P.S.C. text books indicates that you have made slight use of reasoning, hence no originality. Such a thesis is a failure, even if the book review is clever.

Quotations are usually made to support a statement of your own or to be commented on by you. If you make no statement to be supported and no comments upon what is stated, merely depending upon something somebody else has said, then your quotation is out of order.

You will have no trouble in finding something to say and how to say it, if you read the books, digest what you read by thinking it over and then state it in your own language or give your idea of its application.

Not Sciences of Your Own.

Since Philosophy of Chiropractic is the explanation of that science, a philosophy of some science that you invent yourself is no subject for a Chiropractic thesis. Now, it is possible that you have an active, inventive mind and have been working on a phase of psychology, an art or a philosophy of life all your own and are very proud of it. It is a credit to you that you can do this and your "brain child" may have excellent points—but it would not be fitting in a thesis.

Some thesis writers have a mistaken notion that Chiropractic is a specie of psychology, and try to weld the two—it cannot be done. Instead of Chiropractic philosophy being a specie of psychology, psychology is a specie of Chiropractic philosophy.

Rules, Principles and Facts.

In using rules, principles and facts of Chiropractic, use them as taught and as you are expected to give them in examinations. Be sure that you state them correctly for if you do not use them correctly, then they are liable to impair many lines of your thesis. Be sure that the principles you use are the kind approved by the Dept. of Philosophy, and not derived from some "outlawed" source.

When writing upon any point, try to be explicit enough to give as many direct explanations as possible. In many cases it is not possible for any one to do so. In that case it is proper to resort to examples and analogies.

Do not use obsolete theories; it is much better to present your own.

Originality.

It is not necessary to make book reviews or plagiarize, with a field as broad as Chiropractic Philosophy. Even at that, the field has hardly been touched. Much has been done in original research in both clinic and deduction, but more is needed. Chiropractic needs keen and original minds who are ambitious to carry on. The Dept. of Philosophy gladly welcomes new and intelligent ideas of advancement. It will not condemn ideas that will carry on, building up with facts already established as stepping stones. It is certainly like a breath of fresh air to receive a thesis of that kind.

The Title.

The title should tell the subject briefly. It should convey the idea of the subject matter without "denouement." It should hint of what the thesis has in store for the reader. It might possibly be "catchy" or clever, so as to intrigue or arouse curiosity. It is an advertisement; at least it should be attractive. With the dry subjects of sciences, it is well to have some of these mentioned qualities.

At the back of this article is a list of suggested titles and subjects.

It might seem that from the long list of don'ts just given

that the thesis writer is barred from everything; and that this article is written in negative vein. But reader, please notice that nowhere is Chiropractic barred, and the subjects of the don'ts were introduced by former thesis writers. Having been introduced they must be disposed of.

OUTLINING

Listing Topics.

Topics, as used in the technic of composition, are the lesser parts of a subject. They are not limited to any particular number or size. They are small subjects themselves and when they have been written up are small compositions in which the principles of composition should be used when writing. These topics should always say something about the subject directly or indirectly—but the less "indirectly" you have them the better. A subtopic should say something about the topic and through it, of course support the main subject. Subtopics are possible paragraphs, but often you combine two or more into a paragraph.

Make a list of all the things you can say about the subject chosen, keeping the subject in mind all the time you do it. Ask yourself as you jot down a topic, "does this belong to it?" Remember to do that. Do not be stingy with them—jot down more than you need. There may be some that you will find later, do not belong; some you will not need and some that are not important enough to be topics but are subtopics. In the latter case you combine them. This first tentative outline is not to get the complete outline at one stroke or to be done in just a few minutes. Remember that making an outline is a process and that when you have a genuine outline finished, that about two thirds of your thesis work is done. Do not think you can do this amount of work in a short time. The number of topics you will ultimately use, depends entirely upon your knowledge and no one can tell you the size of a topic or a subject, unless he is estimating your mentality. Of course some subjects are larger than others, but they cannot be measured in topics as a unit of measure or in number of words. If a suggestion is worth anything we would say, about fifteen topics averaging a thousand words each would be a good number.

Never mind the order in which you jot them down. Put them down haphazardly as you happen to think of them. Many a fleeting idea can be captured in this way—to get them down on paper is the main thing. This does not pertain to conventionalized learning that can be copied from books, but to your own ideas.

If in making an outline, the process seems to be too abstract and you have difficulty in seeing its application, just remember that the process is not confined to literature; even the plumber makes an itemized specification for your approval and his work. Then he proceeds to make a composition of pipes, joints, elbows, bath tubs, lead and oakum. An artist does not begin at one end of his picture and finish as he goes, he makes a "layout" or a "blocking in" first and all through the job he keeps all parts of the picture going; for a picture is a composition.

Now go over your list again and see if some say the same thing or about the same thing and if they do, combine them. You may find that some things you thought were big enough for topics, could apply as a subtopic to some other topic, if so combine it to avoid repetition.

Numbering.

Now that you have a list of things to say, glance over them and decide which you will say first and number them accordingly. It is easily done with the "bird's eye view" that the outline list gives. This is getting the topics into "time order" or sequence. It enables you to shift your materials here and there like a game.

By this time you will see, what you have written has some time order. The numbers show this. Time order puts your materials in such order that they show what must be said first, to prepare the reader for what comes next. It makes continuity automatic; makes it easier to stay on the subject; lessens chances of omission; keeps a grip on the important parts. You will then have no regrets about "the things I should have said back there."

Estimating Space.

Using the outline properly also enables you to estimate the number of words available and how many pages it will be necessary to have. Assuming that you can write one thousand words on each topic and that it takes from a page and a half to two pages for a thousand words on letter sized paper, then you will have from twenty-five to thirty pages, according to your spacing and paragraphing. Suppose a topic takes a thousand words, then if you have three or four subheads in it, that means possibly you will have three or four paragraphs in a topic.

Copy Outline.

Next, copy your outline afresh, putting your numbered items consecutively. Arrange the lesser items as subtopics to the more important ones.

Outline Each Topic.

Each topic will have a number of lesser subjects in it. These are subtopics, A subtopic, as used in composition is a minute subject about which a number of statements may be made. A subtopic is not as important as a topic, being a part of it. A subtopic is in existence when a topic is too large to be one paragraph. A subtopic is a possible paragraph but if you arbitrarily make paragraphs of subtopics you will find yourself repeating—which should be avoided. If possible make one paragraph of a topic, but if this cannot be done, then make as many paragraphs as the topic has minor parts.

A Bird's Eye View.

You now have the whole thing before you and can see the beginning, middle and the end. You can shift points at pleasure. The shifting will be difficult after you have written the manuscript.

If you use an outline you can easily see that in a composition you should build and not pile up. A thesis is a composition; a composition must be composed. When your outline is completed you have the framework of your building.

Revision of Outline.

Go over the outline again to make revisions, elaborations and joinings. Have your outline as near perfect as you can, before beginning to write. Remember that this preparation is two-thirds of your work done. Rewrite outlines several times if necessary, for it saves time. Go over the outline again and jot down as many as possible your references and authors and names of books, and the pages where you can find what you want, to refresh your memory.

Do your reading and studying, now, before beginning to write. Hunt up your definitions, rules and the like and have them at hand. Remember that **the time to get yourself well informed is while you are making your outline.** It is best not to do this when you write; it cramps your style.

See that everything is in harmony and united to the subject. Mercilessly cut out any thing that does not say something directly or indirectly about the subject. Never assume that your writings are so valuable that you cannot discard.

Better lay out enough in your first draft that you can afford to discard—leaving the best.

If, when you get to writing, you find that you have too much material, cut down by omitting subtopics or even topics. Do not conclude your composition by abruptly chopping off the end leaving some of your outline unfinished.

You are now ready to write.

Place your outline before you. Take up each subtopic as it comes and say all you can about it. Write plentifully. Do not change their time order without good reason; and do not combine topics or subtopics without good reason, lest you disturb your unity and sequence. If you find that you have to do this very much, it is a sign that your outline is not good. In that case stop writing and make a new outline. Write copiously, get enthused. Never mind your handwriting or perfect grammar—get it down.

Assume that each subtopic is the title of a little composition and make a list of sentences about it. This, then, will be a paragraph. The statement of your subtopic is its main idea and the other sentences are modifiers attached to it. If it needs no modifiers or additions, then the subtopic itself, is only a sentence of the topic. Conversely, if a topic is not large enough to have many things said about it, it is because it is not important enough to be a topic and is a subtopic itself. It is permissible to change an outline when writing from it, if this is found to be the case. It is better to have more subtopics than paragraphs, because of so many possible cancelings in this manner. Even topics may be joined when they say the same thing.

Revise, putting the subtopics in good time order within the topic. Much of the work can be done by thinking it out before setting it down on paper.

A good way to write by outline is as follows: Take as many sheets of paper as you have topics and put the names of the topics at the tops of these pages. Then all you have to say about each topic will be by itself. If when writing about, say No. 3 topic it reminds you of something that belongs to No. 8 topic, you get the paper with No. 8 and say it before you forget. This method makes you just as enthusiastic at the end of your thesis as at the first. You can write on any part when you feel like it, for if your outline has been well prepared it cannot fail, and the sequence will be well taken care of. When you have written all you can by this method, you will also find it easy to combine and revise.

In writing, endeavor to cover the framework of your building. Hide the skeleton. Even nature uses frames and covers them with foliage and fruit, or flesh.

Revision of Manuscript.

As you revised your outlines, so should you revise your manuscript. Go over it and look for faults. Good writers are not ashamed or too lazy to rewrite what they have labored hard to write. Be merciless—don't be afraid to throw away—write with that intention and then keep the best. One of the rules of a famous writer is, "write all you can and then boil it down; skim it and boil down the skimmings, and skim it again." Famous writers tell us that the trouble, with inexperienced writers, is that they think everything they have committed to paper is a golden nugget which should not on any account be thrown away. Keep in mind that while you cannot recall spoken words, you can recall written words before you commit them to the reader's judgment.

Revise paragraphing if necessary; revise sentences; see that they are complete and do not contain too many thoughts. Check up your grammar. Be careful of repetition of words. Do not use "pet phrases" too often or too many of them. Do not use hackneyed phrases. Do not use stilted language or quote such. Examine your punctuation for every punctuation mark is shorthand for a word or an idea. Do not try to "sling" big words, for that is only ostentation and is very poor English idiom, according to the masters of English literature.

PRINCIPLES OF COMPOSITION

Kinds of Composition.

Compositions may be spoken (oral) or written. On account of being able to revise the written and in order to indicate by punctuation, idiom and construction, that which is indicated by gestures and expression in the oral, written composition is usually more precise and formal than oral composition.

There are four kinds of composition in either the spoken or written; description, narration, exposition and argumentation. In this article we will give a very brief explanation of these kinds of composition and the principles, but on account of space and the purpose of this article, it will be necessarily sketchy.

Narration.

Narration is all movement. It tells a story or enumerates events. It is used mostly for history and for entertainment. Good examples of narration are: The Bible, histories and Bunyan's Pilgrim's Progress. Because of the fact that time is its chief factor, and its other qualities, narration is unsuited to thesis work.

Description.

Description enumerates objects, tells how things look or feel or smell, etc., etc. It tells how things seem; flashes mental pictures or gives ideation. It may be used in other forms of composition and can be used in parts of thesis work. Alone, however, it is unsuited for thesis work. Good examples of descriptions mentioned are catalogues, travelogues and Washington Irving's books.

Argumentation.

Argumentation is dispute, contradiction, proof of falsity, debate. Logical reasoning is necessary in its use. There must be absolute balance of points and absolute correctness in statements made, for there is danger of making false accusations and statements which weaken, if not discredit the whole composition.

It is possible to use it in thesis work but it requires cleverness and a correct knowledge of debate. There is necessity of being informed correctly on both sides of the question. When used in thesis work there is danger of getting off the subject; this is apt to develop into wrangling.

It requires much more cleverness and more knowledge than the exposition type of composition and does not convey as much information about Chiropractic. At best, it only gives about one-half of fifteen thousand words to Chiropractic and the other half to some other subject which the Department does not care to judge.

Exposition.

Exposition enumerates and describes, but mostly tells why and how; therefore it is most suitable for thesis writing. It explains things. It enumerates and describes in detail, in order to give information or to teach. It must be exact, logical and formal. In it there may be some description, some argumentation and a minimum of narration.

Some good examples of exposition are; recipes, how to build a kite. Explanation of a thing, a science; as, physiology, chemistry, philosophy, etc.

Parts of a Composition.

The parts of a composition are: introduction, body, and conclusion. For convenience or for some other purpose, a composition can be divided into sections or chapters, but there, must be a purpose for it—not done aimlessly. Any composition should have paragraphs and of course they must have sentences and words.

Sections.

Sections are parts of a composition which are too widely different, to be continuous but which are about the same subject. They are not chapters. They should be in perfect unity with the subject and not loosely connected with it. Sections are used in this book.

They can be used in thesis work but there is danger that your sections will be too independent of the subject and may be subjects themselves.

Chapters.

Chapters are parts of a composition or book or story. They are more suitable for narrative than they are for thesis work. They make small epochs and are used when time is a factor as in narration. Best not to try to use them in a thesis.

Paragraphs.

Paragraphs are small compositions. A paragraph has its smaller units—sentences. Being a composition it has its subject, and this subject is usually stated by a sentence which is called the strong sentence. The strong sentence is often the first sentence of the paragraph, the rest of the sentences being its modifiers. Sometimes the strong sentence is the final one. A paragraph usually has a fairly important sentence at the end which is a sort of a summary, and somewhat introductory to the next paragraph.

All this seems complicated to one who has not studied it, but remember this: if you will take enough pains in preparing your outline and get your topics arranged in good sequence, your paragraph construction will automatically take care of itself without undue worry on your part. **At least, it will do for our purpose since we are not grading closely for correct English but for correct Chiropractic.**

For ease in reading, indent the paragraphs, that is, make them start farther in from the margin than the other lines as you see in this paragraph. It is not necessary to put the name of the subtopic on the margin, for the strong sentence takes care of that. Remember this for a test; if you cannot give a group of sentences a name, it is not a paragraph, hence it is not a subtopic.

Sentences.

Sentences are thoughts expressed in words. They are smaller compositions than the paragraph. They have strong parts which are the subject and parts which say something about the subject. Some have words or groups of words attached to them to modify them.

In thesis revision, examine their construction and see that you have capitals and punctuation in their proper places

Punctuation is too long a subject to enter into here, but a good idea is to consider that every punctuation mark is equivalent to a word or a group of words or an idea that says something necessary to the sentence. They express idiom.

Introduction.

The introduction introduces your proposition—your subject. It explains the significance of the title, without necessarily mentioning the title. It conveys to the reader why you have chosen that subject and tells the purpose for which you wrote it (that does not mean that you should say it is for a Ph.C.). An introduction should not be long. Busy yourself with the body of your thesis as soon as possible.

Body.

The body is the bulk of the composition. It is the subject matter. It contains the central idea of your composition. This main point should be evident to the reader before you have finished. Know what you are going to say and say it here in the body.

Conclusion.

The conclusion consists of the closing remarks. It is a summary, a finishing off. It shows that you have fulfilled your obligations, mentioned in the introduction. It shows that the task is finished. It calls attention to the main proposition; exhibits it to the reader so that it leaves no dim edges. It is similar to the "so you see" that nearly every one uses when explaining or telling something.

Climax.

If an exposition or argument could be said to have a climax, the climax in this sort of composition is the clinching of an argument, the proof of a proposition or the final understanding of an idea, which you have been educating the reader to appreciate in the former pages. It is the place where the reader says "Ah! Now I see." It is the main point in your exposition; the "meat" of your subject; the "juiciest portion."

The Principles of Composition.

The thing just said about composition are some of its principles, but there are other principles of a different kind, some of which we will consider. Since a composition must be composed, that is, built, it necessarily must have; unity, cohesion, transition, sequence, balance, truth, and point of view.

Unity.

Unity is the state of union of all topics and subtopics. Everything said in a composition should say something about the subject; to modify or support the subject. Things said in a composition that do not explain the subject directly or indirectly, should not be in the composition. There should be no loose ends. Reject statements that do not apply, for they are foreign matter to the subject. Illustrations, examples or analogies treating of subjects foreign to your subjects are permissible, if they explain; that being the sole reason for giving them.

Cohesion.

Cohesion is the holding together of the parts. To have cohesion, it is necessary to have unity. It is the question of how closely the statements are related to the subject and to each other. Avoid looseness in choosing and putting together of your subjects, for loose composition makes a weak building.

Transition.

Transition is the smooth changing from one topic to another and from subtopic to subtopic, and from paragraph to paragraph and from sentence to sentence. Transition is not difficult if you have good unity and sequence. Abrupt changes are apt to make the reader work harder than is pleasant, to follow your thought, and it is even apt to make the writer get off the thread of his reasoning.

Continuity.

Continuity is the connectedness, due to good transition. It is to avoid abrupt changes in subjects, both large and small. The parts of your composition should be joined together in one chain. It hides the framework of your structure; hides the skeleton. It is like the finishing and painting of a building. It is smooth joining that makes a harmonious whole.

Sequence.

Sequence is good time order; saying the right things first. It is laying the foundation for what comes next. Do not spoil your story by telling the climax first. In an exposition, it is educating your reader step by step; teaches him to understand what follows next. To get the reader prepared for the hard parts.

Balance.

Balance refers to the amount of space given to each part. It is the space proportioned according to importance of the material. It is the harmony of the parts according to their "size" or importance. To give very much space to a part that does not explain very much and is not important is to destroy the proportions of your thesis.

Point of View.

In all composition writing, point of view is important. You should keep in mind to whom you are telling it. In a thesis, assume that your reader understands the fundamentals, principles, rules, technicalities, and terminology but is not yet acquainted with your particular line of reasoning, and your proposition. The attitude, intelligence, education, situation, and location of your reader is always taken into consideration, in any kind of composition. In writing a thesis, you should not use the point of view for the layman but the point of view for some one who is acquainted with your science. This you proceed to show him—"expose" hence exposition.

PREPARATION OF MANUSCRIPT

Typing.

The thesis should be typed on letter size or legal size paper. It may be either single or double space. It should be written on one side of the paper only. Leave a suitable margin, say, an inch and a quarter or more, at the left side. Indent the paragraphs. Head the topics if you wish; in an exposition that is permissible, and often convenient. It is not necessary or desirable to head the subtopics or paragraphs.

Proofreading.

Go over it carefully and see if the typist has made any mistakes even if the typist is yourself. Do not trust any job of typing; see that everything is as you intended it. Do not depend upon the typist to do your grammar, punctuation and to judge what should be put in or left out. Remember they do not always know Chiropractic.

Binding and Finishing.

Bind your pages at the top or left side. It is better to have the thesis covered (bound) with strong cover paper. Be sure to sign your name, serial number, address and when you leave school or out in the field be sure to give your mailing address.

Submitting.

Hand it in or send it to the Department of Philosophy at The P.S.C. After it has been graded, the Dept. will notify you of your success or if revision is necessary, then you can attend to the business of sending your diploma fee, etc.

Grading.

The thesis will be graded on the basis of Chiropractic mostly. Upon the truth or verity of the statements; upon the real knowledge of the writer and of what he has written; upon his principles of composition with moderation, and upon his adherence to his subject. The method of grading is at the discretion of the Department and not according to ruling.

Field Writers.

The same is expected of those in practice as the student in school. When the thesis is sent in, it is graded and then, upon your receipt of the letter advising you of its acceptance, send your cheque. The cheque covers the expense of the sheepskin upon which it is printed and written and for the penman who does the script. Field writers are not exempt from any of the points in grading.

The following are some suggested subjects for thesis writing, which may also be used for titles.

The Serous Circulation.
The Circulations of the Body.
Local and Condition.
Poison.
The Method of Chiropractic Analysis.
Chiropractic Hygiene.
Function.
The General Principles of Chiropractic.
The Specific Principles of Chiropractic.
Intellectual Adaptation.
Immunity.
Cause and Effect.
The Normal Complete Cycle.
Chiropractic Cycles.
The Universal Cycle.
The Sex Cycle. (See Vol. V.)
Evolution and Heredity.
Internal and External Forces.
Inductive and Deductive Methods (an argumentation).
Practical Philosophy.
The Philosophy of Chiropractic Analysis.
The Simplicity of Chiropractic.
Theories and Facts of Chiropractic.
The Philosophy of Adjusting.
The Philosophy of Technic.
The Art of Chiropractic.
The Science of Chiropractic (to show that it is a science).
Chiropractic Veterinarians.
Insanities. (Purely a discussion of soundness, not psychology).
The Philosophy of Restoration.
Transmission.

Abnormal Function.
Coordination.
Deductions of Chiropractic.
Concrete Subjects of Chiropractic.
The Mental Realm.
Germs (man himself, foods, germs as benefactors, etc.).
Innate—Contractor and Builder.
Innate—Caretaker.
Universal Intelligence—Designer.
Clinical Facts.
The Philosophy of Anatomy.
Chiropractic Etiology.
The Seven Point Drill.
As a Man Thinketh. (Take 15 of B. J.'s epigrams from a booklet of the same name.)
The Physical Realm.
The Conductors of Mental Force.
Mind.
The Cause of Dis-ease.
The Law of Demand and Supply.

Choose any one of the thirty-three Principles given in this book and develop it as a subject.

The following is the development of one of the foregoing subjects, chosen at random. It shows the building of the outline from a list of topics jotted down.

First tentative outline, being a mere list as "things to say" as they were written, and then numbered, to give them time order. It is easily seen that they were not thought of in very good time order. The main object being to get them on paper before they "escape."

Innate—Contractor and Builder.

11. Theory of cell expansion.
6. Mitosis.
12. Description of typical cell.
2. Life. Defined and explained.
3. Evolution values.
13. Signs of Life. Explain each.
9. Blastoderm. 4. Sperm. 5. Ovum.
1. Introduction.
7. Mulberry Mass.
8. Primitive Trace. Significance of.

15. Growth of body.
16. Changes of cells. New cells.
17. How bones are lengthened.
14. Expansional Centers.
23. Function.
18. Direction of growth—Innate plans.
19. Amount of Growth—control—maturity.
20. Adaptation.
21. Evidence of Innate's work in every place.
22. Responsive power in tissue cells.
24. A cell able to carry on correspondence with Innate.
25. Conclusion.
10. Primary tissues.

Second tentative outline. Rewritten with numbers in consecutive order.

1. Introduction.
2. Life. Defined and explained.
3. Evolution values.
4. Spermatazoon.
5. Ovum.
6. Mitosis.
7. Mulberry Mass.
8. Primitive Trace. Significance of.
9. Blastoderm.
10. Primary tissues.
11. Theory of cell expansion.
12. Description of typical cell.
13. Signs of Life. Explain each.
14. Expansional Centers.
15. Growth of body.
16. Changes of cells. New cells.
17. How bones are lengthened.
18. Direction of growth—Innate plans.
19. Amount of Growth—control—maturity.
20. Adaptation.
21. Evidence of Innate's work in every place.
22. Responsive power in tissue cells.
23. Function.
24. A cell's correspondence with Innate.
25. Conclusion.

Upon examination this looks like an outline on Physiology, but not so. In every step Innate's work is to be shown, in no unmistakable manner. The next development of the outline is by revision, topic and subtopic building, combining.

1. Introduction.

2. Life.
   a. Definition.
   b. Explanation.
   c. What it means in Chiropractic.

3. Evolution values.
   a. Intellectual adaptation.
   b. Adaptation.
   c. Survival values.
   d. Inherited value.

4. The Germ.
   a. Spermatazoon.
   b. Ovum.
   c. Mulberry mass.
   d. Primitive Trace—significance of. "The Contractor's Shack."
   e. Mitosis.

5. The Blastoderm.
   a. Layers. Beginning of organization made evident.
   b. The four primary tissues.
   c. Description of each and their functions.
   d. Theory of cell expansion.

6. The Signs of Life.
   a. Assimilation.
   b. Excretion.
   c. Adaptability.
   d. Growth.
   e. Reproduction.
   f. Esthetic ability or tendencies.
   g. What Signs of Life really are.

7. Development of the body.
   a. Expansional centers.
   b. Growth of body.
   c. Changes of cells—new cells.
   d. Manner of enlarging organs. Direction. Size, etc.
   e. Innate control of growth, size, direction, amount.
   f. Influence of space allotted on shape of organs.

8. Evidence of Innate's work in every place.
    a. Innate must have organized tissue to Receive.
    b. Responsive power of tissues.
    c. The purpose of body parts.
    d. Coordination.
    e. Function.
    f. Organization.

9. Conclusion.
    a. The body a wonderful machine.
    b. The body a beautiful edifice.
    c. Innate the proud builder.
    d. Innate the jealous owner.
    e. The constant watchfulness of Innate.

Any of the subjects given can be developed in this manner and most of them have been written upon. Many of the subjects were copied from theses That is no reason you cannot use any of them, for what you will say about any one of them will be different from the rest. Do not use this outline necessarily, write your own.

The use of these directions will make better theses in general. It will raise the standard of the Ph.C.; it will lessen the percentage of the rejected ones; it will eliminate "book reviews." This article is calculated to show the error of purchasing theses. It shows that, if you write a thesis, you will perceive a method of instruction and learning unequaled, for it teaches you to think and digest what you have learned in the classroom. Writing a thesis is the best way to learn Chiropractic. It shows that a bona fide Ph.C. will make a better Chiropractor of the candidate. The writer hopes it will encourage the students to better efforts, no matter how good they already are.

Occipito-Atlanto-Axial Region

By

GALEN R. PRICE, D.C., Ph.C.

FOREWORD

THE accomplished purpose of Dr. R. W. Stephenson in his Chiropractic Text was to compile and edit the Chiropractic principles as propounded in Dr. B. J. Palmer's lectures and voluminous writings into a systematized text. A simplified explanation of Chiropractic for the layman. A Text for use in Chiropractic schools and colleges. Teaching the fundamental Chiropractic working principles, and giving an explanatory account of progressive developments in the Chiropractic profession.

Dr. Palmer has recognized the value of this book as a mediator for his advanced research volumes to the developing student mind. The Developer of Chiropractic has published but few of his exhaustive volumes of Chiropractic literature. To the layman, or to the student, these immortal works are impressive but difficult for their complete understanding. They are the works of a savant, the product of a mind capable of reasoning far in advance of present day concepts.

In submitting an additional chapter to the Chiropractic Text, at this reprint, no attempt is made to distract from the merit of former editions. It is with the same spirit with which Dr. Stephenson, my former teacher and instructor, presented the original edition, that I submit an explanation of the more recent Chiropractic developments. This material is based upon practical application, lecture work, statistics compiled in The B. J. Palmer Chiropractic Clinic, and upon Dr. Palmer's more recent lectures and extensive, detailed publications.

GALEN R. PRICE, D.C., Ph.C.

Research in Chiropractic

The material presented in these former chapters has painted a comprehensive picture of the greatness of Chiropractic. Advanced, present-day research, most of which was aimed at the destruction of Chiropractic, is proving beyond scientific doubt, the soundness of our "Old Time Chiropractic Philosophy". More and more the scientific world is turning toward the fundamental principles upon which the practice of Chiropractic is based.

It has remained the life work of Dr. B. J. Palmer to develop the application of, and to systematically arrange, the workable principles; that the world might know and appreciate the greatness of his family heritage, Chiropractic. Although he stands out as the Developer of the Science of Chiropractic, his work is being practically duplicated in many endowed colleges and State universities. I quote one of his most recent publications: "Chiropractic rests upon the premise that vertebral subluxation occludes opening, produces pressure upon nerves, interferes with transmission of Mental Impulse supply between brain and body; this offers resistance to free flow, increases temperature, and makes possible thermo-pile readings". Compare this premise with those earliest Chiropractic premises. You will find them the same. We cannot disprove the facts.

"Chiropractors little realize the extent to which medical men, medical institutions, and medical publications are researching into this problem of Mental Impulse, nerve-energy, human neuro-physiological function.

"We have compiled and tabulated this data to show how extensive it is. We doubt if we have, by any means, secured all literature bearing upon their investigations."

"To date we list 475 medical men who are researching the

neurological interference as the cause of dis-ease, and neurological transmission restoration of that interference as the cure for disease. There are 104 leading medical institutions directly concerned in that research, and 263 medical publications have written articles regarding same. All this research, conducted by medical men, substantiates Chiropractic and establishes jointly the latest research of The B. J. Palmer Chiropractic Clinic."

"Medicine has run the gauntlet of blood and its cause of disease; treatment of blood and its cure of disease, by purifying, cleansing, thickening and thinning, treatments for, etc. They have adopted and adapted stimulation and inhibition, as the plus and minus of drug prescription means and method of eliminating, alleviating, or ameliorating disease; or inhibiting stimulated symptomatology and pathology, or stimulating inhibited symptomatology and pathology. They have woven back and forth with the microscope, observed germs, and advanced the theory that they were the cause of many diseases. They have struggled in laboratories to learn how to kill them and cure disease. They now seek a specific for the cure of disease with vaccines, viruses, and other anti serum injections. They have climbed the heights of various ladders down through history, only to strike bottom and start climbing another. **Now** they are **discarding these** in favor of an approach to the study of **brain, nerves** and **energy flow between brain and body; effect** of **nerve impulse influence** on **physiology, symptomatology** and **pathology.** They are invading a "new field", hoping their research will establish finally, something tangible they can hold to, which explains cause and cure of disease. With all this which is new to them, there are many loose tag frill ends of the old that cling and hang on, that shuttle back and forth and cloud the new picture. But if, in the new, there is the element of fact, then the new which is true will rapidly shed the old that is untrue."

"Old Time Chiropractic Philosophy" is substantiated by the

findings of modern researches in the field of neuro-physiology.

The following are unconditional facts upon which the Science of Chiropractic is based. These facts are well worth repeating time and time again, to facilitate a thorough understanding of the logic and reasoning of Chiropractic, and the soundness of our present day concepts.

The human being is endowed with a given quantity and quality of matter, of which the body organs and tissues are composed.

A given and sufficient amount of energy is assembled in the brain for the specific purpose of controlling the functional activity of this matter thruout life. (Under guidance of Innate Intelligence, present in all living things.)

This energy is transmitted from the brain to the structures and systems of the body by way of the nervous system.

The nervous system manifests both efferent and afferent channels, giving a two-way cycle of communication between source of energy and points of functional distribution. The spinal cord, at foramen magnum, contains the efferent and afferent fibers connecting the brain to all tissues of the body.

Health is a condition in which all the matter of the body receives the proper quantity and quality of nervous energy (Mental Impulses) as a prerequisite to coordinated functional activity.

Dis-ease is due to a vertebral subluxation which occludes an opening, impinges nerve channels, and offers interference to the transmission of mental impulse supply between brain and body.

Development of a Specific

The development of Chiropractic principles and practice has ever been directed toward locating the specific cause of all dis-ease.

Recall mention, in former chapters, the development of the Meric system of dividing the spinal column into zones and meres; the Major and Minor system of adjusting; the development and application of X-ray to the Chiropractic analysis; and the use of the Neurocalometer for the detection of radiated nerve heat.

All these systems and methods of procedure were introduced and used as forward steps in locating the specific cause for all dis-ease.

At present many additions have been made to the list of our Chiropractic research equipment. Namely, the Neurocalograph, the Neurotempometer, the Conturgrafometer, the Side-posture Adjusting table, the Posture Constant Recorder, the Adjustograph, new developments in X-ray technique, and the Electroencephaloneuromentimpograph, which is used in studying the quantity and quality of nerve energy flow in the body.

Present day clinical research and practice has led to the conclusion that the Occipito-Atlanto-Axial region is the only region in the entire spinal column in which we find a single conduit of nerves, containing efferent and afferent nerve fibers, destined to carry Mental Impulses, directly and indirectly, to and from all parts of the body.

Therefore it is the only region in the entire spinal column where a single vertebral subluxation could interfere with the transmission of mental impulses between the brain and any or all parts of the body. It is the only plausible location for "a single specific causative factor" involving **all** physiology, all symptomatology, and **all** pathology.

A thorough knowledge of antagonistic spinal muscles and their relative functional importance in the Occipito-Atlanto-

A List of Twenty Paired Muscles Affecting the Occipito-Atlanto-Axial Area

Muscle	Origin	Insertion	Nerve Supply
Rectus Capitis Posticus Minor	Atlas, post. arch	Occiput	Great and sub-occipital
Rectus Capitis Posticus Major	Spine of Axis	Occiput	Great and sub-occipital
Obliquus Capitis Superior	Atlas Trans.	Occiput	Great and sub-occipital
Obliquus Capitis Inferior	Axis spinous	Atlas trans.	Great and sub-occipital
Interspinalis	Between spines of contiguous vert.		Adjacent spinal ns.
Intertransversalis	Between trans. of contiguous vert.		Adjacent spinal ns.
Multifidis spinae	Trans 7c—sacrum	laminae and spines, axis-5th L.	Cervical plexus and sp. ns.
Biventer cervicis	Trans 2-4th D.	Occiput	Complexus
Complexus	3rd C.-6th D.	Occiput	Great and sub-occipital
Longus colli	Trans 3rd-5th C	Ant tub of Atlas	Lower cervicals
Rectus Capitis Anticus Major	Trans 3rd-6th C	Occiput, basilar proc.	Cervical plexus
Rectus Capitis Anticus Minor	Trans of Atlas	Occiput	Cervical plexus
Rectus Capitis Lateralis	Atlas on ant.	Occiput, jugular proc.	1st C n.
Spinalis Colli	Spines 5C-2D	Axis spine	Cervical branches
Splenius Capitis	Spines 7C-2D	Occiput and Mastoid	Middle Cervical
Splenius Colli	Spines 3rd-6th D	Trans Atlas and Axis	Lower Cervical
Sternocleidomastoid	Sternum and Clavicle	Mastoid	Spinal Accessory
Supra spinalis	Spinous proc. in cervical region		Adjacent ns.
Trachelomastoid	Trans 3rd-6th D; Bodies 3rd-7th C	Mastoid Proc.	Cervical plexus
Semi-spinalis colli	Trans 6th-10 D	Spines Ax-5th L	Cervical plexus

Axial region is the next step in understanding upper cervical adjusting procedure.

In listing the following paired spinal muscles, which affect the position of the structures in the Occipito-Atlanto-Axial region, I do not assume the list to be complete, nor are these the only muscles found in the region. They are selected and listed as having immediate effect and are sufficient to reveal the multitudinous complications confronted in attempting to determine the exact muscle involved in any specific subluxation.

It is well to understand that contracture (P. 219) in any one of these twenty muscles listed, with comparative atonia (lack of muscle tone) in the antagonistic fellow-muscle would be sufficent to lock the Atlas or Axis in its subluxated position.

I refer to the vertebral muscles as "paired antagonistic" spinal muscles in reference to their functional importance. Normally they are coordinated in their antagonistic pull upon the vertebrae. The proper quantity and quality of Mental Impulse supply to the paired antagonistic muscles maintains the supporting muscle tone. This coordinated relationship is retained throughout all normal motion of the head or neck. The motion calls for a specific degree of contraction upon the part of many sets of muscles, while their antagonistic fellows manifest a controlled relaxation. Not a single vertebra, but a series of vertebrae are set into motion at this time.

Refer to the schema of paired antagonistic muscles having immediate effect upon the relative position of structures in the Occipito-Atlanto-Axial region.

Laterality of the Atlas is dependent to a major extent upon the relative pull of the Obliquus Capitis Superior muscles, also upon the related pull of the Intertransversalis found between the transverse processes of the Atlas and Axis. Careful study of their attachments shows that the normal oblique directional pull of these muscles prevents Atlas from sideslipping on its

Posterior View Showing Paired Antagonistic Muscles Immediately Affecting the Position of Structures in the Occipito-Atlanto-Axial Region

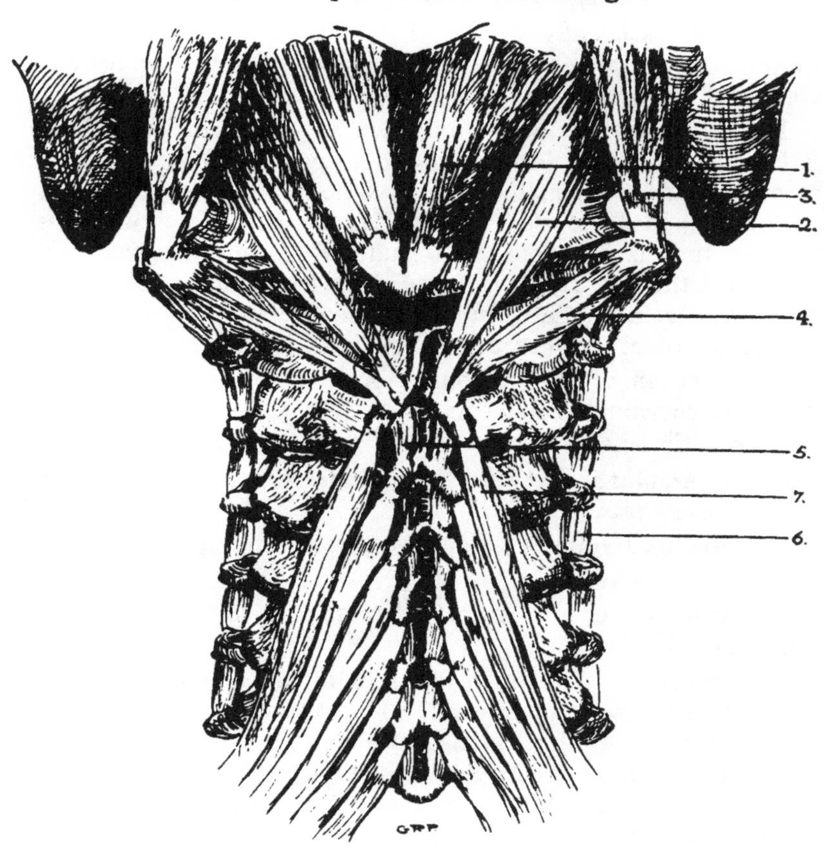

1. Rectus Capitis Posticus Minor
2. Rectus Capitis Posticus Major
3. Obliquus Capitis Superior
4. Obliquus Capitis Inferior
5. Interspinalis
6. Intertransversalis
7. Multifidus spinae

condyle articulation. Such a sideslip would result in sliding the lateral mass upward on the side of laterality and downward on the opposite side, thus forming a wedge on the side to which the Atlas has slipped. The wedge is formed due to the slant in the Occipito-Atlantal articulation which is directed outward and upward.

The numerous variations in sideslips and rotations of the Atlas and Axis are more easily understood in the actual study of normal and abnormal vertebral articulations, together with the arrangement of their muscular and osseous limitations. Such a study is available to all students of the Palmer School, who have the opportunity of spending two hours each day in study of Dr. B. J. Palmer's private collection of normal and abnormal spinal columns and other osseous structures.

The position of the spinous process of Axis is dependent upon the coordinated muscular tone in the following muscles: (Check with schema)

The Interspinalis, between Atlas and Axis and between Axis and 3rd Cervical.

The Rectus Capitis Posticus Major, extending obliquely to the Occipital bone.

The Obliquus Capitis Inferior, extending to the transverse process of the Atlas.

The Multifidus Spinae, leading obliquely downward to inferior transverse processes. The contracture of one set of these strong Multifidus Spinae muscles with the relative atonia in its antagonistic fellow not only brings about laterality in the spinous process of the Axis, but it also draws the spinous to the inferior causing the odontoid process to project backward into the neural canal of the spine.

Probably all the muscles affecting the position of the spinous of Axis also play a part in rotating the Atlas in relation to the adjacent structures. However, I feel that the Obliquus Capitis

Schema of Upper Spinal Nerves with their Branches

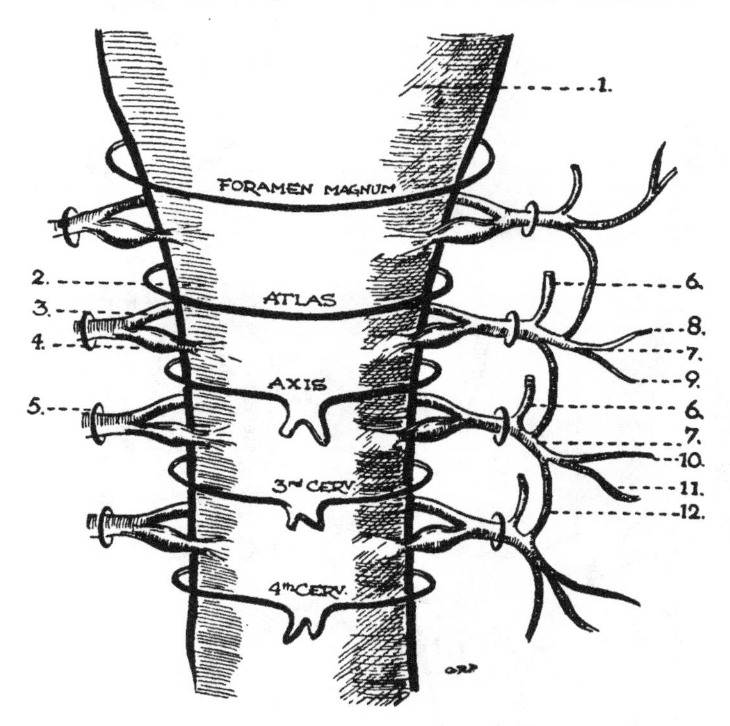

1. Brain Stem
2. Spinal Cord
3. Anterior nerve root
4. Posterior nerve root
5. Intervertebral foramen
6. Anterior Primary div.
7. Posterior primary div.
8. Internal branch (great occipital)

9. External branch (to ms. of neck)
19. Internal branch (least occipital)
11. External Branch (to ms. of neck)
12. Communicating branch, forming plexus.

The anterior divisions (primary) of the upper cervical nerves unite to form the Anterior Cervical Plexus. These nerves supply the viscera of neck and face.

The posterior divisions (primary) unite to form the posterior cervical plexus. These nerves supply muscles of back of neck and head.

Note: Since a plexus is formed before the nerves come to the surface of the neck, superficial, hot, tender nerves need not indicate adjacent impingement.

Anatomical arrangement of communicating fibres between Central Nervous system and the Periphero-Visceral system

Note the recurrent meningeal fibres passing from spinal nerve to spinal canal, supplying adjacent nervous, ligamentous, and osseous tissues.

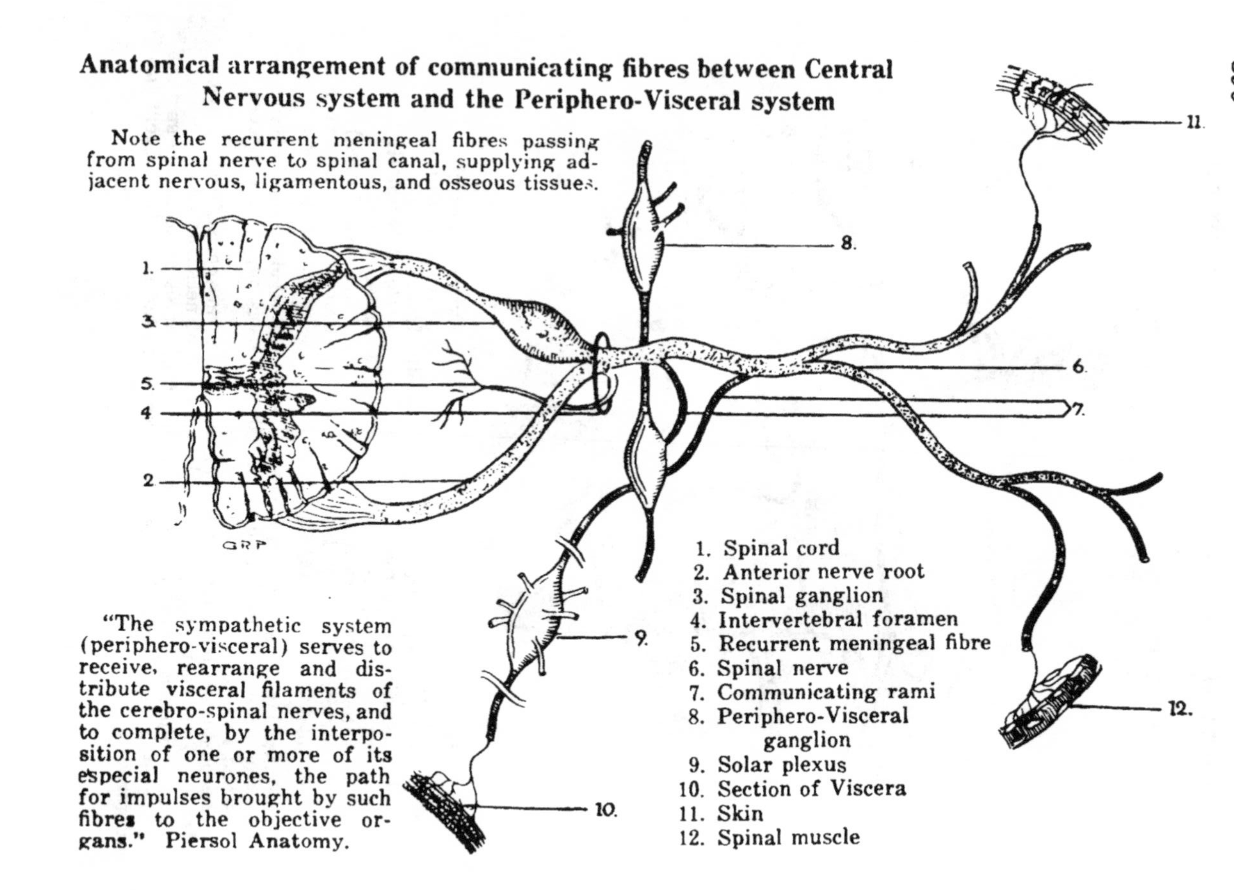

1. Spinal cord
2. Anterior nerve root
3. Spinal ganglion
4. Intervertebral foramen
5. Recurrent meningeal fibre
6. Spinal nerve
7. Communicating rami
8. Periphero-Visceral ganglion
9. Solar plexus
10. Section of Viscera
11. Skin
12. Spinal muscle

"The sympathetic system (periphero-visceral) serves to receive, rearrange and distribute visceral filaments of the cerebro-spinal nerves, and to complete, by the interposition of one or more of its especial neurones, the path for impulses brought by such fibres to the objective organs." Piersol Anatomy.

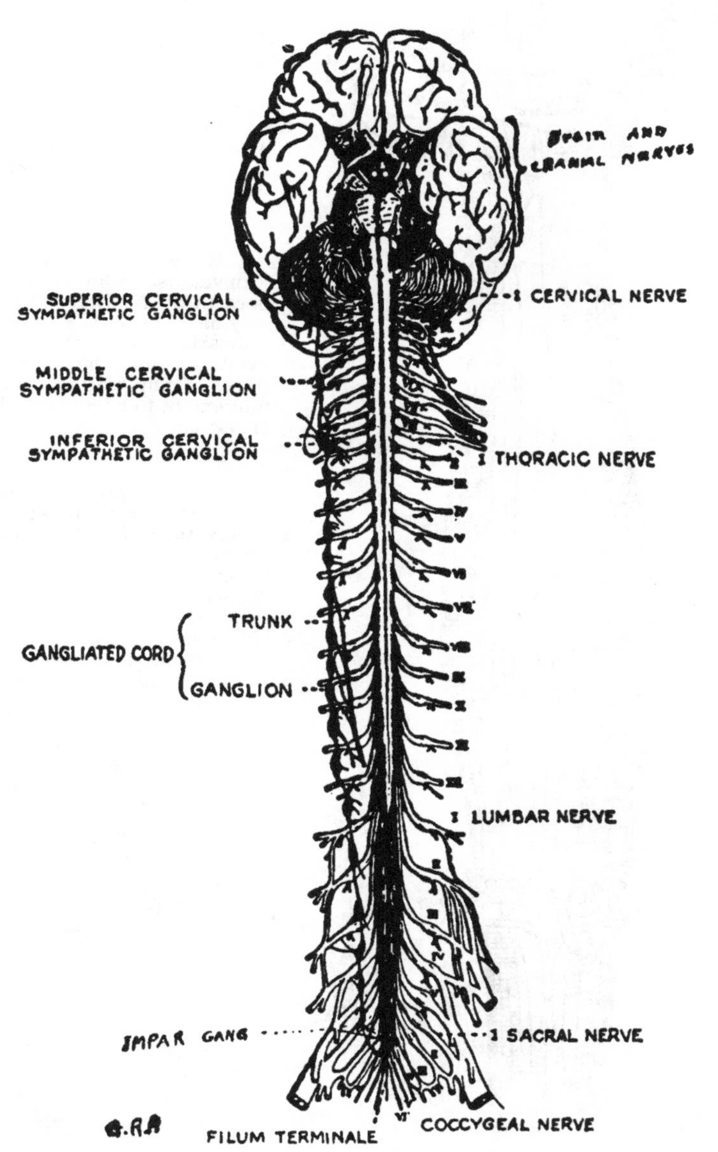
BRAIN AND CRANIAL NERVES
SUPERIOR CERVICAL SYMPATHETIC GANGLION
I CERVICAL NERVE
MIDDLE CERVICAL SYMPATHETIC GANGLION
INFERIOR CERVICAL SYMPATHETIC GANGLION
I THORACIC NERVE
TRUNK
GANGLIATED CORD
GANGLION
I LUMBAR NERVE
IMPAR GANG
I SACRAL NERVE
FILUM TERMINALE
COCCYGEAL NERVE

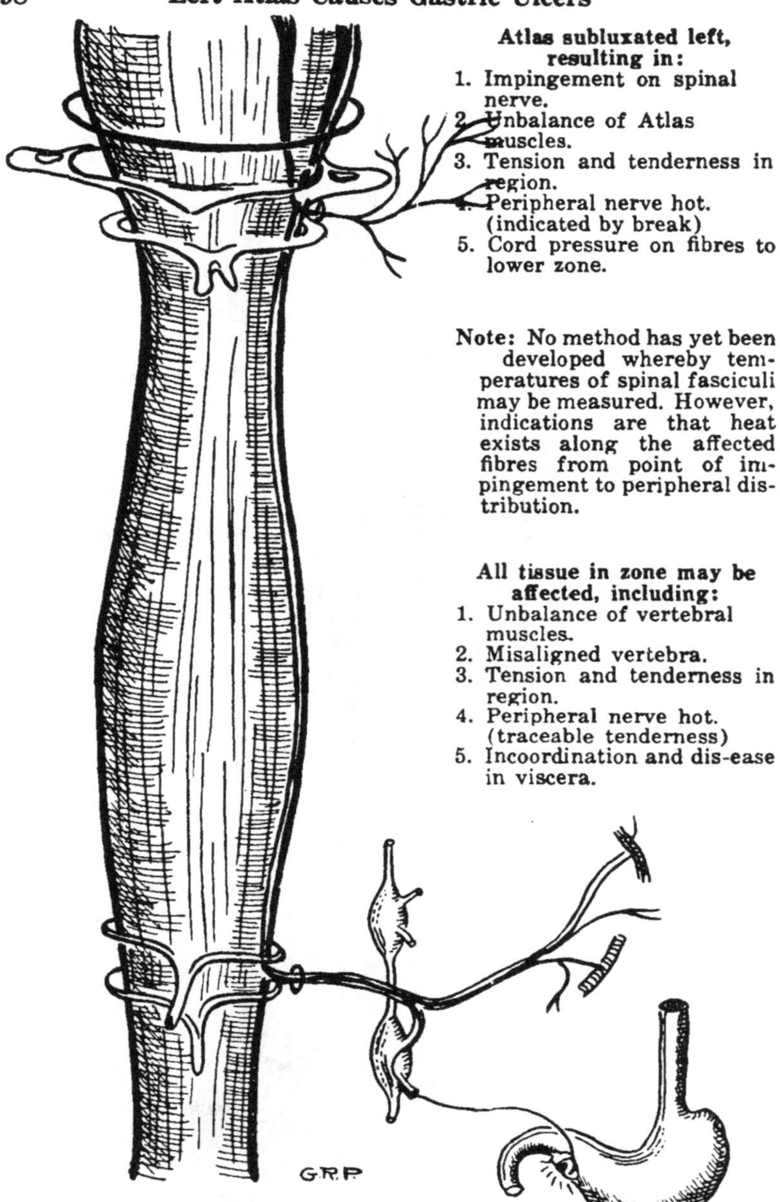

Nerve cells forming the gray matter of the spinal cord are concentrated in the medullary portion of the cord. The white cortical portion of the cord is formed of the ascending and descending spinal fasciculi. These channels carry Mental Impulses between the brain and all parts of the body. Knowing this, it is easy to understand how a subluxated Atlas or Axis causing spinal cord pressure in the Occipito-Atlanto-Axial region may impinge nerve channels destined to emit at any of the inferior intervertebral foramina. This would interfere with nerve supply to all tissue of the inferior zone affected.

Inferior muscles are most important in rotated subluxations of the Atlas.

Following this illustrated example, let us observe the typical clinical picture in such a case. This example is based upon actual records, there being no particular reason for choosing the condition of Gastric Ulcers, as any functional disturbance may result from spinal cord pressure in the Upper Cervical region.

An accidental shock and concussion of forces causes the Atlas to become subluxated sufficiently far to impinge the neuromeric fibers leading to the Atlas muscles. The shock may be general, and cause other body damage, but the Atlas is most liable to be affected for it is the only vertebra which has no osseous limitations to its range of motion.

With interference to normal transmission of Mental Impulses to the Atlas muscles, there is contracture in some of the muscles, with relative muscular atonia in the antagonistic fellows. Thus the Atlas is locked in its misaligned position and is listed as a chronic subluxation. Upper cervical analysis reveals tense, tender muscles, and hot, tender superficial neuromeric fibres.

In the subluxated position, the Atlas occludes the neural canal of the spinal column. The four possible types of occlusions are:

1. Circumferential constriction.
2. Torqued meningeal occlusion.
3. Heat expansion meningeal occlusion.
4. Cicatrical or scar tissue occlusion.

The occlusion of the neural canal in this area results in pressure upon the spinal cord and impingement of spinal nerve tracts, associated with inferior meric zones.

Checking down the spinal column we determine that these impinged nerve tracts were destined, in this particular case, to emit and give Mental Impulse supply to the tissues of the thirteenth meric zone. All tissues of this zone are affected to a greater or lesser degree.

With interference to their nerve supply the adjacent muscles become unbalanced, bringing about a misalignment of the vertebra of the zone. There is tension, pain, heat and tenderness in the region. The visceral organs, supplied via this channel, suffer from lack of coordinating nerve impulse supply, resulting in their functional incoordination. Secretory, Motor, and Reparatory functions are involved. Symptoms of dyspepsia and indigestion appear, followed by ulceration of affected gastric membranes.

Where is the specific causative factor in the condition of Gastric Ulcers? Chiropractically, this question is answered by actual results attained in such cases.

The analysis reveals misalignment of the Atlas in relation to its adjacent structures.

Heat in the superficial nerve fibres gives evidence of actual interference to the transmission of nerve energy to the muscles of the Atlas.

The Chiropractic adjustment of the Atlas releases impingement on its own nerve supply restoring normal functional tone to the muscles. The muscles have a balanced pull with normal nerve supply thus holding the Atlas in the normal position.

The neural canal occlusion is removed (time element dependent upon type of occlusion), restoring normal transmission to affected inferior zone and meric tissues.

Normal nerve supply to spinal muscles of affected zone corrects their misalignment.

The tension, heat, pain, and tenderness at inferior zone are eliminated, as normal function is restored to the muscles and other affected tissues.

With normal transmission of Mental Impulse supply to the affected viscera, the Secretory, Motor and Reparatory functions are restored to normal. Healing and repair take place, relieving symptoms of dyspepsia and indigestion.

The time requirements for complete recovery and health vary with types of tissue involved and with individuals.

Health is a condition in which all body functions are carried on normally, meeting all body demands for adaptation to the environment. Mental Impulse supply is vital to all body function. Therefore, the degree of health enjoyed by each person, is dependent upon the normal transmission of Mental Impulses between the brain and all parts of the body.

Credit is due Dr. Irma Zimmerman for
Art work on my original drawings.—G. R. P.

INDEX

D

E

F

N

U

V

W

Z

CPSIA information can be obtained
at www.ICGtesting.com
Printed in the USA
BVHW030554280721
612886BV00005B/629

9 781626 541993